EVERY VICTORY COUNTS®

Your Go-To Resource of Essential Information and Inspiration for Living Well with Parkinson's

BY THE DAVIS PHINNEY FOUNDATION

AND BY 50 LEADING PARKINSON'S PHYSICIANS, ALLIED HEALTH PROFESSIONALS, AND PEOPLE LIVING WITH PARKINSON'S

SIXTH EDITION, ELEVENTH PRINTING

This publication is supported in part by grants and donations from:

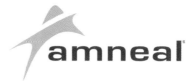

abbvie

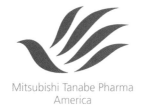

Mitsubishi Tanabe Pharma
America

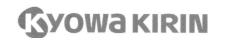

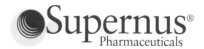

And in part through the generous support from our *Every Victory Counts®* donors:

Ken and Pam Alexander
Barbara and Dale Ankenman
Abby and Ken Dawkins
Bonnie Gibbons
Gail Gitin *in loving memory of Gene Gitin*
Amy Howard and Scott Hunsaker
The Narter Family
David and Stacey Schmid
Carolyn Zeiger *and those who loved and were inspired by Paul Zeiger.*
The fund was started with a generous bequest from Cirsten Carle,
daughter of famed children's book author and illustrator, Eric Carle.

■ TABLE OF CONTENTS

4

Introduction

■ FOREWORD

BY PROFESSOR BAS BLOEM

When the Davis Phinney Foundation invited me to write the foreword for the newest edition of the *Every Victory Counts* manual, I was honored because I know how valuable this resource is to people living with Parkinson's and their care partners. I am thrilled to contribute to it. Now, more than ever, it is time for people with Parkinson's to have hope. Hope for how you can live well today and in the future. While this is officially the foreword to the manual, we could have just as easily called it a forward because that is really what all people with Parkinson's and their families want: to move forward, and preferably at warp speed. One of the essential ingredients of your ability to move forward is to be more knowledgeable about Parkinson's itself as a complex neurological condition and about its many different treatments. Knowledge is power, and I am convinced that this new edition of the *Every Victory Counts* manual will give you that invaluable power.

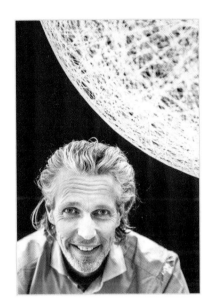

Parkinson's is having its day. Recent work has shown that Parkinson's is the fastest-growing neurological condition globally, which emphasizes the need for immediate action. We need to find better ways of preventing Parkinson's from happening in the first place, and we need to find improved solutions to optimally support all of you who have already developed symptoms. This means that we all must raise our voices to secure more funding and raise further awareness. Fortunately, more people who have Parkinson's are speaking up. More physicians and allied health professionals are being trained to treat it, and more activists than ever are demanding that the Parkinson's community get a seat at the table.

These actions are great news for the Parkinson's community. What's also great news is that today we have a much better understanding of what is going wrong in the brain of people living with Parkinson's. These fundamental insights are beginning to form the basis for innovative therapies that will hopefully be able to slow down or even arrest the progression of Parkinson's, and which may ultimately pave the road towards a cure. Meanwhile, more and better symptomatic and supportive treatments are available than ever before. We have better and more precise medications. We understand deep brain stimulation better, and improved surgical techniques are being developed as we speak. We know how important daily exercise

7

is and what type and intensity deliver the most benefits. Exciting new work is carefully beginning to suggest that regular exercise not only works just like a drug in suppressing the symptoms, but it may even be a way of slowing down the progression of Parkinson's.

We also know, and this may be our most important learning, that there are several million different kinds of Parkinson's because each person's wishes and needs with Parkinson's are different. In a brand-new publication in *The Lancet*, we have made the provocative statement that there isn't just one Parkinson's disease. There are, in fact, seven million different Parkinson's diseases in the world, just as many as there are people living with this condition. This is not just a hollow statement, but one that has very practical implications for the care you receive in daily life. Recognizing that Parkinson's is different for every individual practically means that we need to move from a one-size-fits-all treatment plan into personalized, integrated care to truly crack the code on how to help each person live well with Parkinson's today. And we increasingly recognize that this support does not stop at helping individuals who have Parkinson's. We now understand better than ever before that we should focus our efforts on supporting the entire family and all others affected by it. You don't live with Parkinson's alone!

What does personalized and integrated care look like? In a perfect world, it's a team made up of at least a movement disorder specialist, a primary care physician, and a nurse specialist who directs the show. The second ring of care includes a physical therapist, occupational therapist, speech-language pathologist, rehabilitation specialist, sleep specialist, and maybe a registered dietician. The outer ring of care consists of a urologist, gastroenterologist, ophthalmologist, palliative care specialist, dermatologist, and dentist who understands Parkinson's. This is not to say that all these different professionals should be involved for every individual with Parkinson's, let alone at all times. This long list merely indicates how many professionals are out there to offer support, tailored to your individual needs.

Maybe your own unique experience with Parkinson's means you need ten different people on your medical care team. Or perhaps you are doing well with only two. There's no right way. There's just the way that works for you. But what is crucially important is that each team should always include a well-informed person with Parkinson's and a well-informed family.

In the same paper in *The Lancet*, we emphasized that there are no individual stars within the multidisciplinary team, with one exception, namely the person with Parkinson's. The person living with Parkinson's is the sun surrounded by professionals who are orbiting around that person and offering support whenever needed. But for you to take on that role as the sun within this healthcare universe, you must be informed and knowledgeable. That is why I'm so extremely happy with this incredibly rich sixth edition of the *Every Victory Counts* manual.

Importantly, taking a personalized, integrated approach to care doesn't end with setting up appointments with experts. That's just the beginning. Your mindset, daily exercise regimen, nutritional choices, and the people you surround yourself with are critical pieces of living well. So essential that unless you have those dialed in, medical treatments will only help so much.

As you all know, Davis Phinney was an inspiring, elite athlete. You also know that to be successful in a top sport, where the differences between winning and losing are tiny, every little detail must be optimal, including your sleep, nutritional choices, exercise regimen, et cetera et cetera. In many ways, I think that living with Parkinson's is like being an elite athlete. If you have Parkinson's, you want every possible aspect that you can control to be in optimal shape. That's why I love the *Every Victory Counts* manual. It includes everything you need to know about the motor and non-motor symptoms you may experience with Parkinson's, but it also contains invaluable and incredibly rich information about emotional health, exercise, the importance of connecting, and various other topics that I'd write down on my prescription pad if I could. Use this manual as much as you can to create the optimal circumstances for yourself!

No matter where you are on your path with Parkinson's, this manual and the Davis Phinney Foundation are here to help. Please take advantage of this critical resource and their community so that you can live well today and in the future with Parkinson's. And remember, just like Davis Phinney himself, you are an elite athlete! Use this resource to optimize your chances of being successful in this challenging endeavor.

For more from Professor Bloem, see Chapter 3.

> "*When we attended our first Davis Phinney Foundation Victory Summit in 2012, the first edition of the* Every Victory Counts *manual was brand new. Little did we know how it would change our lives. As Foundation Ambassadors we have shared the manual with numerous individuals who have come back and expressed that this manual is life changing for a person with Parkinson's who is attempting to navigate their diagnosis. Whether you are a care partner or a person with Parkinson's, the* Every Victory Counts *manual is a standard that you can use today and in the future... Welcome!*"

— PAT & CIDNEY DONAHOO

INTRODUCTION

When the Davis Phinney Foundation was established in 2004, Davis wanted its mission to be different from that of other existing Parkinson's organizations. While a cure for Parkinson's is what we all wanted, we also knew that people desperately needed better information about how to live well with Parkinson's right now.

So, the Foundation's mission—then and now—is to help people with Parkinson's live well today. The *Every Victory Counts* manual is an integral part of fulfilling that mission. The manual embraces the Davis Phinney Foundation's philosophy of taking action to improve your quality of life with Parkinson's. Within these pages, we hope you'll feel like you've found your people, your community. Here, we'll acknowledge loss, but we won't dwell on what might have been. Rather, we'll turn our attention to what is yet to be and how we will make the most of today and every day. Most people with Parkinson's will live for many years, and there are things you can do to live well and, indeed, to thrive.

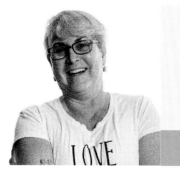

" *The* Every Victory Counts *manual is an active part of my life. It is not something that lives on a shelf."*

— JILL ATER

YOUR ROADMAP FOR LIVING WELL TODAY WITH PARKINSON'S

Parkinson's changes over time, and your experiences, needs, and treatments will change direction from time to time, too. We designed the *Every Victory Counts* manual to provide the information you need to make choices about managing your Parkinson's today and in the future. As your needs evolve, so will your approach. Armed with essential knowledge and inspired by the successful experiences recounted in these pages by clinicians and people with Parkinson's alike, you can create your own wellness plan and build in the flexibility to adjust your course over time. Though your symptoms will inevitably change, your commitment to living well is constant. Remember, whatever your current situation, it is possible to live well with Parkinson's *today*.

> *I appreciate the manual's fundamental perspective, which is to empower people to live well with Parkinson's today. I routinely recommend this manual to my patients, whether they are newly diagnosed or have been living with Parkinson's for years."*
>
> — AARON HAUG, MD

Think of this manual and the additional material located on the *Every Victory Counts* website (dpf.org/evc-hub) as a living resource to help you take steps to preserve or improve your quality of life after a Parkinson's diagnosis. Please don't feel that you must read it front to back to benefit from its contents. Dig into the sections that are most meaningful to you and remember that it is a resource you can read in any order and at any time. You can turn to it when you need a little extra motivation or hope or when you want to dig deeper into a specific topic that is especially important to you right now. Keep the manual out where you will see it and where it will serve as a daily reminder of your commitment to living well with Parkinson's.

The key to living well with Parkinson's today is actively choosing to do what will result in your best quality of life. Be informed, be engaged, be connected, be courageous, and be active. Each day will bring new challenges and opportunities for positive change. Remember, your daily triumphs, large or small, are worth celebrating: *Every Victory Counts*!

> *I can't tell you how impactful the manual has been. Families constantly testify to how useful the manual has been in their own Parkinson's journey. In fact, it is rare to find a publication that has such a profound consumer impact."*
>
> — AL CONDELUCI, PHD

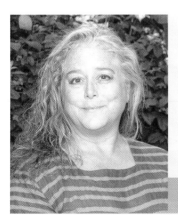

> *We get the life we are given; it is finite, progressive, and degenerative for us all. We only have our choice about how to LIVE. I believe that finding joy and gratitude is possible for anyone no matter the challenge."*
>
> — KAT HILL

■ UPDATES FROM THE FIFTH EDITION

First published in 2010, the *Every Victory Counts* manual broke new ground as the only resource of its kind, devoted solely to the principle of proactive self-care and a holistic approach to managing Parkinson's. In subsequent editions, it has gained international recognition as a superb and comprehensive resource for changing the way people live with Parkinson's.

Like Professor Bas Bloem explained in his foreword, Parkinson's is a rapidly evolving field. Our latest edition of the *Every Victory Counts* manual reflects that. This manual is the cornerstone of our new *Every Victory Counts* suite of resources, a robust collection of printed and digital manuals, each tailored to specific audiences. The suite includes the following:

- *Every Victory Counts* Print Manual (the one you're holding in your hands)
- *Every Victory Counts* Digital Manual
- *Every Victory Counts* Care Partner Print Manual
- *Every Victory Counts* Care Partner Digital Manual
- *Every Victory Counts* Worksheets and Assessments
- *Every Victory Counts* Discussion Guides
- *Every Victory Counts* Companion Website (dpf.org/evc-hub)
- And more to come!

Through this expanded collection of Parkinson's resources, we hope to provide even more accessible and comprehensive materials to people affected by Parkinson's, their care partners, their friends and family; Parkinson's physicians, nurses, and other healthcare professionals; community health workers and support group leaders; and more.

In this new edition of the *Every Victory Counts* manual, you will find updates on everything from surgical therapies to research, nutrition, self-care, medications, and more. There are new stories from people living with Parkinson's who share how they're living well, and new contributions from Parkinson's experts about how you, too, can do so. We also reorganized the content so it's easier to follow and digest and made simple changes to font color, font size, and paper to make it easier to read. To make the manual more physically accessible, we moved the worksheets and handouts to the ⌂ *Every Victory Counts* website, where you can also find printable discussion guides and a continually updated collection of Parkinson's articles, videos, webinars, and more.

WHY ISN'T X IN THIS MANUAL?

While we wanted to create a Parkinson's resource that was as comprehensive as possible, we chose to include in this printed manual only information that applies to most people living with Parkinson's. If we left out a specific topic, it's because there is insufficient scientific evidence to support its use for Parkinson's, it's not something we've had experience with, or it is not necessarily relevant for most people who are living with Parkinson's. In the latter case, we put content on less common experiences on the ⤤ *Every Victory Counts* website (dpf.org/evc-hub). In addition, for this sixth edition, we pulled out most of the content related to care partners and created the *Every Victory Counts Manual for Care Partners*. Care partners play such a critical role for people living with Parkinson's that we wanted to give them their own resource. You can order our manual for care partners, free of charge, at ⤤ everyvictorycounts.org. We hope the new *Every Victory Counts* suite will be your go-to collection for everything Parkinson's. We want to educate you and your loved ones not only about Parkinson's and all the ways you can treat it but about how to become your own best advocate, stay connected, and live well TODAY.

> *Your life and hopes and dreams may appear to have completely changed, and that may even be for the better... eventually. Take a deep breath. And another. Allow yourself time to grieve what you feel you have lost. It's okay to be in denial (I certainly was!), to get angry, to bargain, to feel sad and depressed. Just don't allow yourself to get 'stuck' in one or more of these stages. Find your own way to living life well with Parkinson's. Don't overload yourself with information and misinformation. Find a reputable source, like the Davis Phinney Foundation. Exercise! Find a support group or a mentor. Take it a day—or hour—at a time and work to surround yourself with positive and supportive people. Develop your own individualized plan for managing your life with Parkinson's. I'm not sure any of us truly get to acceptance, but we continually work towards living our best life with Parkinson's."*

— MARTY ACEVEDO

13

A MESSAGE FROM DAVIS PHINNEY

My background is one of sport; cycling, specifically. The Olympics and the Tour de France are my former domains. I learned a lot about myself through years of competing successfully in tough, demanding events. I came to understand the importance of focus and purpose and that paying attention to and being engaged in the process is just as important as achieving goals. I came to understand that victory—that elusive, electric moment of triumph—was not exclusive to those who crossed the finish line first.

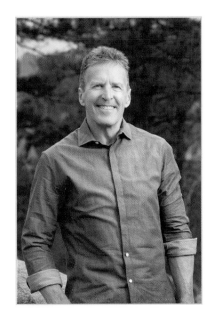

These are lessons that are rooted in me, and they help me now in the much more challenging race against Parkinson's. This race is a no-holds-barred winner-take-all type of event. It demands everything from me. If I let down my guard, it'll knock me flat. But, when I refuse to give in by exercising daily, eating well, and most importantly, maintaining a positive attitude, I always find ways to win.

I've had Parkinson's since 2000 (plus another 10 or so years pre-diagnosis), and what I know is this: We CAN improve our quality of life. It takes work and commitment. It takes patience and support. It takes education and understanding. And it takes a roadmap, which is precisely what this manual is.

If there's an upside to Parkinson's, it's that I'm constantly meeting members of the Parkinson's tribe who are exploring new ways to live well and better than they ever imagined. I know people with Parkinson's who climb mountains, run marathons, and even ride their bikes across the country. Others find victory in spending time with their loved ones or walking around the block. I've met singers and songwriters, painters, and poets. The commonality is their motivation to keep living an inspired life. Ultimately, it's not the size of victory that counts, but the acknowledgment of every victory and the incentive it provides us to keep seeking ways to win. It's about what we can do today to improve our lives. And that is a victory in itself.

— DAVIS PHINNEY

Living with Parkinson's

▮ CHAPTER 1 – YOU HAVE PARKINSON'S. NOW WHAT?

OVERVIEW

Hearing the words, "You have Parkinson's," is life changing. For some, a Parkinson's diagnosis marks the end of a long and frustrating search to explain a collection of seemingly disconnected symptoms. For others, a Parkinson's diagnosis is a complete shock, filled with feelings of disbelief and despair. For everyone, a Parkinson's diagnosis brings a new and unexpected journey.

" *I didn't choose to get Parkinson's, but I did choose who I would fight it with. When I first received my diagnosis, I tried to identify African Americans who had it. The only African Americans I identified were my sister Caroline and Muhammad Ali. What a frightening revelation to think that I might be one of the few African Americans to get Parkinson's. I was always under the impression that this was something only white people get.*

To effectively fight Parkinson's, I needed to find out the real impact of Parkinson's on the African American community. My research led me to the Every Victory Counts manual and other books. What was clear to me was, there was little information on African Americans who had Parkinson's as well as African Americans who worked in the care and treatment of Parkinson's.

In the early stages of Parkinson's, I learned the importance of establishing a good care team. I have been blessed with the resources to put together a quality care team starting with my wife April. My neurologist, physical therapist, and Rock Steady Boxing coach are all African Americans. The importance of my care team is, we all work with a common passion and a set of goals that allow me to live well."

— RON SMALL

The good news is that there are numerous ways you can take action to make the journey a great one. Just a decade ago, researchers, clinicians, and people living with Parkinson's alike did not stress the importance of exercise, stress management, nutritional choices, and other positive life choices on Parkinson's. Today, we know your experience will be impacted positively by your choices and actions.

Think about your life with Parkinson's as a designer would think of a project. When designers encounter a problem, rather than think their way forward, they *build* it. They build it by reframing the problem and then taking action. In the nearly two decades we have spent working with people living with Parkinson's, we've seen that the people who take this design approach—the people who refuse to let Parkinson's define them—create for themselves meaningful, joyful journeys. These people have learned how to reframe the problem.

Without question, the members of our community who are living well with Parkinson's take action consistently. They attend support group meetings and exercise classes, connect with and encourage others, give back, serve as advocates, host fundraisers, and live life to the fullest. They don't see themselves as people with Parkinson's; they see themselves as multi-faceted people who also happen to live with Parkinson's.

Your design plan is yours to make. We, and many others, are here to help. We hope the information, advice, tools, and stories in this manual will show you that you can live well with Parkinson's today and in the future. We hope they will empower you to take action and to design your best life with Parkinson's. Be active. Be engaged. Be informed. Participate actively in your own care. Take control of your destiny. And know that you hold the power you need to live well.

INTEGRATED CARE: BUILDING YOUR PARKINSON'S CARE TEAM

As you set out to design your best life with Parkinson's, remember that you are not in this alone. Many people can make your life with Parkinson's better. Some you'll want to bring onto your medical care team now (such as a movement disorder specialist and physical therapist), and some you may need a bit down the road. Shape your care team in a way that best suits your needs and goals. Here are the types of providers you may consider.

NEUROLOGISTS AND MOVEMENT DISORDER SPECIALISTS

A neurologist is a physician specializing in the conditions of the nervous system (the brain, spinal cord, and bundles of nerves that transmit information to and from them). They can confirm your diagnosis and establish an appropriate treatment plan.

16

A movement disorder specialist (MDS) is a neurologist with additional training in movement disorders. Your MDS will most likely be the person on your medical care team who is most familiar with the full spectrum of Parkinson's medications and treatments. They see thousands of people with Parkinson's every year; so, they have probably helped people with issues like yours before.

" *Your care team begins and ends with you! Those focused on your care and your journey could include your care partner, your movement disorder specialist (MDS) (don't settle for less than an MDS), physical therapist, occupational therapist, speech pathologist, perhaps a neuropsychologist, pharmacist, registered dietitian, trainer. You may not need all of the members of the team at first and members will come and go. But you always remain at the center of your team, and you need and deserve to have team members you trust and who understand and listen to your concerns."*

— MARTY ACEVEDO

Finding an MDS close to you isn't always possible, but because you may only need to see your MDS in person once or twice a year, driving a few hours to these appointments will be time well spent. And with current advances in technology, you may be able to add an MDS to your care team through telemedicine, which is becoming more mainstream every day. If you don't have an MDS close to home, and you aren't able to see one via telemedicine, find an empathetic neurologist or primary care physician who will listen to you and your family, work with you to define your needs and goals, and be open to your suggestions and ideas. If your local care team doesn't include an MDS, but you can occasionally travel to see one in another city, your MDS and local physician can work together to address your needs.

Before you see your physician, review the Worksheets and Assessments on our ⟳ *Every Victory Counts* **website**. We designed these to help you get the most out of your appointments and make sure you communicate with your providers effectively. The 🖹**Goal Summary for Physician Visits** and 🖹**Parkinson's Care Questionnaire** can help you record important information to make your time with your physician more productive.

PRIMARY CARE PHYSICIANS

In addition to your MDS or neurologist, your primary care physician (PCP) will be a critical part of your team over the coming years. Not all health problems are related to Parkinson's. For example, fatigue is a common Parkinson's symptom, but it can also be caused by thyroid disease, anemia, vitamin deficiencies, malnutrition, diabetes, or heart and lung disease, to name a few. Your PCP can check for these and other conditions during your regular check-ups and can help you with medical issues that are unrelated to Parkinson's.

NURSES

Nurses are potent team members and can be strong liaisons between hospitals, medical offices, and the community, helping create and maintain an integrated approach to care. For many people, nurses are the first line of access and can address many health issues that arise. If your question or concern is a problem they cannot solve, they know who on the team can. They can also educate people living with Parkinson's and their families about medication schedules, care team members, and what to expect throughout a Parkinson's journey.

NEUROPSYCHOLOGIST

Neuropsychologists specialize in the relationship between behavior and brain function. Cognitive impairment and behavioral complications such as depression, anxiety, and apathy can be some of the earliest symptoms people with Parkinson's notice, often before they even get an official diagnosis. Most people with Parkinson's will experience these issues at some point. If you do, a great first step is to get evaluated by a neuropsychologist who specializes in neurological disorders. They can assess your thinking skills, including memory, attention, reaction time, language, and visual perception. They will also evaluate your emotional functioning. They will then combine your results with the rest of your medical record to develop a diagnosis and recommendations for improving your quality of life. One of the benefits of getting an evaluation like this is that you will see how your Parkinson's is progressing and act quickly to manage your symptoms.

SOCIAL WORKER, COUNSELOR, THERAPIST, OR PSYCHOLOGIST

Professionals who focus on emotional health and well-being will be beneficial throughout your Parkinson's journey. Counselors, social workers, therapists, and psychologists are trained to assess emotional difficulties and work with you to promote good mental health. They can help you cope and stay positive. They can also help you manage the stress that can make Parkinson's symptoms worse, causing additional strain on you and your family. They serve as guides, helping you to respond with resilience to changes you hadn't anticipated.

PSYCHIATRIST

Psychiatrists are physicians who specialize in mental health. They are qualified to assess both the psychological and physical aspects of psychological problems and prescribe medication. If you experience emotional symptoms such as anxiety, depression, or apathy, a psychiatrist can work with you to adjust your medication regimen in ways that can help.

> **"** *If you focus on Parkinson's, then you will be depressed, anxious, apathetic. If you focus on what you can do to live well and be happy, that changes things. You've got to think about what makes you happy and then go make that happen. You have to be the one who initiates the action."*
>
> — EDIE ANDERSON

SPIRITUAL ADVISOR/CHAPLAIN

If faith is part of your life, a pastor, chaplain, rabbi, or other spiritual advisors can help you find peace, discover meaning, and accept life changes within the comfort and context of your beliefs. Whether within the construct of traditional religions or through other forms of spiritual expression, many people rely on these advisors to provide the support and hope they need to embrace the future.

PHYSICAL THERAPIST

Physical therapy (PT) can help you improve strength, flexibility, and mobility, and it can also decrease stiffness and pain related to Parkinson's. Many people with Parkinson's don't realize how valuable a physical therapist (PT) can be in the early days (especially if you find one who specializes in working with people with neurological disorders); however, those who have worked with them consistently have received tremendous value from doing so, both physically and emotionally.

When you begin seeing a PT early after your diagnosis, they can teach you exercises that address current weaknesses, which will allow you to stay stronger and mobile for longer. If you are new to a daily exercise routine, your PT can offer tailored exercises to build stamina and strength. Maybe you ride your bike every day or run multiple 5ks (or marathons) a year; maybe exercise is new to you. Either way, there may be gaps in your flexibility or mobility that physical therapy could close. Also, by getting an assessment early, your PT will see how your Parkinson's is progressing over time and recommend exercises to address areas that may be getting weaker.

OCCUPATIONAL THERAPIST

Occupational therapy (OT) is the only profession that helps people across the lifespan do things they want to do through therapeutic activities (occupations). Occupational therapists (OTs) enable people of all ages to live life to its fullest by helping them promote health and prevent or live better with injury, illness, or disability.

Occupational therapy interventions focus on adapting the environment through modifications, modifying the task, teaching a skill, or educating the person, care partner, and family to increase participation and perform daily activities. Occupational therapy is practical and customizable, focusing primarily on activities that are important and meaningful to you.

SPEECH-LANGUAGE PATHOLOGIST

As Parkinson's progresses, some people find it difficult to speak loudly, pronounce words clearly, speak fluidly, and show facial expression. However, it is possible to improve all these symptoms by working with a speech therapist or speech-language pathologist (SLP). These rehabilitative professionals can also help you with eating, swallowing issues, saliva management, dry mouth, drool, and more.

PHARMACIST

If you see a pharmacist regularly (instead of ordering medications through an online service), they can be a valuable part of your care team. Because they will know all the medications you take—those related to Parkinson's and those that aren't—your pharmacist will be on the lookout for medication interactions that your primary care physician may not always be aware of. Whenever you are prescribed a new medicine, be sure to ask your pharmacist (in person or if you order medication online, via phone) if there's anything you need to know about how it might interact with other meds you are taking. Pharmacists can also advise about crushing pills, splitting doses, and easy-open bottles.

REGISTERED DIETICIAN

When it comes to nutritional plans, what works for you may not work for someone else. And for every article (peer-reviewed or otherwise) on why diet X is the best, there is another that claims Y is better. To find the best nutritional strategy for you, see a registered dietician (RD) specializing in working with people with Parkinson's or other neurological disorders. RDs are usually the most qualified health professionals on nutrition and dietetics, unless your primary care physician, neurologist, or MDS specializes in that field.

DENTIST

Regular dental exams are an important part of preventive care for everyone, and for a person with Parkinson's, good dental care is even more critical. That's because Parkinson's can impact the mouth and jaw and make dental care more challenging. Regular dental exams and cleanings are important to ensure you have healthy teeth and gums. At these appointments, often scheduled every six months, your dentist can check for cavities, plaque, tartar, and gum disease and ensure that you are properly caring for your oral health.

DERMATOLOGIST

Melanoma, one type of skin cancer, has been consistently linked to Parkinson's. Because melanoma is treatable if caught early but can be dangerous if not detected until the later stages, it's crucial that people with Parkinson's focus on skin protection and regular skin cancer screenings. During these screenings, a dermatologist will check your skin for moles, birthmarks, or other marks that are unusual in color, size, shape, or texture. If skin cancer is suspected after a screening, your physician will perform a biopsy to remove cells from the suspicious mark on your skin. A pathologist will then study the cells or tissue under a microscope to check for damage or disease.

EYE CARE PROFESSIONAL

Regular eye exams with an eye care professional should be part of your preventative care routine. These exams are essential for screening for eye diseases and preserving your vision. There are several different types of eye physicians: ophthalmologists, medical physicians who have completed four years of medical school followed by four years of residency training in ophthalmology; optometrists, healthcare providers who complete physician training in optometry but who have not attended medical school; and neuro-ophthalmologists, who are neurologists or ophthalmologists with expertise in visual symptoms from neurologic disease.

CARE PARTNER

Your care partner is an essential member of your team. While most care partners are spouses, children, siblings, parents, and even friends can play an integral role on your care team. This role is so important that we created a separate resource just for care partners called the *Every Victory Counts* **Manual for Care Partners**, which you can find on our website.

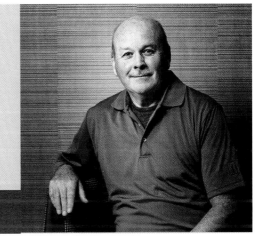

> " *I've only missed one appointment in my wife's six years with Parkinson's. I find it very beneficial to be there and fully involved in the discussion. Our neurologist will ask Edie a question and I'll chime in with my opinion so he gets both sides.*"
>
> — SCOTT ANDERSON

FAMILY AND FRIENDS

Your family members are also living with Parkinson's and will be key partners throughout your journey. They can work with you to assemble the rest of your care team and be the record keeper of therapies and outcomes. Look to your friends and community as sources of healthy social connectivity and for support.

YOU

Then, of course, there's you. YOU are the most critical member of the team. Think about the role you want to play as the primary team member. Be an active participant in managing your condition. Being engaged and empowered in your care gets results. Use this manual to learn what you can do to partner with your medical and wellness teams and how you can keep yourself on track.

You, your care partner, and your family need a support system that will be in place for the duration of your time with Parkinson's; so, do not wait to reach out and start adopting a holistic approach. Create a team of providers who can offer expertise in many different areas. Be an advocate for yourself as you build a team of providers who listen, respect your input, and with whom you feel comfortable. Being a strong self-advocate will give you a solid foundation and help you to live well with Parkinson's today and for many years to come.

"How Can I Build or Strengthen my Self-Efficacy to Live Well with Parkinson's?"

By Diane G. Cook

Self-efficacy is the belief that we can achieve influence over the conditions that affect our lives. It is a concept increasingly used by people living with Parkinson's to help us take a proactive role in its management. Research shows that people who can exert some control over their lives fare better and experience a better quality of life. Virtually everyone has some degree of self-efficacy. The challenge for people like you and me who live with Parkinson's (either as a person with Parkinson's or a care partner) is to strengthen our self-efficacy and channel it in ways that help us better cope.

HOW SELF-EFFICACY CAN HELP

Building belief in our capabilities increases our level of self-efficacy and influences what we can do. This increasing belief in our own power to effect change is a catalyst for a range of new, healthy behavioral patterns. For example, we can maintain a more positive attitude that positively impacts our emotional state and motivation level. We can find the strength from within to accept setbacks as challenges and to persevere more easily in the face of difficulties. For instance, while exercise may be challenging for us (and in some cases, it may seem entirely too difficult), by applying self-efficacy principles, we can, particularly with the help of others, reinvigorate our exercise regimen and gain the quality of life and symptom improvement exercise can bring.

ENHANCING YOUR SELF-EFFICACY

A scientifically-based process for enhancing self-efficacy was developed by renowned psychologist Dr. Albert Bandura of Stanford University in the 1970s. The first step is to set a series of ever more challenging goals; each enhances the belief that we can achieve the next. This creates an experience of mastery, which is the foundation of a strong sense of self-belief. The second step is to identify models to which we aspire, such as one or more people living with Parkinson's who are managing their Parkinson's well. Seeing others in a similar situation succeed through their determined efforts raises the belief that we, too, can overcome the specific challenges we face. The third step is to seek positive reinforcement and encouragement, strengthening our belief that we have what it takes to succeed.

WHAT IS YOUR CURRENT STATE OF PARKINSON'S-RELATED SELF-EFFICACY?

The questionnaire below can help you determine the extent to which you are currently exhibiting self-efficacy related to managing your Parkinson's. It can also give you some sense of where you could improve those behaviors to support your efforts better.

On a scale of 1 to 5, rate your current level of confidence that you can perform the activity described, where 1 = "not at all confident," 3 = "adequate," and 5 = "very confident."

Develop Knowledge about Parkinson's and Its Treatment

- ☐ I can accurately describe my Parkinson's in depth
- ☐ I can describe in detail my specific motor and non-motor symptoms
- ☐ I keep a complete and updated list of my medications and dosages
- ☐ I know and follow the nutritional guidelines for Parkinson's
- ☐ I understand the precautions and interactions of my medications and supplements
- ☐ I know the range of available complementary therapies
- ☐ I know techniques to address my stress and anxiety

Create Critical Partnerships

- ☐ I have a strong and supportive relationship with my care partner
- ☐ I have discussed my support needs with my family
- ☐ I have established an open and trusting relationship with my physician(s)
- ☐ I have sought out other healthcare specialists to assist, as needed
- ☐ I know where to go for help
- ☐ I am aware of national and local Parkinson's resources
- ☐ I attend a Parkinson's support group or similar group

Proactively Manage My Parkinson's

- ☐ I accept responsibility as the manager of my well-being
- ☐ I set increasingly difficult goals and make progress toward them
- ☐ I actively replace any unhealthy habits with healthy ones
- ☐ I track all my symptoms on a regular basis
- ☐ I keep thorough and up-to-date healthcare records
- ☐ I prepare for appointments with my physicians
- ☐ I communicate my concerns openly with my healthcare team
- ☐ I advocate for myself rather than letting others speak for me
- ☐ I follow a regular Parkinson's-specific exercise regimen

Maintain a Self-Efficacious Attitude

☐ I stay firm in the belief that I can positively influence my Parkinson's

☐ I focus on possibility rather than loss

☐ I practice evaluating available options to solve problems

☐ I put setbacks in perspective

☐ I reframe to help manage any negative emotions

☐ I persevere in the face of difficulties

☐ I remain hopeful and focus on the positive

The resulting snapshot from the survey should give you a sense of where you are on the Self-Efficacy for Parkinson's Scale. If you have any 1s or 2s, these are areas to focus on. If you have 5s, give yourself credit and build on this to be more successful in the areas you need to strengthen. For example, suppose you gave yourself a low score on "setting increasingly difficult goals" but had a high score on "attending a support group." In that case, you could ask the group leader to incorporate some regular goal-setting activities into the meetings. Suppose you gave yourself a low score on understanding your medications' precautions and interactions but a high score on seeking healthcare specialists to assist. In that case, you could use that skill to find a pharmacologist with whom to consult.

As you build your level of self-efficacy, you will find a renewed focus and energy that will support you in achieving your goals and positively impacting the course of your Parkinson's.

Every part of you is connected to and influenced by the other parts of you. Design your life with Parkinson's, keeping in mind the whole picture: goals, needs, lifestyle, nutritional choices, exercise, stress management, medication, relationships, personal and spiritual care, and growth. Living well means living well in all aspects of life. It means asking for help from people who can make your life better. And it means taking action to shape the future you want for yourself and those around you.

About Diane G. Cook

Diane Cook was diagnosed with Parkinson's in 2008 and has founded and facilitated many groups for newly diagnosed people with Parkinson's. She has participated in 15 clinical trials, serves as a patient consultant to several studies, and is an active advocate for greater patient participation in the clinical research process.

»

Nationally, Diane serves as a patient representative to the FDA, a Parkinson's Foundation research advocate, and has just completed terms as a member of Parkinson's Foundation's People with Parkinson's Advisory Council and the Steering Committee of the Clinical Trials Transformation Initiative (CTTI).

Diane pioneered the science of self-efficacy to newly diagnosed Parkinson's patients and has presented in that regard at the Montreal World Parkinson's Congress, the Sydney and Berlin International Movement Disorders Congresses, and the New York Academy of Sciences. The Colorado Neurological Institute (CNI) Foundation funded her initial research on the impact of self-efficacy on disease outcomes in newly diagnosed people with Parkinson's, and she has since trained people with Parkinson's/ healthcare professional teams to deliver the PD SELF (Self-Efficacy Learning Forum) program she developed in ten metropolitan areas across the US. Parkinson's Foundation designated PD SELF as one of their national pilot programs.

■ CHAPTER 2 – PARKINSON'S 101

OVERVIEW

When you are first diagnosed with Parkinson's, the sheer amount of information and the uniqueness of your experience can be overwhelming. We're here to help. This chapter is designed to be a starting point for people newly diagnosed with Parkinson's, answering some of the most common questions asked within the first year following diagnosis. It also provides some adaptive strategies to set you on the best path for living well with Parkinson's, including staying engaged and informed about your health and about the actions you can take to improve your quality of life.

WHAT IS PARKINSON'S?

Parkinson's is a brain disorder associated with a loss of dopamine-producing nerve cells (neurons) deep inside the brain. Dopamine is a neurotransmitter (a chemical substance) that helps regulate your body's movement. Less dopamine in the brain means less control over movement and less mobility in general. Parkinson's is both chronic and progressive, which means symptoms will change and worsen as time goes on. The rate of progression will vary from person to person. No two people living with Parkinson's will experience its symptoms or progression in the same way.

Because it involves damage to the areas of the brain that affect the speed, quality, fluency, and ease of movement, Parkinson's is officially classified as a movement disorder. Motor (or movement-related) symptoms, which we will cover in Chapter 3, are usually the most visible elements.

Although the effects of Parkinson's on movement often get the most attention, non-motor symptoms, which we will cover in Chapters 4-6, can have an even more significant impact on your quality of life.

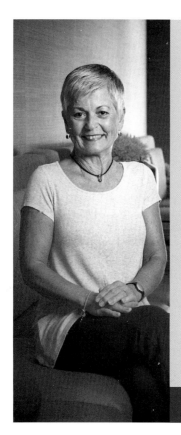

“ *Looking back, I was in a pity party for about a year after I was diagnosed. I didn't spend the whole year huddled in a corner feeling sorry for myself, but I went through the motions with no drive, no goals, no purpose. I felt empty and alone. Even though I had the support of a lot of family and friends, none of them could truly understand what I was dealing with. Finally I went to a local support group meeting and there was a person in the group who recognized my struggle. She'd been living with Parkinson's for about eight years and said something very profound to me. She said, 'Look, these are the cards you've been dealt. Play your cards, and play to win.' That's when it clicked that living well was up to me. Nobody could fix me, but I could make it better.*”

— **EDIE ANDERSON**

HOW IS PARKINSON'S DIAGNOSED?

The diagnosis of Parkinson's is usually made clinically, based on the symptoms a person is experiencing and signs that a neurologist or other health care provider detects on physical examination. Parkinson's typically has four cardinal motor symptoms:

- Slowness
- Stiffness
- Resting tremor
- Postural instability

Physicians determine you have Parkinson's after reviewing your medical history, asking you about your symptoms, and performing a clinical examination.

To support the diagnosis, your physician will also look for other signs:

- Micrographia (small handwriting)
- Facial masking (reduced facial expression)
- Decreased arm swing or leg drag on one side of your body while walking

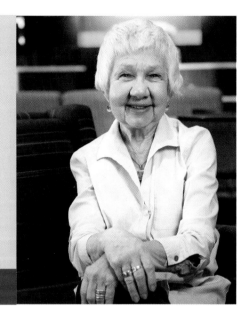

" *I was officially diagnosed at 72, but I started noticing changes when I was trekking in the Himalayas at 70. I would stumble on hikes or struggle to get my leg over the crossbar during a long bike ride. I made up all kinds of excuses until one day I collapsed on the trail and was taken to the hospital. It took a year before I saw a movement disorder specialist and was officially diagnosed with Parkinson's.*"

— **BRENDA**

After diagnosis, many people with Parkinson's look back and realize they had non-motor symptoms many years before their motor symptoms began. Early non-motor symptoms, which are often called pre-motor symptoms, can include:

- Rapid eye movement sleep behavior disorder (RBD): May begin 15-20 years before motor symptoms; the temporary paralysis most of us experience when we sleep that prevents us from acting out our dreams is disrupted in people with RBD, so they physically act out their dreams
- Constipation: May begin up to 20 years before motor symptoms
- Depression and anxiety: May begin up to 20 years before motor symptoms
- Loss of smell: May occur years before motor symptoms appear

SUPPORTIVE DIAGNOSTIC TESTING

In many cases, history and physical examination by an experienced clinician are sufficient to make a diagnosis of Parkinson's. However, there are several circumstances in which additional testing may be helpful. These circumstances include if a person has early, subtle symptoms, or if there are symptoms that are unusual for Parkinson's. Also, some medications, such as neuroleptics used for mental health like aripiprazole or risperidone, can cause drug-induced parkinsonism, for which physical symptoms may be indistinguishable from Parkinson's.

Levodopa Challenge Test

Levodopa is the gold standard treatment for Parkinson's. It was one of the first Parkinson's drugs, and it is still the main drug prescribed to treat Parkinson's for many people. It acts to help with slowness, stiffness, and tremor. Levodopa can be used in conjunction with other medications to address the same symptoms. Carbidopa is now always combined with levodopa to enable more levodopa to reach the brain rather than the bloodstream.

A levodopa challenge test can help confirm a Parkinson's diagnosis if your symptoms improve while taking the medication. If your symptoms do not improve while on levodopa, you likely have a different neurological condition. For people with prominent tremor, the dose of levodopa may need to be fairly high, up to 1500 mg of levodopa per day.

> *Originally, I was diagnosed by a general neurologist. He was a great doctor, but what he did initially... it was a little haphazard, to tell you the truth. Part of my diagnosis was a drug challenge, and he used the wrong meds, in the wrong dosage and the wrong order to come to the conclusion that I wasn't responding to meds. Then I went to a movement disorder specialist, and he put together a drug challenge that was clinically effective and found that I did respond to the medication after all and had young onset Parkinson's. One of the benefits to me was a whole lot less mental anguish going to someone who had specific experience with movement disorders."*

— COREY KING

DaTscan

A specialized brain scan called a ⌗ **DaTscan** can help in the diagnosis of Parkinson's. This test determines if you have a normal amount of cells that make dopamine. If the amount of cells that make dopamine is low, you may have Parkinson's, but you may have another neurological condition such as multiple system atrophy (MSA) or progressive supranuclear palsy (PSP). The test can help determine that one of these conditions is present, but it cannot distinguish among them.

Drug-induced parkinsonism is a condition caused by dopamine-blocking medications; in this condition the amount of cells that make dopamine in the brain is still normal, so a DaTscan would be normal. For a similar reason, DaTscan results are not affected by taking levodopa, as levodopa increases the amount of dopamine available in the brain, but does not affect the amount of cells that make dopamine in the brain. Certain medications such as bupropion or methylphenidate can affect the results and are often held for several days in advance of the test.

Skin Biopsy and Spinal Fluid Analysis

Parkinson's involves a misfolded protein called alpha-synuclein. For this reason, Parkinson's is sometimes called a synucleinopathy. In recent years, specialized analyses of skin biopsies and spinal fluid have become available that can detect the presence of misfolded alpha-synuclein. These tests can be used to confirm the presence of a synucleinopathy, and may soon be use to distinguish Parkinson's from other synucleinopathies, such as dementia with Lewy bodies (DLB) and MSA.

The skin biopsy is known as Syn-One®. This is an outpatient procedure that takes about 15 minutes and requires local anesthetic. The spinal fluid analysis is known as SYNTap® and requires a lumbar puncture.

Insurance coverage for these tests varies and hopefully will improve over time. This is an evolving area. Please see the ⟳ **Davis Phinney Foundation website** for additional details about diagnostic testing for Parkinson's.

DETERMINING WHICH TESTS ARE RIGHT FOR YOU

Consult your medical care team to determine if any of these tests might be helpful for you.

As technology and research progress, tests may become more helpful and informative. Some of these tests are being looked at in people with nonmotor/ premotor symptoms to see whether earlier initiation of new or old medications may help slow the development of Parkinson's.

> ❝*Don't look into the future, take one day at a time. And take the word CAN'T out of your vocabulary. You can accomplish any goal with patience and a little extra time.*"
>
> — MICHELLE LANE

WHO GETS PARKINSON'S?

Parkinson's is second only to Alzheimer's as the most common neurodegenerative disease in the United States, affecting between one million to 1.5 million nationwide. More people are living with Parkinson's in the US than the number of people living with multiple sclerosis, muscular dystrophy, and amyotrophic lateral sclerosis (ALS) combined.

Nearly 90,000 Americans are annually diagnosed with Parkinson's—a 50% increase from the previously estimated 60,000. More than 10 million people are estimated to be living with Parkinson's around the world.

> *"When I got the diagnosis, it wasn't like when I was diagnosed with breast cancer. Nobody said, 'We can fix this.' There is an action plan, it's just different. You don't focus on fixing Parkinson's. You focus on how to live with it so you can enjoy life."*
>
> — EDIE ANDERSON

Men are roughly twice as likely to be diagnosed with Parkinson's than women; however, women often see a quicker progression of Parkinson's and have a higher mortality rate. Most people living with Parkinson's are 60 years or older, though 5-10% of people are diagnosed before the age of 50. These individuals are referred to as having young onset Parkinson's disease (YOPD). One percent of the population over age 60 is estimated to be affected by Parkinson's, which increases to 5% of the population over age 85.

While these statistics give a high-level picture of Parkinson's, the reality is that Parkinson's affects many different populations, and it affects them in different ways. Here, we'll take a quick look at some of the different populations of people with Parkinson's.

> *"Don't be your own worst enemy. Instead of climbing up a ladder and risking a fall, ask for help. I am fiercely independent, and it was hard for me to admit I have some limitations. It isn't a sign of weakness. It takes wisdom to realize you need assistance and courage to ask for it."*
>
> — JULIE FITZGERALD

YOUNG ONSET PARKINSON'S DISEASE (YOPD)

The emotional, social, physical, and psychological needs of people diagnosed with YOPD are different from those diagnosed at an older age. While YOPD is characterized by the four common motor symptoms of Parkinson's (rigidity, slowness of movement, tremor, and postural instability), these symptoms often progress more slowly. The most common initial symptoms for YOPD are rigidity and painful cramps, while the most common initial symptoms for older-onset Parkinson's are tremor and instability with balance while walking. Another significant difference is that YOPD has a strong genetic component. For example, one gene abnormality, called PARK2 (Parkin gene), is found in up to 15% of younger individuals with Parkinson's.

Motor symptoms of both young and older-onset Parkinson's respond well to medication. Over time, motor complications such as end-of-dose wearing OFF and carbidopa/levodopa-induced dyskinesia can become a problem, leading to fluctuations in response to medications throughout the day. Both motor fluctuations and dyskinesia occur earlier in the disease progression and tend to be more severe in YOPD than in older-onset Parkinson's.

Despite earlier problems with motor complications, YOPD progresses more slowly, and other issues, such as dementia, are less common in YOPD.

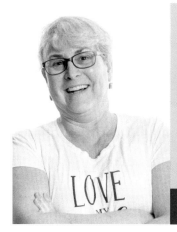

" *Especially when you have young onset Parkinson's, you realize so clearly that life is short. Because of Parkinson's, I act more quickly. Let's take that trip. Let's do that move. Let's retire way before we ever thought we would. The value of living fully right now is something that we as a family have really emphasized."*

— JILL ATER

People with YOPD will live with Parkinson's for many years and need to find ways to adapt to its effect on their lives. For some, this means adjusting to changes in physical abilities over time. For others, coping with the impact of Parkinson's on work, hobbies, family, and relationships is most important. It is vital to understand that you can affect how you change and feel with Parkinson's over the years. It is critical to take control, tend to your health, and proactively take the steps needed to do your best with Parkinson's. Using this manual to help you navigate Parkinson's and take the actions necessary for your wellness is an essential step toward lifelong health.

31

" *I was diagnosed with essential tremor and Parkinson's at age 44. The movement disorder specialist said, 'Your husband needs to keep his job, because you'll need the insurance. And you'll be bedridden in 10 years.' Determined to prove her wrong, I decided I would increase the frequency and intensity of my exercise regimen. Denial worked for a short time. Work became increasingly more challenging as my gait issues and internal tremor worsened and other symptoms (fatigue, bladder issues, pain) creeped in. I felt two steps slower than colleagues in meetings, and I feared that my work performance would suffer. Accepting the inevitable, I scheduled an appointment with a different doctor. We had a great relationship and communicated effectively. A decade after that initial diagnosis, my movement disorder specialist and neuropsychologist encouraged me to stop working and to leave my toxic work environment because stress was worsening every symptom. That last drive home from work was AWESOME! My symptoms immediately improved — no more 10- to 12-hour workdays in a very busy leadership role, and my husband and I hit the road to travel. Sure, there have been challenges with financial concerns, worry about healthcare insurance, and adjustment to the end of a 35-year career. I benefited from earlier decisions related to private long-term disability insurance plans that, after much angst and drama and lots of documentation, were approved. I have no regrets related to my medical retirement; this decision has allowed me to find my true purpose in my life — to help others to find their way to living life well with Parkinson's."*

— MARTY ACEVEDO

Because of the unique challenges of living with YOPD, we want to increase awareness of its common characteristics, provide resources, and share stories to help people with YOPD live better today. Our *Every Victory Counts* **website** has a section dedicated solely to YOPD, with videos, advice, webinars, and YOPD spotlights.

WOMEN

In general, women and men diagnosed with Parkinson's experience many similar issues with Parkinson's, ranging from sleep problems, cognitive impact, responses to surgery, medication benefits and side effects, emotional health, and the care partner experience. However, when a woman is diagnosed with YOPD, you can add possible challenges related to contraception, pregnancy, menstruation, menopause, and hormones. There is a growing body of content on this topic, and we share many of those resources on the *Every Victory Counts* **website**.

PEOPLE WHO LIVE ALONE WITH PARKINSON'S

Many people with Parkinson's may not reside with a spouse acting as a care partner or have children or other family members nearby who can help. When you live alone, staying informed, being engaged in your own health, and remaining connected to your friends and community become even more critical. There are numerous ways to stay connected and involved (for more on that, see the chapter about social connection), create a safe living environment for yourself, find the help you may need, and more.

Throughout this manual, we stress the importance of self-advocacy. This is even more crucial to living well with Parkinson's if you live alone and far away from family and loved ones. Ask for help when you need it. Accept help when it is offered. Recognize your boundaries and limits but also your strengths and abilities. Make choices that will keep you living well with Parkinson's far into the future and reach out to those who can help you do so. Many can! For strategies on living well with Parkinson's when you live alone, see the *Every Victory Counts* **website**.

❝ *I don't have a spouse or children; I live alone. I have lots of friends, but I'm on my own to determine how to live and handle Parkinson's. Living alone has actually given me strength to handle this diagnosis."*

— BRENDA

WHAT CAUSES PARKINSON'S?

BACKGROUND

The complexity of the brain has made the search for the underlying causes of Parkinson's challenging. We know that the pathological hallmark of Parkinson's is the aggregation of misfolded alpha-synuclein protein. These form so-called Lewy bodies and other changes in brain tissue that can be seen with a microscope. However, there is no known single cause of these changes that cause Parkinson's. Scientists and researchers believe a unique combination of genetics, environment, lifestyle, and other factors are at play for each person who develops Parkinson's.

GENETIC FACTORS

In the January 1999 issue of the *Journal of the American Medical Association*, researchers first concluded that genetic factors play a role of varying degrees in the development of Parkinson's. In October 2003, scientists at the National Institutes of Health discovered that mutations in the alpha-synuclein gene could cause Parkinson's. These findings suggest that genetic components could play a more significant role in Parkinson's than initially thought. By 2020, researchers were linking approximately 15% of Parkinson's cases to a direct genetic cause. Studies are ongoing that explore Parkinson's and genetics, with hopes of discoveries that lead to improved, personalized treatments.

Abnormal genes have been identified in some people with Parkinson's, especially younger individuals, and those with gene mutations whose Parkinson's "runs in the family." However, no single genetic abnormality has been found for the majority of people with Parkinson's. Researchers have identified more than a dozen gene abnormalities associated with Parkinson's.[1] Unlike the alpha-synuclein gene mutation, most of these genes are referred to as "susceptibility genes," meaning that while they do not necessarily cause Parkinson's, they do increase the risk of developing it. Variants in the GBA gene are the genetic factor most commonly associated with Parkinson's. Inherited cases of Parkinson's can also be caused by mutations in the LRRK2, PARK2, PARK7, DJ-1, PINK1, or SNCA genes or by mutations in genes not yet identified.

> ❝ *My mom and sister both have Parkinson's — we have the LRRK2 gene — so when I was diagnosed, I understood what it meant. I'm not a doctor, but with my family experience and doing my own reading, I knew this was a progressive disease that doesn't get better. I didn't know what our future would hold, but I knew things were never going back to 'normal.' That said, not being 'normal' is a gift in itself! The Mack truck has hit us. The worst has already happened. Parkinson's has forced me and my family to make so many changes for the better."*
>
> **— JILL ATER**

After receiving a diagnosis of Parkinson's, many people are concerned about passing it along to their children. Remember that genetic factors play a role in only a small number of cases, and even if your children inherit an abnormal gene from you, they may not automatically develop Parkinson's. While genetic testing is available, it does not necessarily offer answers to many pressing questions people may have about their condition. If you have a family history that includes many people with Parkinson's, you may wish to talk with your physician about testing. If you decide to be tested, it is important to see a genetic counselor before and after receiving the results. These specialized counselors, available in many large medical centers and university programs, will help you understand the results, their potential impact on your family, and how they may influence insurance qualification and other issues you may not have considered.

ENVIRONMENTAL FACTORS

Epidemiological studies based on large populations suggest that certain toxins increase the risk of developing Parkinson's. For instance, there is an increased risk for people living in rural communities or who drink well water. This may be due to ingestion of or exposure to certain pesticides proven in the laboratory to be toxic to dopamine neurons. Other chemicals, such as solvents used in the industrial dry-cleaning industry, have been implicated, suggesting that certain environmental toxins increase the risk of developing Parkinson's.

In a report co-authored by the Science and Environmental Health Network consortium of advocacy groups based in Iowa, a summary of 31 population studies examined the possible connection between pesticide exposure and Parkinson's. According to the report, 24 of those studies found a positive association, and in 12 cases, the association was statistically significant. In some studies, the group found there was *as much as a sevenfold greater risk* of Parkinson's in people exposed to pesticides than those who were not. Also, scientists at the University of California, Los Angeles, published a provocative study in April 2009 connecting Parkinson's to occupational pesticide exposure and living in homes or going to schools close to a pesticide-treated field.[2]

The *Collaborative Health and the Environment* states that "pesticide exposures as defined by occupational exposure (vineyard worker, agricultural worker, farmer, animal breeder, pesticide applicator) or inferred by rural residences or well water as a source of drinking water has been associated with PD. Several population-based case-control studies have identified a 3-4-fold increased likelihood of PD with past herbicide or insecticide exposure."[3]

LIFESTYLE FACTORS

A study published in 2015 identified many possible lifestyle factors that may increase or decrease a person's risk of developing Parkinson's. This list included habits that may negatively impact the risk of Parkinson's, such as drinking alcohol, well-water ingestion, and exposure to anesthesia, manganese, solvents, and farming chemicals. Habits found to potentially protect against developing Parkinson's include drinking coffee or green tea; a diet rich in vitamins, minerals, unsaturated fatty acids, and flavonoids (found in many plant-based foods); and exercise.[4]

A September 2016 analysis conducted by the *Journal of the American Medical Association*[5] of three major studies that used autopsy data to examine the association between traumatic brain injury (TBI) and neurodegenerative diseases found that TBI with loss of consciousness is associated with increased risk for Lewy body accumulation, progression of parkinsonism, and development of Parkinson's. While important information highlighting the need for head injury prevention, this research supports one potential lifestyle factor cause and does not explain how people who have never experienced TBI (or have genetic or environmental factors) develop Parkinson's.

WHAT TREATMENTS ARE AVAILABLE FOR PARKINSON'S?

For most people, the first line of treatment is medication. (And exercise.) Many will later opt for surgical and complementary therapies as well. Here's a brief breakdown of treatments; we will explain each in more depth in later chapters.

> " *Life is incurable, life is progressive, life is degenerative, and all of us have to come to terms with that and live life to the fullest anyway. I don't feel like I'm any different than anybody else, I just have more insight into my challenges."*
>
> — COREY KING

MEDICATIONS

There are many different types of medications that can help manage symptoms of Parkinson's. It may take some trial and error to find the combination of medications that work for you, and your ideal combination will continue to change over time. Please do not let the challenges of finding the right type, timing, and dose frustrate you. This happens, but it will get better.

Sometimes medications impact other symptoms of Parkinson's or cause bothersome side effects; so, it is important to communicate your symptoms and your medications' impacts with your physician. Often, adjusting the dosage or changing the medication can help. For an in-depth look at the latest in Parkinson's medications, be sure to explore Chapter 7 of this manual, along with our online medication guide on the ⟳ *Every Victory Counts* **website**.

EXERCISE

In the last decade, research studies and clinical experience have upgraded the importance of exercise to treat people with Parkinson's from a "nice to have" activity to an essential way to help manage symptoms and maintain quality of life. Exercise can improve everything from your mood to fatigue, muscle stiffness, tremor, constipation, and more. Learn all about the power of exercise for Parkinson's in Chapter 9.

SURGICAL THERAPIES

As Parkinson's symptoms progress, increasing medications to address them can bring significant side effects. One of the most common and bothersome side effects of Parkinson's medications is dyskinesia, which is characterized by uncontrollable, involuntary movement. Surgical therapies are often explored after medications have been optimized and the side effects of adding more medications begin to outweigh the benefits that medications provide. Current surgical therapies include deep brain stimulation (DBS) and enteral suspension of carbidopa/levodopa. In Chapter 8, we'll take a close look at these and other innovative therapies currently being researched.

REHABILITATIVE THERAPIES

Rehabilitation specialists include physical therapists, speech-language pathologists, and occupational therapists. Your rehabilitation team can help you prevent or delay problems, minimize the impact of symptoms, and maintain daily functioning as Parkinson's progresses. In Chapter 10, we'll explore the many benefits of having these specialists on your care team.

COMPLEMENTARY THERAPIES

Complementary therapies are used alongside traditional medical treatment. Various complementary therapies can help you manage and reduce your Parkinson's symptoms. Complementary therapies include everything from acupuncture to art, music, dance therapy, tai chi, mindfulness exercises, and more. Chapter 10 is dedicated to these and other complementary therapies that people in our community have tried and found to help them live well with Parkinson's.

HOW DOES PARKINSON'S CHANGE OVER TIME?

Everyone's experience with Parkinson's is different, so much so that anticipating its progression can be terribly frustrating. Physicians rarely try to predict the exact course of your Parkinson's or how severe or mild your symptoms will be. Each person's symptoms change at different rates and present different variations. Sometimes things change for the better in one area, but a new symptom will crop up elsewhere. Age and overall health can also influence the progression of Parkinson's.

That said, there are similarities most people with Parkinson's experience over time. Symptoms typically evolve slowly. Many times, you may not be aware of a change in mobility or certain other symptoms until someone else points it out. In the beginning stages of Parkinson's, symptoms such as tremor, slowness, and rigidity typically begin on one side of the body, then spread to the other side over time. Walking, speech, or swallowing problems can occur, too, though these symptoms usually progress slowly over many years. For most people, balance problems occur in later stages, leading to concerns about falls and serious injuries.

> **"** *In the beginning, I really didn't have a whole lot of challenges. Now, a decade into living with Parkinson's, I have to be really cognizant of sleep, my schedule, and medicine. If I'm not, I might be okay today, but I'll have an off day tomorrow. I need to manage Parkinson's more hands-on and consciously."*
>
> — STEVE HOVEY

How your Parkinson's progresses and the different symptoms you experience will be unique to you. Remember that the actions you take today and every day can significantly impact both, so choose those that help you live well in the moment and set you on the strongest path for the future.

WHAT ARE THE STAGES OF PARKINSON'S?

As we have explained, everyone's experience with Parkinson's is different, and your symptoms and stages may look different from those others experience. In general, however, the stages of Parkinson's tend to look something like this:

Early Stage

- Symptoms on one side of the body
- Decreased arm swing on one side when walking
- Decreased stride length
- Dragging your foot while walking
- Scuffing your toes, especially when tired
- Change in leg coordination when cycling or running
- Sense of muscle fatigue or heaviness in your arm or leg on one side of the body
- Difficulty completing repetitive movements due to sense of muscle fatigue
- Trouble with hand coordination, especially on one side. This is often apparent doing tasks that use both hands, like shampooing your hair
- Reduced range of motion in your shoulder, shoulder pain, or frozen shoulder
- Mask-like face or change in facial expression (hypomimia)
- Decreased or small handwriting (micrographia)

Mid Stage

- Symptoms on both sides of the body

- Soft speech (hypophonia)

- Mild swallowing problems, such as difficulty swallowing pills

- Flexed or bent posture and shuffling gait

- Motor fluctuations and dyskinesia

Advanced Stage

- Postural instability with balance problems and falls

- Walking problems, with increased shuffling, freezing of gait, and festination

- Significant speech and swallowing problems

- Drooling

- Rigidity in the neck and trunk parts of the body

> *The best thing I could do to accept my diagnosis was to get involved in activities within the Parkinson's community. I have met wonderful people who will be my friends for the rest of my life. Their stories have encouraged me to tell my story, which is something you can't really do unless you accept it."*
>
> — CAROL CLUPNY

As you journey through the different stages of Parkinson's, remember to reach out to current and new members of your care team who can help you manage changing symptoms. Remember, too, that at every stage there are many actions you can take to live well and maintain a high quality of life. Self-advocate during appointments, ask for referrals, try new exercises and therapies, and take time for self-care.

WHAT ABOUT PARKINSONISMS? ARE THEY THE SAME AS PARKINSON'S?

Parkinsonism, also called atypical Parkinson's or Parkinson's plus, is the umbrella term used to describe a group of neurological problems. Interestingly, Parkinson's represents only 10-15% of all diagnosed cases of parkinsonism. Parkinson's is caused mainly by the degeneration of nerve cells in the brain. In contrast, the causes of parkinsonism are numerous, ranging from the side effects of medications to metabolic diseases, toxins, and neurological diseases.

Parkinsonism is considered a clinical syndrome in which a person may have some but not all Parkinson's motor symptoms and other symptoms related to an additional condition or cause. These indications can range from low blood pressure to the inability to move one's eyes up and down to dementia.

The clinical features of parkinsonism and Parkinson's are similar and often indistinguishable. If you have movement problems including tremors, slow movement, or stillness and wonder whether you have Parkinson's or parkinsonism, you're not alone; it's a challenge to identify. People are often diagnosed with Parkinson's when they have another form of parkinsonism. On the other hand, people can be diagnosed with the general umbrella term parkinsonism when they have Parkinson's. Because the root cause and treatment for each form of parkinsonism is different, it's critical to obtain an accurate diagnosis, and working with a movement disorder specialist is undeniably your best option to ensure you get one. For more information on all the different types of parkinsonisms and treatments, visit the ⌁ *Every Victory Counts* website.

"How Can I Move from Diagnosis to Acceptance?"

By Amy Montemarano, JD

I learned some things about acceptance on a summer day just a couple of months after my Parkinson's diagnosis at age 48. It was supposed to have been a fun outing—kayaking with a few friends and, collectively, our six middle-school-aged daughters for a last hurrah before their school year started. We rented kayaks and set into the Mullica River in Southern New Jersey, about an hour and worlds away from where I live in Philadelphia. I grew up near the Mullica, deep in the Pinelands, and joining us was one of my closest childhood friends, Tracy, the kind of person who drops effortlessly back into the comfort of a longtime friendship even though it had been years since we'd last seen each other.

As we started out in the gentle tributary that wound through the pines, for the first time in my life, I was nervous about whether I was physically strong enough to spend an active day outdoors. That nervousness turned into despair about an hour into the three-hour journey, as the sky and the river both widened, and my arms started to shake uncontrollably from the repetitive movements of paddling. My daughters noticed; one of them paddled close to me and laid her hand on my arm to try to keep it still. Then everyone noticed. I fell behind and could not keep up, exhausted from the paddling and the energy of trying to seem normal.

The Mullica runs to the Atlantic Ocean, and the part of the river we were kayaking that day is tidal, which meant that about a mile from our ultimate landing spot, the river suddenly became more powerful. The current began to switch directions with the ocean tide. We would have already finished by that time had I not been so slow. Paddling harder didn't work because my arms wouldn't obey me. I fell even farther behind and couldn't imagine how I would paddle another mile like that. I struggled so hard against the mighty current, only to find myself moving backward. Every ounce of strength and confidence was slipping away, right there on the river of my childhood.

All I had wanted was for my daughters to have a fun day. Instead, they had to watch me fall apart.

That's when Tracy intervened. She kicked into overdrive and paddled ahead to a house on the river where a friend lived, and with charm and cheer, he tied all our kayaks together and towed us with his powerboat the last mile up current to our landing spot. We were in awe of how he navigated our connected kayaks through the twists and turns of the river without any of us getting stuck, tangled, or separated. He understood angles better than an MIT math professor. The girls were thrilled.

We all learned a lot that day, but I didn't really understand my lesson until much later. After my diagnosis, I immersed myself in reading everything I could get my hands on about mind-body medicine, meditation, brain health, epigenetics, spirituality, and holistic health. I made lists of best practices for living well with Parkinson's. I tried different diets and supplements and visited all kinds of medical practitioners. I incorporated hypnosis and tapping and deep breathing, hot and cold therapy, infrared light therapy, music therapy, and, of course, many forms of exercise. I called my first year after diagnosis The Year of Living Experimentally (and expensively)

It's been six years since that day on the river. A few months ago, a guided meditation randomly showed up on my playlist. The teacher spoke of a principle of Taoism called the water way. It's a principle that teaches how to live life without suffering so much, and the gist of it is this: be like water.

Water flows wherever the path of least resistance leads. It takes the shape of whatever container it occupies, from a pot to a pond to the wide-open ocean. And while it changes appearance when frozen into ice or heated into steam, it never changes its true nature. This makes water more resilient to outside circumstances. When it hits an obstruction, it is patient, and through its soft grace and gentle steps, it eventually finds a way around, often leaving beauty (like the Grand Canyon) in its wake.

Being like water means having the ability to flow in whatever direction and into whatever container our life situation hands us. It doesn't change anything about our lives' difficulties, but it allows us to stop struggling and deal with any situation from an authentic place. And that is where our power lies because it comes to us effortlessly. If we constantly fight our life situation and try to force it into the shape we want, we get frustrated, angry, anxious, and scared because we are relying on a form of power that ultimately doesn't work. That's what the Mullica taught me. When the current switched, and I struggled to be the person (and mom and kayaker) I wanted to be, I fell farther behind and suffered more. But when I let go and gave up any sense of control and ego, what filled that space was the kindness and love of both friends and strangers, and what was delivered to me were awe and gratitude and a bunch of delighted girls who had the time of their lives that day.

This lesson, of course, is not easy, and it's not learned once and done. It requires active, daily practice (and if ever you need inspiration, consider watching (or re-watching) *The Shawshank Redemption*, an excellent story of being like water). Now, as I approach my seventh year after diagnosis—the end of a period that many people call the honeymoon stage of Parkinson's—if the current takes me over the cliff into the well of despair, I need to remind myself that if I fight it, I will drown. I hope I have the strength of mind not to struggle and instead wait patiently for the next nourishing spring rain to raise the water and lift me out.

About Amy Montemarano

Amy Montemarano was diagnosed with young onset Parkinson's at age 48. Through the strong medical and support networks for people with Parkinson's in the Philadelphia area, she learned how to rely on exercise, stress management, and other wellness tools to help her live well with her diagnosis. To her, living well with Parkinson's means not giving up your enjoyment of life and fully engaging with the world in a way that uses your own special purpose and energy to its highest potential. Finding purpose and meaning in her own life post-diagnosis has led Amy to help people with Parkinson's and their care partners navigate employment, as well as find volunteer work or creative projects to discover their own personal adventures.

Amy finds enjoyment in writing, traveling, lifelong learning, and listening to live music. Since her diagnosis, Amy has traveled to New Zealand, Europe, Canada, and other states within the US. On a perfect Sunday morning, you can find Amy going on a hike with her dog Dylan, meeting her husband in a café, and ending the day spending time with her two teenage daughters.

41

■ CHAPTER 3 – MOTOR SYMPTOMS

OVERVIEW

Although the motor symptoms of Parkinson's tend to get the most attention and treatment, they often don't appear until many of the brain's nerve cells that produce dopamine have already stopped working. In this chapter, we'll help you identify and learn about the primary Parkinson's motor symptoms. Even though you may not experience all of them, knowing about common motor symptoms will help you be proactive in managing the motor symptoms you do experience so you can live well.

WHAT MOTOR SYMPTOMS MIGHT I EXPERIENCE?

The four primary motor symptoms of Parkinson's include tremor, rigidity, slowness of movement (bradykinesia), and postural instability. Early motor symptoms can also include a mask-like face or loss of facial expression, small and cramped handwriting (micrographia), and decreased natural arm swing. Other movement symptoms of Parkinson's can include reduced manual dexterity, severe muscle cramping or contractions (dystonia), and, though not common, a deficit in the motor aspect of expression called the pseudobulbar affect, which presents as frequent, short, uncontrollable outbursts of crying or laughing that is contradictory to a person's emotional state.

TREMORS

Even though other health conditions can cause shaking hands and feet, approximately 70% of people with Parkinson's experience tremor. A tremor is an involuntary, rhythmic shaking or quivering movement which can occur in the hand, arm, foot, leg, and chin, with the most common being in a person's hands.

Imbalances in neurotransmitters cause tremors. As dopamine cells disappear because of Parkinson's, a neurotransmitter called acetylcholine becomes overexpressed, and this excess results in involuntary shaking movements. In the early stages of Parkinson's, tremor is typically seen on one side of the body, often starting in a hand; however, as Parkinson's progresses, tremor may impact both sides and affect more body regions. The patterns, forms, and progression of tremors are individual to each person.

> " Since I have Parkinson's, I dazzle my doctor by threading the needle on my sewing machine while it is still running! I put the thread in the hand that has tremors and as my hand tremors, it puts the thread in the needle eyelet multiple times."
>
> — BARRY BRANSON

Tremors can cause complications with many activities of daily living that involve fine motor skills, such as brushing teeth, shaving, bathing, getting dressed, writing a letter, and eating. If you have a tremor, activities can also take longer to accomplish than they once did. The good news is that although a tremor is bothersome and can be embarrassing, it is not incapacitating or life-threatening.

TYPES OF TREMOR

There are many different types of tremor. Here, we'll discuss those that are most common for people living with Parkinson's.

Pill-Rolling Tremor

This type of tremor, often one of the first symptoms of Parkinson's, occurs in the fingers. Finger twitching is a movement that looks like a person is rolling a pill between their thumb and fingers. In medical jargon, it is fittingly defined as a "pill-rolling" tremor.

Resting Tremor

The most common tremor in Parkinson's is the resting tremor, which occurs when a person is at rest or (paradoxically) under emotional or physical stress. When the affected part of the body is actively moving, resting tremors often subside. For example, when a person holds a spoon while eating, the thumb and index finger muscles are held in one position, and a resting tremor can transpire; consequently, the food on the spoon may spill. The resting tremor lessens when the muscle is in action. For example, if a person's hand is shaking while sitting, once that person moves the hand to shake hands with someone, the shaking will often disappear. Similarly, resting tremor in the legs occurs when a person is lying down or sleeping or when one's feet are dangling. Again, if one starts moving, the tremor disappears.

Action Tremor

An action tremor, of which essential tremor is a type, is the shaking motion that occurs when a limb or body part is being moved. While action tremors are much less common in people with Parkinson's, more than 25% of people with Parkinson's experience them.

Internal Tremor

Even though others cannot see an internal tremor, many people with Parkinson's report a shaking sensation inside the chest, abdomen, or limbs. Because this internal tremor is difficult to explain to others and is often upsetting to the person with Parkinson's, it can distract and interrupt the flow of what they're doing. While internal tremors can be extremely difficult to identify and describe, they often respond to medications in a similar way that external tremors do.

STRATEGIES TO MANAGE TREMORS

Medications

Routine. Routine. Routine. It is critical to take your medications consistently and on time, even if you don't currently feel a tremor. Having a constant medication level in your body by following your physician's medication schedule can help prevent OFF times. OFF times are when your medications aren't working optimally, and your tremor returns or worsens. Create a habit of taking your medications at the same time each day and of taking your carbidopa/levodopa on an empty stomach with a full glass of water. Drinking a full glass of water when taking your pills helps flush the medicine quickly from your stomach to your small intestines, where it is absorbed. If you need help with medication management, talk with your physicians about wearable technologies that can help monitor movement fluctuations and determine proper medication dosages.

Exercise

Exercise can help manage many motor symptoms of Parkinson's, including tremor. Learn about the many benefits of exercise on Parkinson's tremor in the "Taking Action" section of this chapter and Chapter 9 of this manual.

Reduce Multi-Tasking

Doing just one thing at a time can lessen tremors. For example, when eating, place your elbows on the table to stabilize your arms. Sit down when you brush your teeth, so you only need to focus on your upper body muscles. Hold your arms as close to your body as possible when writing a check. When you walk, keep your hands and arms free.

Reduce Stress

Not completing tasks as efficiently as you could before you experienced tremor can be disheartening, stressful, and fatiguing. The next time you feel frustrated while trying to accomplish a task, take a few deep breaths to help rebalance your nervous system and allow your muscles to relax. Then, try the action again.

Consider Assistive Technologies and Products

To help you everywhere—from the kitchen to the bathroom, bedroom, golf course, swimming pool, sidewalk, and more—there are tools, gadgets, and equipment designed especially for people who experience tremor, and new ones are invented all the time. Whether it's stretchy elastic shoelaces or a long-handled shoehorn to help you put on socks and shoes, an adaptive mouse for computer work, weighted silverware to help decrease tremor while eating, or Velcro buttons, a wide variety of devices can help you feel safe, become more confident when attempting various tasks, gain more independence, and increase self-efficacy.

Although some adaptive products are covered by insurance, many are not. Still, a written prescription from your physician for any changes in your home, from grab bars in the bathroom to a ramp inside or outside your home, can help with potential tax deductions.

RIGIDITY (STIFFNESS)

Stiff or inflexible muscles are often seen as symptoms of arthritis or normal aging; however, stiffness or rigidity of the limbs and trunk are cardinal symptoms of Parkinson's. Muscles become rigid because they lose the ability to relax and stretch, which not only feels uncomfortable but can also cause pain.

Like tremor, rigidity in Parkinson's usually appears first on one side of the body and spreads to both sides over time.

"Cogwheel rigidity" is stiffness at the joints, so named because the movement at a joint, such as at the elbow, causes ratchet-like start and stop movements similar to cogs on a cogwheel. Rigidity can also impact the muscles of the face. If they become stiff, you can develop a fixed, "mask-like" facial expression. Rigidity can impact sleep quality because stiffness in the late evening can cause aches and pains, and you may have problems turning over in bed. Also, because stiff muscles can impact how you walk, rigidity can cause problems with walking or gait abnormalities and put you at an increased risk of falling.

STRATEGIES TO MANAGE RIGIDITY

Move Frequently Every Day

Frequent movement can help relieve stiff and achy joints and muscles. Whether it's standing up and marching in place during TV commercials, setting the alarm on your phone to remind you to stretch your arms above your head and walk around the house for five minutes, or parking your car at the farthest spot from the store, regular movement breaks can minimize stiffness. To help with walking problems or gait abnormalities, look straight ahead and not at your feet. Focus on the size rather than the frequency of your steps. Sometimes, smaller steps will get you to your destination faster. Retrain your brain by telling yourself to land with your heel first and not the ball or front part of your foot.

Change It Up

Try to mix up your exercise routine so that you are consistently using and strengthening different muscles. See how many different activities you can do in one week that make you feel great physically and bring you joy.

Track Your Steps

For those with a competitive spirit, use a fitness tracker to track your steps, compete with others, and provide an objective way to measure your goal. Even increasing by five to ten steps or 100 steps per day follows Davis Phinney's philosophy that "Every Victory Counts."

Join a Class

Not only will joining a movement or exercise class help improve your mood, but it can also help you decrease rigidity by strengthening your muscles and improving your flexibility.

Consider a Complementary Therapy

Evidence supports the use of music-based movement therapy for people with Parkinson's to improve motor function. In 2018, a review of 27 different studies supported this finding. It demonstrated that music therapy has beneficial effects on the nonpharmacologic treatment of motor and non-motor symptoms and quality of life for people living with Parkinson's.

In addition to music therapy, art therapy, meditation, and massage, physical therapy is very effective in helping people with Parkinson's maintain strength, improve mobility, and stay active longer. Speech-language therapy can help keep facial muscles flexible to optimize your speech and swallowing efforts.

BRADYKINESIA (SLOWNESS OF MOVEMENT)

Bradykinesia means slow movement, and it can be problematic for many people who live with Parkinson's.

Bradykinesia can show up as:

- A change in walking from a normal gait to shuffle-like steps
- A change in handwriting from large letters to increasingly smaller letters
- Difficulty getting in and out of bed
- Fatigue because tasks take longer to accomplish
- Movement that starts fine but slowly deteriorates
- Change in speech and vocal projection

STRATEGIES TO MANAGE BRADYKINESIA

Regular exercise, physical therapy, and medication are some of the ways you can manage slow movement. Under the supervision of a physical therapist, some of the tasks you may try include walking faster than you usually would, traversing different surfaces, and walking with your eyes closed and then open. By challenging your normal gait, these exercises can improve your ability to walk.

POSTURAL INSTABILITY (POOR BALANCE AND COORDINATION)

Balance is a state of equilibrium. When you can control your body's center of mass over its base of support, you remain upright and steady. However, Parkinson's can cause a loss of reflexes needed to maintain an upright posture, causing some people with Parkinson's to feel unstable while standing upright. Parkinson's impact on the brain can also cause delays in a person's reaction time, speed of movements, and postural "righting reflexes." (This means if your body sways off its base of support, it might take too long to "right" itself.) All of these increase the risk of falling.

One way that physicians test for postural stability is by using the "pull test." In this test, a physician will stand behind a person and give a tug to pull back, then watch how well the person reacts and how many steps it takes to recover balance. Usually, a person without postural instability takes a quick backward step to prevent themselves from falling. However, a person with Parkinson's is often unable to recover and would fall backward if the physician weren't there to catch them.

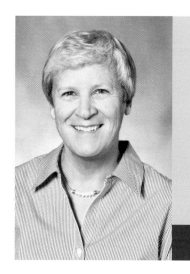

> " *For my Parkinson's friends with a closet full of shoes that contribute to a less-than-stable walking experience: did you know that athletic shoes come in many styles and can look great with most outfits? Yes! And, on those occasions when casual shoes really won't work, try a low-heeled dress shoe so you can look good and have fun while staying safely on your feet.*"

— LORRAINE WILSON

STRATEGIES TO MANAGE POSTURAL INSTABILITY

With practice, you can improve your postural stability and even regain some of your automatic reflexes. Exercises that focus on balance, strength, agility, and flexibility are keys to improving balance and coordination.

Balance

The most effective balance exercises are high intensity; challenging and cognitively engaging (requiring your sustained attention to perform them well); repetitious (taking place every day or most days of the week); progressive (demanding more work and attention as your skills improve); meaningful (improving your quality of life); and enjoyable.

Activities that incorporate balance elements such as yoga, tai chi, Pilates, boxing, and dance are ideal for people with Parkinson's because they relieve stress and help build balance control.

The key to building balance control is practice. Just like when you first learned to stand and walk, keep practicing and incorporate balance control exercises into your daily life.

Strength

Strength exercises challenge your muscles to remain strong. To build strength, you need to use your muscles repeatedly in a specific and controlled way. This is especially important in your trunk muscles, which help hold you upright so you don't stoop forward. Lifting weights and using machines at the gym can be effective, but you can also do strength training at home using everyday household items such as milk jugs filled with sand, soup cans, or broomsticks.

Agility

Agility, or the ability to move quickly and easily, is essential to efficiently change one's body position. The goal of agility exercises is to gain greater control of your body when it is in

47

motion. These exercises can condition your lower body to stand and move in ways that offer you more stability. As a result, your improved muscle memory can help you avoid falls. The most effective agility drills are designed to enhance your response during moments of split-second locomotive decisions.

Flexibility

Flexibility and stretching exercises are essential for maintaining a good range of movement in joints and muscles. If you lose flexibility, you lose range of motion and mobility. If you improve your flexibility, you will have an easier time with everyday movement such as walking.

Other Strategies

- Assess and improve your posture by standing against a wall, ensuring that your lower back and shoulder blades touch the wall. Do this a few times a day to keep your posture in check

- When you're standing, plant your feet shoulder-length apart instead of close together to create a more stable base for your body

- Use a bum bag or belt bag to carry things so that your hands are kept free and unrestricted. With both hands free, making a conscious effort to swing both arms can help you maintain balance

- If you have difficulty changing directions or with quick movements, try making a wide turn that looks like the letter "U" instead of a quick and potentially risky pivot that looks like the letter "V"

DYSTONIA

One of the other common motor symptoms you may experience is dystonia. Dystonia is an involuntary muscle contraction in which the brain tells the muscles to tighten and move even though you don't want them to. These involuntary movements can cause painful and awkward postures, writer's cramp and calf cramps, curled and clenched toes, and excessive eye blinking. The contractions can range from mild to severe and can be sustained or intermittent. They can also be so painful that they interfere with accomplishing your day-to-day activities. When people with Parkinson's talk about pain, it's often due to dystonia.

Dystonia, however, is not only a symptom of Parkinson's. It is also the third most common movement disorder. People can have dystonia with Parkinson's and Parkinson's without dystonia. An estimated 17% of people with Parkinson's experience dystonia.

For some people, dystonia feels like a Charlie horse, which can be so painful that it wakes you up at night. For some, it feels like opposing muscles, muscles that work in pairs, are competing. For example, when your bicep muscle contracts, your tricep muscle relaxes or elongates. In dystonia, both muscles want to contract simultaneously, and it feels like they're fighting. For some people living with Parkinson's, dystonia is the most distressing symptom they experience.

What Parts of the Body Can Be Affected by Dystonia?

Muscle contractions can occur in a single area of your body (focal dystonia), in two or more adjacent areas (segmental dystonia), or all areas of your body (general dystonia). Parts of the body that can be affected include:

- **Jaw and tongue.** You might experience involuntary opening and closing of your jaw and difficulty chewing or swallowing. Dystonia of the tongue can also cause drooling and slurred speech

- **Eyelids.** Even though spasms in the eyelids are generally not painful, rapid blinking and involuntary contractions of the muscles around the eyes can affect your vision. Using "sensory tricks," such as putting pressure on your eyebrows, singing, laughing, or chewing, seem to distract the brain and may relieve dystonia on your eyelids

- **Vocal cords.** Contractions in your vocal cords can cause you to have a breathy, whispering voice, making you sound hoarse or tight. Yawning may ease dystonia in your vocal cords

- **Neck.** Overactivation of your neck muscles can cause your head to turn repetitively side to side or back and forth, which can cause pain

- **Hands.** Sometimes involuntary cramping and spasms are brought on by task-specific movements, such as playing an instrument (musician's dystonia) or writing or typing (writer's dystonia)

- **Legs and feet.** A common manifestation of dystonia in people with young onset Parkinson's causes the toes to curl and the foot and ankle to turn in (inversion). This may occur when you're walking or running or doing some other type of movement

- **Trunk.** Though this is less common, twisting of the trunk can cause contorted posture and pain

- **All over.** Even though the prevalence of pain in people with Parkinson's is high, it's often underreported and underrecognized. People are often embarrassed to mention pain because they think it's "all in their head" and that discussing it will sound like complaining. However, dystonic pain can decrease your quality of life; so, don't be afraid to talk to your physician about it

STRATEGIES TO MANAGE DYSTONIA

Different treatment approaches are available. Most of them involve a combination of self-care (focusing on exercise, sleep, and healthy eating), medication adjustments, and physical therapy.

Strategies:

- **Keep a diary.** By tracking the onset of dystonia and medication timing, you can determine if there's a pattern between the two. Keep your tracking current and show the diary to your physician. Dystonia symptoms can be relieved by adjusting the dose and frequency of your medication and/or adding another medication that targets dystonia

- **Exercise, stretch, and strengthen.** Even if you don't feel like it, exercising every day increases flexibility in your muscles and joints, reduces pain and discomfort, and improves circulation

- **Trick your body.** Using the sensory trick called "geste antagoniste," lightly touch a part of your body that is *not* cramping or curling. Sometimes this can quiet the dystonia. For example, touching your chin may prevent your neck from twisting

- **Try Botox.** If dystonia is in one easily accessible muscle, injections of botulinum toxin (Botox) in the contracted muscle can cause it to relax and return to a normal state

- **Consider muscle relaxants.** Since dystonia is due to the contraction of muscles, physicians sometimes prescribe muscle relaxants as a treatment

- **Talk to your physician about deep brain stimulation.** If dystonia is generalized all over your body and affects muscles that are inaccessible, and you have tremor and dyskinesia, you may want to discuss deep brain stimulation with your neurologist or movement disorder specialist

- **See a rehabilitation specialist.** Many people who experience dystonic pain find that meeting regularly with a physical therapist, occupational therapist, and/or speech-language pathologist is another good way to manage their symptoms

Dystonia and the pain associated with it are often underreported and not addressed because people ignore the symptoms. However, because dystonia can affect your quality of life, it's essential to educate yourself about managing your symptoms and not dismiss them as just a part of getting older. From exercise, sleep, medication adjustments, and healthy eating, there are many actions you can take today to live better with dystonia and Parkinson's.

TAKING ACTION TO MANAGE MOTOR SYMPTOMS

As you have probably noticed, one common strategy to help improve the cardinal motor symptoms of Parkinson's is exercise. While studies show regular exercise can improve heart health, increase strength, improve endurance, reduce fatigue, and positively impact mood and self-esteem in all people, research illustrates the incredible impact exercise can have on both the motor and the non-motor symptoms of Parkinson's.

Research also suggests exercise may even help protect the areas of the brain affected by

Parkinson's from getting worse (a phenomenon known as neuroprotection), which may slow the progression of Parkinson's. Research studies have found that people with Parkinson's who participated in high-intensity exercise experienced noticeable improvement in their overall movement and even reduced tremor after exercising. Also, individuals with Parkinson's who exercised more often required less additional medication and had the slowest rate of change over a year.

Of course, talk to your physician before starting any exercise program, but once you receive the go-ahead, find a form of movement that you enjoy. Whatever movement activity brings a smile to your face will help manage the motor symptoms of Parkinson's, boost your mood, and help decrease anxiety and depression.

Also, a physical therapist or occupational therapist can be incredibly helpful if you experience the motor symptoms we just discussed. Physical therapists and occupational therapists can asses your ability to do activities of daily living and your gait and balance. They are also experts at recommending assistive devices and exercises to prevent falls and improve safety. We talk about these care providers more in Chapter 10.

You can begin managing your motor symptoms today by practicing all the tips we just shared. The key to managing your motor symptoms is to take action now. The more you do as soon as you're diagnosed, the more vital, more mobile, and happier you will be while living with Parkinson's.

"My Balance Seems Off. What's Happening?"

By Helen Brontë-Stewart, MD, MSE

Balance is a general term that refers to our ability to stay upright, whether seated, standing, or moving. If we can't balance, we fall. Imbalance is an inevitable complication in Parkinson's and leads to falls in more than 50% of people living with Parkinson's. Falls may result in severe injuries and have a major impact on activities of daily living.

People with Parkinson's fall most frequently when changing position, turning, moving in dim light, and/or on an unstable surface. All of these movements challenge their dynamic balance control. Thus, activities like bending, standing up from a squat, moving from a seated to a standing posture, moving on a thick carpet at night, and walking on a rocky trail may lead to falls from imbalance.

Why does Parkinson's affect balance? It is thought that the brain has difficulty recruiting learned templates of how to maintain balance when incoming orientational sensory information is incongruent or absent. Another problem in Parkinson's that makes a fall more likely is that postural "righting reflexes," reaction time, and movement speed are all delayed or slow.

Your Balance Can Improve

The key thing to understand about the balance system is that it is learned. If we hadn't spent our first year or two of life falling over and getting up again, we would not have been able to balance as we know it. Learning is constant in the balance system, but most of us don't even think about it as we challenge our balance every day by our activity. The hopeful aspect of this for people with imbalance is that it can get better with training.

Training the Deficit: The Athlete Model for Improving Balance in Parkinson's

Balance is one of the most vulnerable yet one of the most re-trainable mechanisms we have. If you don't use it, you lose it—familiar words if you live with Parkinson's, but true.

Consider athletes: Their static and dynamic balance is superior to what they need in daily life because they practice specific aspects of balance for their sport. Studies have shown that gymnasts have exceptional static balance, soccer players have better dynamic balance than swimmers, and judo athletes have better static balance than ballet dancers (probably because they practice kicks and balance with their bodies at angles rather than only straight upright). Gymnasts practice on the balance beam, dancers do pointe classes, cyclists ride on rough ground at high speed, and yoga participants practice one-legged poses. Footballers lift weights while balancing on balance balls. These are just some of the focused balance exercises athletes do in addition to general conditioning and aerobic training.

Therefore, it makes sense for people with Parkinson's to "train up" imbalance by training into the deficit. The goal is to bring balance back to normal.

The first step is identifying your specific balance deficits. I recommend getting a comprehensive assessment of your static and dynamic balance with a physical therapist. The sooner you know the problem, the sooner you can start to fix it.

 Once you know the specifics, you can work alone or with a physical therapist, a personal trainer, or a sports or movement disorder specialist to develop a focused training program to address your balance deficits.

As with athletes, focused balance retraining should be one part of an overall wellness routine. You also need to maintain the health of other systems, like keeping muscles and bones strong and your heart healthy.

Measuring Progress

An important component of balance training is measuring progress; the more specific, the better. If you have access to a center with dynamic posturography and gait analysis technology, then, by all means, take advantage of it. If you don't have the technology to help you, you can effectively measure your progress at home using a journal and charting specific observations.

The days of sitting on the couch and giving up because of imbalance are over. It's time to get out and practice balance. If you don't know where to start, just stand up. If that is easy, close your eyes. If that is still a simple task, make it a bit harder. Try putting a firm pillow on the floor beside a wall where you can hold on if necessary. Now stand on the pillow. You are on your way to training your balance.

Talk to your neurologist about getting a balance assessment and retraining program, and then do it every day. It works, it is usually free, it's fun, and it has no side effects!

About Helen Brontë-Stewart

Helen Brontë-Stewart is the John E. Cahill Family Professor in the department of neurology and neurological sciences and in the department of neurosurgery (by courtesy) at the Stanford University School of Medicine, Stanford, California. She received her bachelor's degree in mathematics and physics at the University of York, England and a master of science in bioengineering (MSE) from University of Pennsylvania School of Engineering in Philadelphia, PA. Dr. Brontë-Stewart received her MD degree from University of Pennsylvania School of Medicine.

Dr. Brontë-Stewart's research goal is to understand how the brain controls movement. She is also very interested in balance and gait disorders and maintains an active research program in this area. With a ballet and modern dance background, she initiated the idea and helped design a dance studio in the Stanford Neurosciences Health Center. She has also authored and co-authored more than 90 peer-review manuscripts, book chapters, and other materials on Parkinson's-related issues.

She has held many teaching positions throughout her career, beginning during her undergraduate years with directorships of two dance companies. Her research has been supported by numerous foundations devoted to Parkinson's awareness. She currently serves as a member of the Davis Phinney Foundation's Board of Directors.

"How Can I Prevent Falls?"

By Jorik Nonnekes, MD, PhD and Bastiaan Bloem, MD, PhD

Falls are common and can be debilitating in people with Parkinson's. They can have devastating consequences, often leading to injuries, reduced mobility, loss of independence, and a lower quality of life.

To manage falls in Parkinson's, it is important to appreciate the complexity and the multiple factors that can contribute to their occurrence. Deficits in balance and gait disorders are common in Parkinson's, and both can lead to falls. Environmental factors in your home and other places in your daily life can also lead to falls and include slippery floors, loose rugs, and poor lighting.

Freezing of gait is one of the leading causes of falls, presumably because freezing events typically occur suddenly and without warning. Recent research has underscored the additional importance of cognitive impairment (for example, difficulties with handling complex situations or sudden changes) as a key factor contributing to both falls and freezing.

Preventing falls might seem difficult, but it is not impossible. Given that there are so many factors that can contribute to falls, a multidisciplinary approach aimed at the specific factors in your situation is important. Crucial elements for minimizing falls include optimizing Parkinson's medication, stopping any sedative medications (such as sleeping pills or anxiety drugs), and tailoring physical therapy based on evidence-based practice guidelines.

Fall prevention is possible when the solution is tailored to your unique situation and considers environmental, cognitive, and physical factors.

INDIVIDUALIZED ASSESSMENT

Each person with Parkinson's deserves a careful and systematic approach to identify all factors contributing to falls. Your physician should emphasize testing you for freezing of gait; rapid turning on the spot is the best test for this. You should also tell your physician if you feel afraid of falling again, which is common. Fear of falling is not only a risk factor for falling again; it can also lead to decreased mobility. Balance and gait training to improve confidence might be an option for you if you experience these fears. Preventing osteoporosis through exercise, nutritional choices, and/or medication also reduces the chance of fracture if a fall does occur.

OPTIMIZE YOUR MEDICATIONS

Most balance deficits are not improved with dopaminergic medication; however, some gait problems—including freezing—can improve. Higher or more frequent doses than those typically needed to increase hand functioning due to tremor might be required. Again, sedative drugs should be stopped whenever possible.

PHYSICAL THERAPY

The evidence-based guidelines on physical therapy for Parkinson's were recently updated, providing a menu of treatment options designed to improve mobility and reduce falls.

Designing and implementing specific interventions requires the expertise of a trained physical therapist who can tailor the approach to your unique situation and needs. Examples of evidence-based physical therapy strategies include cueing techniques, cognitive movement strategies, and exercise. Rhythmic auditory or visual cues can improve gait and freezing difficulties. Listening to music with a strong beat and appropriate tempo can also help improve gait.

Another promising approach, especially for people experiencing freezing of gait, is cycling. This skill can be remarkably preserved in some people with Parkinson's, even when gait has become very difficult. If outdoor cycling has become too difficult or if your climate or geography aren't conducive, you can still benefit by riding a stationary bicycle at home. Various other exercise programs—walking, tai chi, and dancing—can improve strength, endurance, and balance, and several controlled trials have shown they lead to a significant reduction in falls.

Physical therapists can also teach you to make safer transitions (e.g., from sitting to standing or rolling over in bed) and to increase overall fitness (with an individually tailored exercise program).

Promoting the use of walking aids also deserves specific attention. Many people do not use them, either because their physician has not recommended them or because they are ashamed or embarrassed. This is unfortunate because, for those who cannot improve their stability adequately through physical therapy alone, the benefits of regained confidence, mobility, and independence that walking aids can provide far outweigh the cons.

OCCUPATIONAL THERAPY

Home visits by occupational therapists can reduce hazards in your living space. An occupational therapist can screen for behavioral risks during their visit and assess the appropriateness of your preferred footwear. Sometimes, people are reluctant to make changes to their homes or behaviors or doubt that doing so will reduce their fall frequency. Remember, for any preventative measure to succeed, your cooperation and agreement to make changes are important.

Many people fall more often at night when rooms are dark. If you frequently make nighttime visits to the bathroom, you might consider installing proper lighting to help get you there safely. Choosing a red-light nightlight (one that emits red light wavelengths) can help light your way without interfering with your circadian rhythm and waking you too much to fall back asleep easily. A commode next to the bed (or a condom catheter for men) can provide peace of mind for those with limited mobility. For an in-depth home safety checklist, visit the ⤤ *Every Victory Counts* **website**.

The key to successful preventative intervention is cooperation from the person living with Parkinson's.

YOU AND YOUR PHYSICIAN

Your neurologist should ask you about falls and their impact on daily functioning as a standard part of their medical evaluation. As a person living with Parkinson's, you can also initiate the conversation by asking your physician to build a multidisciplinary team approach to tackle the vexing problem of falls.

About Bastiaan Bloem

Bas Bloem is a medical director and consultant neurologist at the department of neurology, Radboud University Nijmegen Medical Centre, the Netherlands. He received his MD degree (with honors) at Leiden University Medical Centre in 1993. In 1994, he obtained his PhD degree in Leiden, based on a thesis entitled: "Postural reflexes in Parkinson's disease." He was trained as a neurologist between 1994 and 2000, also at Leiden University Medical Centre.

He received additional training as a movement disorder specialist during fellowships at The Parkinson's Institute, Sunnyvale, California (with Dr. J.W. Langston), and at the Institute of Neurology, Queen Square, London (with Prof. N.P. Quinn and Prof. J.C. Rothwell).

In 2002, he founded and became medical director of the Parkinson Centre Nijmegen (ParC), which was recognized from 2005 onwards as a center of excellence for Parkinson's disease. Together with Dr. Marten Munneke, he also developed ParkinsonNet, an innovative healthcare concept that now consists of 66 professional networks for people with Parkinson's covering all of the Netherlands. Because of the evidence-based quality improvement and significant cost reduction, ParkinsonNet has received multiple awards, including the prize "Best Pearl for Healthcare Innovation" in 2011 and "Value Based Health Care" prize in 2015.

»

In September 2008, Professor Bloem was appointed as professor of neurology, with movement disorders as a special area of interest. He has published more than 550 publications, including more than 400 peer-reviewed international papers. He recently co-authored Ending Parkinson's Disease: The Book *with Drs. Michael Okun, Ray Dorsey, and Todd Sherer.*

About Jorik Nonnekes

Jorik Nonnekes is a consultant physiatrist at Radboud University Medical Center and Sint Maartenskliniek Nijmegen in the Netherlands. His focus is on improving the quality of life of people with gait impairments. Both his clinical and scientific work focus on diagnosis and personalized treatment of complex neurological gait disorders. By working as a clinician and researcher, he can bridge the translation gap between (fundamental) research and daily clinical practice. Specifically, he focuses on gait impairments in three groups of neurological disorders: Parkinson's, rare and hereditary movement disorders (such as spinocerebellar ataxia and hereditary spastic paraplegia), and stroke.

Dr. Nonnekes earned his MD degree in 2010 and PhD degree in 2015, with his thesis entitled "Balance and gait in neurodegenerative disease: what startles tell us about motor control." His thesis was awarded the European Academy of Rehabilitation Medicine Prize, and thesis prizes of the Dutch Society for Movement Sciences, and the Dutch Society for Rehabilitation Medicine. Dr. Nonnekes has published more than 50 papers in international peer-reviewed journals, including first-author papers in Lancet Neurology, Nature Reviews Neurology, JAMA Neurology, and Neurology. He has received several international awards for his scientific work, and in 2018, obtained a prestigious VENI-grant to study mechanisms underlying compensation strategies for gait impairments in Parkinson's.

■ CHAPTER 4 – NON-MOTOR SYMPTOMS (EMOTIONAL)

OVERVIEW

As we explained earlier, Parkinson's is classified as a movement disorder because it involves damage to the brain, nerves, and muscles that influence the speed, quality, fluency, and ease of movement. While the effects of Parkinson's on movement are often the most visible, non-motor symptoms, including emotional and cognitive challenges, can have an even more significant effect on your quality of life.

The effects of Parkinson's not related to movement are called non-motor symptoms. Non-motor symptoms of Parkinson's may outnumber motor symptoms and can appear years before motor symptoms. Non-motor symptoms include those that fall into three categories: emotional, cognitive, and autonomic. This chapter will discuss the most common non-motor symptoms related to emotional health, including depression, anxiety, and apathy. We'll also explain how therapy, medication, and lifestyle changes can help you manage and treat these symptoms.

DEPRESSION

Depression is a medical illness caused by an imbalance of chemicals, such as dopamine, serotonin, and norepinephrine, in the brain. Depression causes a persistent feeling of sadness and is associated with a lack of pleasure in things you might have once enjoyed, as well as changes in sleep and, possibly, thoughts of suicide. There's nothing you're doing unconsciously or consciously that causes depression; instead, it is due to a chemical imbalance that, for the most part, can be treated.

> **"** *I'd always been able to juggle a lot of things at once and ideas about what I was doing next, but I became unable to cope with that volume of information after Parkinson's. Things came into my mind, very dark things. A lot of feelings of loss of control and feeling depressed, down, sad. A lot of days, I'd go to work, and it was very difficult to concentrate or feel productive and to deal with the volume of work I had at the time."*
>
> — TIM

About 40-50% of people with Parkinson's experience depression. Because in addition to its impacts on mood and mental well-being depression can make the physical symptoms of Parkinson's worse, it's critical to identify and treat symptoms of depression right away. However, because symptoms of Parkinson's and symptoms of depression can present similarly, it's often difficult to diagnose. Parkinson's and depression share symptoms that include slower movement, slower speech, flattened expressions, and downcast eyes. If you experience these symptoms, be sure to talk with your physician to determine the cause and appropriate treatment.

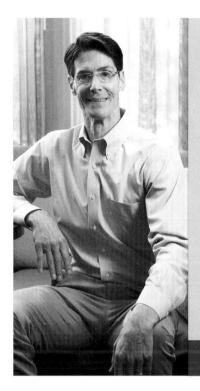

" *About five years into my journey with Parkinson's, I realized that I was getting really run down and it was hard to keep up. I was still working full-time and that meant long days, evening networking events, etc. It was starting to really affect how I felt. I loved doing all that stuff, but it was just killing me. I made the difficult decision to sell my business and went from being ultra-busy to just nothing. I quickly found out that wasn't good either. Depression was 'something that happens to other people,' but suddenly I realized that I was feeling really lonely. I got involved with volunteering and mentoring, and now life feels balanced.*"

— STEVE HOVEY

STRATEGIES TO MANAGE DEPRESSION

Seek help. Asking for help is a sign of strength. Talking with a qualified therapist or psychiatrist can help you manage depression and give you strategies for dealing with triggers that worsen it. By being proactive, you can also find support groups and connect with others experiencing similar challenges, giving you strength and ideas to cope with your situation.

Create a regular exercise routine. You may have heard of the "happy hormones" called endorphins. When you exercise, your body releases these hormones, which trigger a positive reaction and make you feel better. Make it a habit to incorporate exercise into your daily routine. This way, even when you may not feel like exercising, your habit will give you the boost needed to get moving. Also, if you join an exercise class and make friends who expect you to show up, you'll feel more motivated to go. Look to see if special Parkinson's exercise classes are offered in your community that can meet your needs cognitively and physically, such as a dance class. If you are 65 years or older, look for Silver Sneaker classes in your community. These classes are designed for seniors, are affordable, and are often paid for by your insurance. You can also find countless exercise classes available online at no cost, which feature everything from aerobics to yoga, cycling, tai chi, dance, and more. You will feel much better physically, mentally, and emotionally after exercising.

Stay socially connected. Research suggests that social connections positively impact your physical *and* mental health. People who feel more connected to others have reported lower levels of depression and anxiety than those who feel less socially involved. Looking for ways to maintain or build your social connections? Volunteer, attend support groups, phone a friend, or join a new group to explore a new hobby.

ANXIETY

Anxiety is another common non-motor symptom of Parkinson's caused by changes in the chemicals in the brain. Anxiety is more common in people with Parkinson's than the general public and is more common in people with Parkinson's than those living with other neurological diseases. About 50% of people with Parkinson's will experience various levels of anxiety at some point. In most cases, depression is accompanied by anxiety, and many medications treat both. However, it's still important to understand the difference. If you're diagnosed with depression, you should ask your physician to screen for anxiety as well.

Anxiety may present as jitteriness, nervousness, or worry. Feelings of panic, fear, tension, or feeling keyed up are also signs of anxiety. Though worry is an understandable reaction to the diagnosis of Parkinson's, if it turns into anxiety that affects your ability to function and complete your day-to-day activities, it is important to communicate these concerns to your physician.

Many people with Parkinson's find that medication significantly minimizes the symptoms of anxiety. Treating anxiety is like treating motor symptoms; even though exercise helps, you wouldn't move well without dopamine. Without some form of medication, your anxiety will probably not be alleviated.

One problem with not treating anxiety is that it can negatively affect your social life because you may *avoid* social situations that cause anxiety. Isolation can have a domino effect of increasing anxiety and depression and decreasing the brain stimulation you need for improved cognition. Anxiety can also increase your dependency on your care partner and add pressure to their routines; so, even if you don't want to treat anxiety for yourself, do it for them. Speak to your physician about treatment options that could work well for you.

STRATEGIES TO MANAGE ANXIETY

Practice relaxation techniques. Deep breathing, such as breathing in for four seconds, holding your breath for four seconds, and then breathing out for four seconds, is just one example of a breathing technique that can help restore a sense of calm. Meditation, yoga, and listening to classical music or nature sounds can help you relax and enjoy the moment.

Turn off the news, mindless TV, and violent video games. Watching events that you have no control over can create tension and worry. Turn off the TV, read a book or some poetry, learn a new hobby, or play a game.

Laugh. You have heard that "laughter is the best medicine." When trying to decrease or eliminate anxiety, keeping a sense of humor helps. Watch a funny video, read a comical book, or talk to an amusing friend who can help keep your anxiety in check. Or, take a laughter yoga class. It's a thing.

Cognitive behavioral therapy (CBT). Cognitive behavioral therapy is based on the idea that individuals with anxiety hold distorted thoughts. CBT aims to provide a structured approach to help people identify the thoughts that contribute to emotional discomfort and replace them with more empowering choices. Speaking with a therapist trained in CBT can teach you new ways to deal with triggers that increase your anxiety. See more on CBT at the end of this chapter in Dr. Roseanne Dobkin's article.

Make smart nutritional choices. While treatment of anxiety primarily consists of medication and psychotherapy, healthy nutrition can work in tandem with more traditional treatments to improve mood and reduce anxiety. How? Proper nutrition impacts the effectiveness of medication. It alleviates symptoms of Parkinson's by helping your body work more efficiently, which gives you more energy. By eating well, you make conscious choices that will help improve your sense of overall well-being and counter anxiety symptoms. Check out Chapter 11 to learn more about how healthy eating can help you live well with Parkinson's.

APATHY

Apathy is a loss of motivation, desire, and interest. It can occur separately from depression and may be misinterpreted as laziness, disinterest, or lack of initiative. Though the cause of apathy in Parkinson's is unclear, research indicates that it's due to a chemical imbalance and structural changes in the brain.

Not only can apathy affect your attitude, but it can also negatively affect the treatment of Parkinson's. If you have lost the incentive to take your medicine, it can exacerbate your motor symptoms. If you have lost the desire to exercise, work on hobbies, or attend social engagements, it can cause social isolation and affect your personal and work life.

Often apathy is more frustrating for the care partner than the person with Parkinson's. The adage, "You can lead a horse to water, but can't make him drink," holds for your care partner when apathy is part of your lives. If you're a care partner of someone experiencing apathy, be sure to check out the *Every Victory Counts Manual for Care Partners* for ideas on how to best manage apathy in your person with Parkinson's.

WHAT IS THE DIFFERENCE BETWEEN APATHY AND DEPRESSION?

One day a care partner brought her husband to see psychiatrist Dr. Greg Pontone because she was worried that he just sat on the couch all day and did nothing. Dr. Pontone asked him, "Do you know the difference between apathy and depression?" He replied, "I don't care." This is a perfect example of apathy—he did not care. Usually, with depression, there is a negative component of hopelessness, sadness, and possibly suicide. However, like this man with Parkinson's demonstrated in his apathetic reply, he felt nothing and was emotionally flat.

Another person Dr. Pontone worked with was a lifelong baseball fan. One day when he was watching the seventh game of the World Series, the power went out. When the power came back on, the screen showed snow. An hour went by, and he continued to watch snow on the screen rather than the seventh game of the World Series. Again, he was not frustrated, upset, or depressed. He was apathetic and just didn't care.

DIAGNOSIS

It is critical to work with your physician to obtain an accurate diagnosis since treatment for depression is often different from treatment for apathy. Apathy seems to parallel cognitive decline in that it impacts disorganization and memory loss more than depression does. The best evidence that apathy is more linked to cognitive decline than to depression is the medications' effectiveness based on the diagnosis. Medications for cognitive problems appear to work better for apathy than medications used to treat depression.

STRATEGIES TO MANAGE APATHY

Like all the symptoms of Parkinson's, apathy requires that you make active choices to achieve your best quality of life.

Get out of the house daily. Create a weekly plan, or at least a plan for the day ahead, of leisure activities you want to do outside the home. If you plan the activity ahead of time, you don't even have to think about it, and you can just step into it.

Ideas include:

1. Try a new restaurant
2. Meet a friend for coffee
3. Check out your public library
4. Walk around the mall
5. Go to a thrift store or second-hand store
6. Window shop
7. Look up weekly events in your town
8. Explore a new hobby
9. Attend a poetry reading
10. Join a local club (chess, book, knitting, jazz, quilting, gardening)
11. Make yourself accountable by planning to meet a buddy
12. Join a Parkinson's exercise class

Practice good "sleep hygiene." Sleeping enough each night can affect how motivated you are to get out of bed and do something. One of the side effects of Parkinson's is sleep disturbance. Lack of sleep can cause fatigue the next day, which can cause you to be apathetic. In addition to the basics of good sleep hygiene of getting up and going to bed on a set schedule, keeping your mind active during the day can help promote a more restful night of sleep. We'll explore more about sleep and Parkinson's in Chapter 6.

"How Can I Manage my Depression and Anxiety?"

By Roseanne D. Dobkin, PhD

Depression and anxiety are very common in Parkinson's and can significantly impact physical and cognitive functioning, quality of life, and relationships. But, despite these detrimental effects, there is good news: you have control over depression and anxiety. You didn't have a choice in your Parkinson's diagnosis; however, you do have a choice in how you cope. A powerful way is through cognitive behavioral therapy.

COGNITIVE BEHAVIORAL THERAPY (CBT)

Cognitive behavioral therapy is a skills-based, non-pharmacological treatment that teaches practical strategies to help people living with Parkinson's and their family members more effectively navigate the challenges of living with Parkinson's. It is a kind of psychotherapy or "talk therapy" that focuses on examining the connections between thoughts, feelings, and behaviors to provide individuals with the skills needed to change thinking patterns (e.g., negative thoughts about self, world, and future) and behaviors (e.g., procrastination, social isolation and withdrawal, lack of structure in the day) that may be related to uncomfortable feelings like depression or anxiety. Unlike some other talk therapies, CBT is highly instructive and involves active one-to-one collaboration between the person living with Parkinson's and the therapist. Sessions are usually structured, and specific techniques and coping skills are explained during each session. CBT is tailored to each person's unique goals, and people are encouraged to practice their newly acquired coping skills between sessions to work toward their goals.

CBT is generally a brief, time-limited treatment (three to six months). However, the number of sessions varies, depending on the needs of each individual. With ongoing practice, you can continue to benefit from your newly acquired coping skills long after your therapy sessions have ended.

Learning new information is not enough: change requires putting different coping skills into action in daily life. Here's an analogy: If you fill your prescription for your Parkinson's medication but don't open the bottles and swallow the pills, your tremor and stiffness likely will not improve. Similarly, if you learn innovative tools to combat depression and anxiety in the face of Parkinson's but do not use them daily, they will not help you. Consistent practice over time is key.

You can use several different CBT strategies to help you cope more effectively with depression and anxiety, as well as with the daily stress of living with Parkinson's. Some tools focus on what you are doing or not doing in response to the current challenges that you are experiencing, while others focus on how you are thinking about yourself and your changing life circumstances. Behavioral tools include:

- Daily goal setting
- Increasing involvement in meaningful, pleasurable, and social activities
- Safely increasing daily exercise

All the people living with Parkinson's with whom I work are encouraged to set three realistic, achievable goals per day: one exercise goal, one social goal, and one other goal, which might be something productive like paying a bill or doing some self-soothing like taking an Epsom salt bath. An example of a realistic social goal could be answering the phone when your sister calls instead of letting it go to voicemail. Effective behavioral goal setting often involves collaborative problem-solving and thinking outside the box to meet the challenging demands of Parkinson's. This point is nicely illustrated in the case of Howard (Table 1, below).

Managing Your Thoughts

Regaining control of your thoughts is another necessary ingredient for improving your mood. In the CBT model, negative feelings like depression and anxiety don't come out of the blue; feelings come in response to your thoughts and interpretations of the situations you face. Often, thoughts might come so quickly that you might not even be aware that you have them, yet they linger long enough to have a negative impact on how you feel and how you act. Importantly, the negative thoughts we observe in depression (and anxiety) are often not as accurate as they feel and are guided more by emotion than by fact.

To further illustrate this point, let's consider the fictional case below. "Mary" and "Joe" are newly diagnosed with Parkinson's and experience similar physical symptoms and comparable levels of impairment. They both experience tremor when they eat in public and struggle to button their clothes. Mary thinks, "My life is ruined, and I have no control." In response to this thought, Mary is likely to feel scared and isolate herself. She may avoid eating out and decline social invitations from friends. She is unlikely to be proactive regarding her own self-care.

Joe, on the other hand, thinks, "I wish this didn't happen, but I know I can still have a meaningful life even with Parkinson's." While Joe is certainly not happy about his diagnosis, he is likely to feel more hopeful than Mary and remain active and engaged in his life. The likelihood that he obtains all the multidisciplinary services recommended to optimize his health and well-being is very high, and he may proactively seek referrals from his physicians.

This vignette highlights that different thoughts about the same situation can lead to different feelings and behaviors. A primary goal of cognitive therapy is to "press pause" on negative thoughts, evaluate them to determine if they are as accurate as they feel, and replace them, as appropriate, with more balanced, realistic thoughts. Several different tools can be used to facilitate these efforts. Tables 2 and 3 illustrate examples of two common techniques you can use to test your thoughts and see if they are as accurate as they feel or if modification is necessary. The goal of "cognitive restructuring" (revising your thoughts after further examination) is not to think more positively; the goal is to turn excessively skewed and negative thoughts that impede successful coping efforts into balanced and realistic thoughts that fuel healthy responses to life stress.

Table 4 presents a sampling of self-assessment questions. If you suspect that you are suffering from depression or anxiety, and/or that there is room for improvement in your mood and coping efforts, there are resources and practical strategies you can implement to help you manage these symptoms. You have the power, control, and inner strength to make the changes necessary to improve your health and quality of life today!

Table 1: Behavioral Activation Example

Howard was a volunteer firefighter for more than 40 years. He stopped responding to calls when he felt he was no longer physically able to do so due to the worsening of his Parkinson's symptoms. At this point, he became quite depressed and no longer went down to the firehouse to spend time with friends. He also stopped participating in all firehouse-related activities, including those that required no physical exertion, like the monthly chili dinner.

Part of Howard's treatment included reconnecting with the local fire department. He began to bring coffee down to the station and visit his friends one evening per week. He slowly began to explore ways he could remain connected to this organization that was near and dear to his heart. Four months later, he reported that he was spearheading all fundraising efforts for the fire department and his mood greatly improved. Even though Howard was no longer in the physical condition needed to fight fires, he found an alternative way to make a meaningful contribution to the cause.

Table 2: Examining the Evidence

This technique involves examining the "facts" that support and do not support your negative thoughts. Use the evidence that is gathered to come up with a more balanced thought, as appropriate.

- Situation: Freezing in the bathroom

- Automatic Thought: I'm helpless

- Evidence For: I was alone in the bathroom in the middle of the night and was unable to move

- Evidence Against: This happens quite a bit, so I planned for it. I had my cell phone in my pocket. I called my wife on the house phone, and she helped me back to bed

- Rational Response: Even though I was physically unable to move my feet, I was able to help myself out of the situation. I am not helpless

Table 3: Behavioral Experiment

This technique involves engaging in a specific behavior designed to test out a negative prediction and evaluate the outcome.

- Negative Thought or Prediction: It will be impossible to have dinner in a restaurant because of my tremor

- Experiment: I will go out to dinner with my spouse on Saturday

- Outcome: I was able to eat dinner at our favorite restaurant. I ordered food that did not need to be cut and requested a straw and lid for my drink. I enjoyed getting out of the house and had a fun evening

Experiment results suggest that the negative prediction was not accurate.

Table 4: Self-Assessment Questions

- Is your mood as good as you would like it to be?

- Think about your average day. Which of these activities are you engaged in?

  - Socializing with family members and friends

  - Exercising

  - Engaging in hobbies

  - Engaging in other leisure activities

  - Volunteering

  - Working

- Describe activities that you engage in that bring you meaning, joy, and pleasure.

- Since your Parkinson's diagnosis, are you as actively involved in things you used to enjoy? Explain.

- Have you decreased the time you spend on any of your activities? Have you stopped any activities altogether? Explain.

- What does a Parkinson's diagnosis mean to you?

- What strategies are you using to cope with the daily challenges that Parkinson's presents?
- Does fear often guide what you do or don't do?
- Do you predict the future in a negative light?
- Do you often focus on the worst-case scenario?

Newly diagnosed and early Parkinson's
- Do you overestimate the extent of your physical and functional limitations?

More advanced Parkinson's
- Do you underestimate your ability to cope effectively with the challenges Parkinson's presents?

As with all aspects of Parkinson's, your experience may or may not include all (or any) of these symptoms related to emotional health. The good news is that if you experience depression, anxiety, or apathy, you now know that you can take action to manage and treat them. Talk to your care team about the best strategies for you, and whatever you do, remember that you are not alone. Be compassionate with yourself. Be committed to exploring ways to manage these symptoms. Be prepared to live well...today and every day.

About Roseanne Dobkin

Roseanne Dobkin is an associate professor of psychiatry at Rutgers-Robert Wood Johnson Medical School in Piscataway, NJ. She is also a licensed psychologist in New Jersey and Delaware. Dr. Dobkin received her PhD in clinical psychology from the Medical College of Pennsylvania-Hahnemann University in Philadelphia, PA, in August 2002. She completed a postdoctoral fellowship in clinical psychopharmacology in the department of psychiatry at Robert Wood Johnson Medical School in September 2003.

The principal goal of Dr. Dobkin's research program is to help people with Parkinson's and their family members cope as effectively as possible with various challenges to enhance overall physical and emotional health and quality of life. She explores the interactions between physical and mental health in Parkinson's and the impact of their intricate associations on quality of life and functional disability.

She's also very interested in examining barriers to mental health care use in Parkinson's, the use of telemedicine to leverage access to specialized mental health

»

care in Parkinson's, and the impact of successful depression treatment on key outcomes such as cognition, physical disability, quality of life, and caregiver health.

The National Institutes of Health have funded her research, as have the Patterson Trust Awards Program in Clinical Research, the Michael J. Fox Foundation for Parkinson's Research, the Parkinson's Unity Walk, the Parkinson's Disease Foundation, and the Health Services and Research Development Division of the Veteran Affairs Administration.

■ CHAPTER 5 – NON-MOTOR SYMPTOMS (COGNITIVE)

OVERVIEW

From memory problems to problem-solving challenges, cognitive changes are something that approximately 50% of people with Parkinson's will experience.

Cognition is a general term used to describe the mental ability to process information and apply knowledge. Not only can Parkinson's slow down movement (bradykinesia), it can also slow down your ability to think and process information (bradyphrenia).

Because Parkinson's affects many regions of the brain, it can change cognition to varying degrees. In mild cognitive impairment, which is estimated to occur in 20-50% of people with Parkinson's, a person may still be able to work and complete day-to-day tasks, just at a slower pace. Many people with mild cognitive impairment can think and analyze, communicate, remember information, and function normally.

" *During the year and a half it took me to get diagnosed with Parkinson's, I went to my primary care doctor and told him I thought I had Parkinson's. He said, 'No, you don't. You only have a tremor on one side.' It shows me he didn't know much about Parkinson's. Since I've been diagnosed, I have been teaching him about Parkinson's so he can help other patients."*

— EDIE ANDERSON

A person with Parkinson's may have difficulty retrieving information, but it's very uncommon for them to forget who they or their family members are. However, over time they may develop more severe cognitive problems that affect their ability to function in everyday life. Though it generally occurs many years after initial onset, some people experience dementia in later stages of their Parkinson's.

Because changes in cognition can have other causes, it is essential to tell your physician right away if you notice changes in your ability to pay attention, make decisions, form thoughts quickly, or remember details about events. Other medical conditions, such as a vitamin B12 deficiency, thyroid disease, urinary tract infection, pneumonia, stroke, and side effects of medications, can also cause confusion, hallucinations, and sleepiness. It's critical to rule out those causes and/or treat those first rather than simply assuming that the changes in cognition are caused by Parkinson's.

THE PRIMARY AREAS OF COGNITION AFFECTED

Because Parkinson's alters many regions of the brain and the dopamine system, it can affect executive function, language, and memory.

EXECUTIVE FUNCTION (PROBLEM-SOLVING)

Think of executive function as the CEO of an organization. The CEO's role is to direct the tasks of a group. This job involves making decisions, solving problems, initiating change, and keeping the organization on task to meet goals. Executive function helps us do similar tasks in our daily lives. A change in the brain's executive function is one of the most common cognitive changes in Parkinson's and can make problem-solving and decision-making very difficult.

LANGUAGE (COMMUNICATION)

When under pressure, you may feel frustrated when you try to speak, follow, and understand conversations.

SPEECH

The most common language problem in Parkinson's is called the "tip-of-the-tongue" phenomenon. You may know what you want to say, but you have difficulty finding the right words to say it, such as naming an object. A person once remarked that the worst thing for him about Parkinson's is that he can still think of funny things to say, but he can't say them at the right time. In addition to this phenomenon, you may begin to lose volume and speak quietly. It can be increasingly frustrating when you want to express a feeling or thought, and people can't hear you and therefore don't respond or communicate with you.

COMPREHENSION

You may have difficulty following explanations with too many details. Everyday conversations may seem overloaded with information. Your thoughts might get stuck on a single topic, and you may have trouble shifting your thoughts to another.

MEMORY

You may struggle to remember things and to keep your train of thought, or you may zone out in the middle of an activity. This challenge may change from minute to minute or week to week. You may feel clear as a bell one minute, then fuzzy the next. One man with Parkinson's told us that he would put on one shoe, then zone out, and need to be reminded by his care partner to put on the other shoe. You may also have difficulty with everyday tasks with many steps, such as making coffee or balancing a checkbook.

STRATEGIES TO MANAGE CHANGES IN COGNITION

Remember that life is a journey, not a destination. Give yourself more time for everyday activities and tasks. You will better manage cognitive changes and challenges if you avoid rushing to complete jobs quickly. Stay present and focus on what is happening in the moment.

Initiate the conversation about cognitive changes early. Your physicians may be so focused on your motor symptoms that they put cognitive changes on the back burner. Therefore, it might be up to you to start this conversation early on in your diagnosis. Cognitive changes are never too mild to address with your provider. If you feel it's a problem, it's a problem. Usually, changes in cognition in a person with Parkinson's are gradual, not sudden. If a sudden change does occur, it could be something else, such as the side effect of a medication. Be sure to address that as soon as possible.

> *As we age, we're told that word finding, attention deficits, and memory loss are part of the aging process. Nevertheless, it's hard to accept the feeling of losing ground mentally. I've found things like music, reading, Sudoku, and engagement on projects with others make a difference. The real danger is pulling back from meaningful social engagement because of shame or self doubt. Talking to friends and family members about your experience and specific cognitive challenges allows them to adapt in ways that make it easier for you. Asking questions for clarification, requesting that information be repeated, or summarizing what you've heard in your own words can help ensure comprehension. I found that a neuropsychological evaluation was helpful in separating fear from reality. Adequate sleep and exercise also are key."*

— RICH WILDAU

Consider visiting a neuropsychologist. As we mentioned in Chapter 1, although it can be expensive to see a neuropsychologist (a healthcare professional specializing in understanding the relationship between the brain and behavior), it can be beneficial. A neuropsychologist can give you a cognitive evaluation and offer recommendations for maintaining or improving your thinking skills and emotional functioning.

Engage in mental exercises. In the same way physical activity improves movement and strength, brain exercises can help improve your cognitive functioning. Many games and puzzles are designed to boost the brain's fitness, from traditional crossword puzzles to interactive brain teasers modeled after video games. Creativity can also enhance cognition, and many people with Parkinson's discover a newfound enjoyment in various art and music projects. (More on this in Chapter 10.)

Trying new things creates new pathways in the brain and helps keep your brain healthier and active. Embrace and seek out new and novel adventures and activities to continually challenge your brain. Find new ways to exercise, different types of brain teasers, or even a new path for your daily walk. You're also keeping your brain engaged and strong when you:

- Take a class that challenges you
- Study a new language
- Try out improv (a favorite among many people in our community!)
- Run, walk, or ride a new route every week
- Get your coffee at different locations
- Rearrange the apps on your phone
- Reorganize your kitchen cabinets
- Learn all of the countries of the world

Do something you've never done at least once a week. It doesn't take much to shake up the circuits in your brain, but the effects can be long-lasting and powerfully beneficial.

Build aerobic exercise into your daily life. As neuropsychologist Mark Mapstone, PhD, explains later in this chapter (and as we discuss in detail in Chapter 9), exercise has been proven, again and again, to improve motor symptoms of Parkinson's *and* cognition. Talk to your care team about ideal exercise routines for you, find those you enjoy, and regularly move your body.

> ❝ *I used to be a technology teacher, but I've lost a lot of my ability to multitask and do math because of Parkinson's. However, recently I've taken up building and it's fired me up in a way I haven't been since I retired from teaching. I'm outside creating something and even though it takes me a lot, lot longer to do things, it's new and challenges my brain. I don't care how long it takes me to finish; I care that I did it.*"
>
> — BRIAN

Remember that thinking and processing can be improved in many enjoyable ways. Visit your community center, senior center, Parkinson's support group, or local community college to see what programs are available to you and your family. Many libraries, universities, school districts, and online outlets also offer adult learning programs covering a wide range of interests. Ask your healthcare provider to refer you to an occupational, recreational, art, music, dance, or physical therapist for more focused cognitive wellness programs. (We take an in-depth look at the many benefits of these and other complementary therapies in Chapter 10). Commit to doing activities that challenge your brain. Choose activities you enjoy, pace yourself, and have fun.

For cognition checklists and other helpful resources, be sure to check out our ⤤ *Every Victory Counts* website.

PARKINSON'S DISEASE PSYCHOSIS

Parkinson's disease psychosis (PDP) is a non-motor symptom of Parkinson's that causes people to experience hallucinations and/or delusions. Approximately 50% of all people living with Parkinson's will experience some form of hallucinations or delusions, and the longer you live with Parkinson's, the greater the likelihood you'll experience them.

HALLUCINATIONS

A hallucination is something someone sees, hears, smells, tastes, or feels that's not there. Essentially, hallucinations are tricks the brain plays on the senses. Most of the time, these hallucinations are visual. For example, one person told us he often sees tiny people along the floorboards in his kitchen. Another person said he sees people who aren't there when he walks into a particular room of his house. One physician told us about a person with Parkinson's who regularly mistook her laundry piles for a person.

These hallucinations appear clear as day to the person with Parkinson's but cannot be seen by anyone else. In some cases, the visions may be disturbing and cause emotional distress, but that's not always the case. They may be friendly and not bothersome at all.

" *It was hard to talk about hallucinations with my family and friends because their immediate assumption was that I was losing my mind."*

— **COREY KING**

When people with Parkinson's first start experiencing hallucinations, they typically experience them with insight. This means the person knows that what they're seeing isn't real, and they're able to recognize it as a symptom of living with Parkinson's.

When people lose this insight, however, they begin to believe that hallucinations are real. They may start talking to them, interacting with them, and even try to draw their care partner into the scene with them. When their hallucinations reach this stage, they can go on for a very long time and cause hyper-agitation and aggressiveness, which can be very difficult for the care partner to witness and manage. Whether the hallucinations are distressing or not, interacting with them can pose a potential risk of harm to the person with Parkinson's and anyone else in the room.

DELUSIONS

Delusions are specific and fixed beliefs that are very real and true to the person experiencing them, even though they are contradicted by what is generally accepted as reality or reason. They can contradict all semblance of reality and rational thought, but nothing can convince the person experiencing them that they are untrue. Additionally, if you try to convince someone experiencing a delusion that it's not true, they can become suspicious and doubt you, making an already difficult situation even worse.

Delusions occur much less frequently than hallucinations. Only a small percentage of people with Parkinson's experience them, but because they're often ongoing, involuntary, and feel very real to the person who experiences them, they can be much more challenging to manage and treat.

The most common delusions people with Parkinson's experience are:

- The belief that their partner is being unfaithful
- The belief that their care partner is poisoning them with their medications
- The belief that people are stealing from them or planning to

Fortunately, many people with Parkinson's have found ways to treat and manage Parkinson's disease psychosis symptoms.

HOW TO TREAT PARKINSON'S DISEASE PSYCHOSIS

The single most important thing to do when it comes to Parkinson's disease psychosis is to tell your care providers and partners the minute you notice changes in your vision, hearing, thinking, and behavior. The earlier they know what's going on, the sooner they can begin interventions to help you feel better.

Once you bring your concerns up to your physician, they will typically do a clinical evaluation, review your medications and dosage, assess your lifestyle, and determine your symptoms' severity. Depending on what they find, they may refer you to counseling or therapy, adjust your medication, change your medication, eliminate a certain medication, or do all of the above. If none of those strategies work, they may try antipsychotic drug therapy to see if they can adjust the brain's chemical levels. This can bring with it an entirely different set of problems, so it's crucial to be invested every step along the way and be sure you're well-informed before you move in that direction.

Later in this chapter, movement disorder specialist Cherian Karunapuzha, MD, will explain more about hallucinations and delusions in Parkinson's and additional information about managing these possible symptoms.

IMPULSE CONTROL DISORDERS AND PARKINSON'S

Impulse control disorders (ICDs), including compulsive gambling, sexual behaviors, shopping, and eating, are common in people with Parkinson's who take dopamine agonists, a class of drugs sometimes used to treat the symptoms of Parkinson's.

In one study, 411 people diagnosed with Parkinson's were followed for five years. During that time, the risk of developing ICDs among those who took dopamine agonists was 52%. The risk of developing ICDs was only 12% for those who had taken only medicines other than dopamine agonists. Because ICDs can be common in people with Parkinson's and have a profound effect on quality of life, it's essential to become more educated about them and how they may affect living well.

WHAT ARE IMPULSE CONTROL DISORDERS?

According to *Psychiatric Times*, impulse control disorders are characterized by:

- The perpetuation of repeated negative behaviors regardless of negative consequences
- Progressive lack of control over engaging in these behaviors
- Mounting tension or craving to perform these negative behaviors before acting on them
- A sense of relief or pleasure in performing these problematic behaviors

People who experience impulse control disorders may or may not plan the acts; however, the acts themselves nearly always fulfill their immediate wishes, even if they are ultimately distressing to the person and make them feel out of control.

The most common ICDs reported in people with Parkinson's are pathological gambling, hypersexuality, compulsive shopping, and compulsive eating. More than 25% of the people who have ICDs have two or more of these behavioral addictions.

WHAT ARE DOPAMINE AGONISTS?

Dopamine agonists mimic the effect of dopamine in the brain. They stimulate dopamine receptors just as dopamine does. Dopamine agonists are one of the most common medications used to treat the early stages of Parkinson's. One of the main reasons for this is that compared to carbidopa/levodopa, dopamine agonists are less likely to cause motor complications such as ON-OFF fluctuations and dyskinesias. In the middle and later stages of Parkinson's, carbidopa/levodopa and dopamine agonists are often taken in conjunction. We'll discuss this further in Chapter 7.

What makes someone more susceptible to developing ICDs?

Besides taking dopamine agonists, there are a variety of factors that put someone at a higher risk of developing impulse control disorders, such as:

- Being male
- Younger age at diagnosis (YOPD)
- Longer duration of living with Parkinson's
- History of drug abuse
- History of gambling
- Impulsive sensation personality traits
- Family history of psychiatric disorders
- Depression
- Overuse of dopaminergic medications due to dopamine dysregulation syndrome

HOW DO IMPULSE CONTROL DISORDERS IMPACT PEOPLE LIVING WITH PARKINSON'S?

ICDs have the potential to reduce the quality of life for people living with Parkinson's. In some severe cases, it can cause loss of employment, divorce, and financial ruin.

ICDs can cause people to feel ashamed, embarrassed, and weak. They may lie to hide their addictions, act in secrecy, and withdraw from their care partner or family members for fear of being found out. In some instances, someone who has developed an ICD must also reconcile that they get some level of satisfaction and pleasure from their addiction, even though it could be wreaking havoc on their lives and their most important relationships.

When we spoke to one of our community members about this symptom, she shared how her husband felt shame and guilt for his sudden interest in pornography and his overspending. Fortunately, he came to her and told her what was going on. They worked with his physician, and though it's an ongoing issue to make sure the balance of medications is best for him, the silver lining is that their relationship is strong, and they're working through it together.

We spoke to another woman whose husband had become a compulsive spender, put them in significant debt, and refused to get help. It led to the end of their marriage and many of the dreams they'd once had. While this is an extreme example, it illustrates what is possible if ICDs are left unreported and untreated.

Fortunately, being knowledgeable about ICDs, risk factors, and causes is the first step in recognizing them and seeking treatment.

WHAT'S THE TREATMENT FOR IMPULSE CONTROL DISORDERS?

The most important thing to remember about impulse control disorders is that it's a medical condition, not the result of personal weakness. If help is sought, it is possible to get better.

All ICDs are at some point on a continuum of severity, and where they fall on that continuum will indicate the kind of treatment needed.

For example, a man taking a dopamine agonist may become much more sexual. This isn't necessarily a problem. However, it could be a problem if he wants to have sex far more often than his partner wants or if he goes outside of a previously committed relationship. If it is a mild change in behavior, then discussion and possibly marriage counseling may be all that are needed. If the sexual behaviors are pathological and destructive, then medication adjustment would be necessary.

The first line of treatment when the behaviors are severe and destructive is to reduce the offending medication. In most cases, reducing or discontinuing the dopamine agonist reduced or eliminated the severity of the ICD.

Some people experience withdrawal symptoms when they stop taking their dopamine agonist, called dopamine agonist withdrawal syndrome (DAWS). The risk of DAWS is higher with higher doses of dopamine agonists and with more abrupt discontinuation. Symptoms may include panic attacks, sweating, nausea, and generalized pain. These can be challenging to manage. Another challenge is that reducing the dosage of a dopamine agonist or eliminating it can cause other distressing symptoms for the person with Parkinson's, such as decreased motor control or increased non-motor symptoms. In these situations, physicians will often put the person back on the dopamine agonist and then slowly titrate them off. This can take a long time, and controlling the ICD in the meantime can be a significant challenge.

One of the physicians we spoke to told us about a person in his 80s that he worked with. Managing his ICD ended up being a choice between the lesser of two evils. When he was on a dopamine agonist, he was very engaged in his life but also addicted to pornography. When he was on a lower dose, he became apathetic. His wife decided that she would rather he be engaged in his life and watch pornography than be shut down and apathetic. In that instance, they put in safeguards to make sure he was being monitored.

Like treatment for many addictions, the therapies designed to curb or eliminate ICDs involve finding a replacement for the time previously spent engaging in destructive behavior. It's critical to find something else to fill that time. Part of doing that is finding a support system while looking for something new to focus on during your most vulnerable times. If you have a primary care partner who lives with you or nearby, they can be a significant help during this time. More on their role can be found in the *Every Victory Counts Manual for Care Partners*, which you can find through our *Every Victory Counts* website.

If you are experiencing impulse control disorders, please work closely with your movement disorder specialist to assess your unique situation and create a treatment plan that's right for you. No two people experience ICDs in the same way, so it's critical to understand and evaluate all of your potential options. Throughout the process, be sure to note how you feel, how you behave, and how medications or therapies impact you so your physicians and care partners can keep an up-to-date record of your experience.

> *Early on in my life with Parkinson's, I determined I would constantly try to expand my horizons. I always loved playing the piano, but quit playing when I was first diagnosed. I committed to playing a certain amount of time every day, and even bought a new piano to make my playing more enjoyable. Every now and then I will add a metronome to assist in my Parkinson's rhythm weaknesses. I also decided to learn Spanish and have taught myself nearly every day for the last six years. I also got some Paint by Number kits to improve my manual dexterity. I really enjoy painting and am excited to continue hanging my 'works of art' in our nursery for the grandsons. My next challenge will be to relearn playing the flute. I played at a competent level as a child but have not played for decades; and, since my daughters bought me a flute, it's time to start again."*
>
> — PATTI BURNETT

WHAT'S NEXT?

Remember, while changes in cognition or thinking abilities can happen at any time, they typically tend to come as we age. In many situations, these challenges do not significantly impact daily life. For some people living with Parkinson's, these changes will never progress beyond mild cognitive impairment. Others experience a prolonged cognitive decline over time. If you or your care partner and family members notice changes in your cognition, discuss them with your physician. Many cognitive challenges may be treatable or even reversible. Physicians can perform objective tests to measure your thinking and memory to identify when cognitive impairment should be addressed. Keep in mind that the progression of cognitive challenges that can come for some people in the later stages of Parkinson's, such as dementia, can be influenced when caught early and managed proactively.

Often the most challenging part of dealing with these Parkinson's cognitive symptoms is the fear of the unknown. As a person with Parkinson's, you may worry that you'll experience cognitive decline and be unable to do anything about it. The good news is you now have information about these symptoms, the risk factors to look out for, biological and environmental triggers that can bring them on, and how to manage them if they show up.

The diagnosis of a chronic illness in and of itself requires a lot of adjustments. When you add something like Parkinson's cognitive symptoms into the mix, it's vital that you also add another level of self-care to your everyday life. Here are a few ways you can do just that.

- Join a Parkinson's support group if you don't already belong to one. Talk about your experiences, ask for help if you need it, and share what has worked and not worked for you
- Make time to exercise and get outdoors every day
- Communicate frequently with your physicians and discuss the possibility of tweaking your medications if your symptoms become worse
- Rest when you need it
- Plan a day trip or a vacation and get away from your normal surroundings
- Take control where you can and keep authoring your own story
- Practice meditation, yoga, or tai chi to relax and calm your mind
- Start a new project that you're excited to work on every day
- Communicate with your care partners and let them know how they can best help you

"What Cognitive Changes Should I Expect with Parkinson's?"

By Mark Mapstone, PhD

Have you ever considered what a remarkable and delicate piece of biology our brains are? They are truly amazing. This three-pound organ orchestrates everything from the movement of our bodies to making complex decisions, communicating thoughts, remembering past events, feeling sad or happy, or even just paying attention to things going on around us. These complex abilities are the product of many different brain regions working together in large networks and synchronized harmony. However, when one or more brain regions are not working the way they should, whole networks may be affected, and problems can result. Because Parkinson's causes a specific brain region to slowly stop working, people with Parkinson's often experience thinking or cognitive changes due to a decline in particular brain networks.

Most of the cognitive problems that people with Parkinson's experience are linked to bradyphrenia (brady means "slowed" and phrenia means "thinking"). This is the consequence of slowed signals moving through these brain networks, so some information is delayed or even lost as it moves through the brain. In many ways, bradyphrenia is the cognitive equivalent of the slowness that also affects physical movement in Parkinson's. These slowed signals can affect many cognitive abilities that rely on the speedy transfer of information. Some cognitive changes may be significant, but it's essential to realize that most are typically limited to specific cognitive abilities. While your ability to process information might be different than it was in the past, that doesn't mean you have a global decline in intellect.

Some of the most common cognitive changes associated with Parkinson's involve executive function. These include difficulty making complex decisions, keeping multiple things straight in your mind, organizing actions or ideas, or doing tasks in a specific sequence. Like calculating a tip at a restaurant or having a conversation on a cell phone while grocery shopping, executive tasks may become next to impossible for the person living with Parkinson's because of these brain-network changes. These executive problems can be particularly frustrating because we rely on these very abilities to navigate our complex and fast-paced world.

Another cognitive change that people living with Parkinson's may experience involves memory. The most common memory problems affect short-term recall, especially the ability to come up with information from things you have just seen or heard or to recall information on the spot. Word-finding problems, when we search for a word that just won't come to us, are common for people living with Parkinson's and can be frustrating or embarrassing. Long-term memory is less likely to be affected by Parkinson's.

Any change in thinking can be concerning. Understandably, most people living with Parkinson's, especially those recently diagnosed, want to know if they will experience significant cognitive changes. This is an important question that will affect you and the people around you, including care partners, family members, and communities at large. It isn't easy to make predictions about what your experience will be. We don't have reliable ways to predict cognitive changes for an individual or tell them which cognitive symptoms they will develop or how severe cognitive symptoms may be. That said, most people with Parkinson's will experience some cognitive changes like those described above while living with Parkinson's, but not all will have the same combination or severity of symptoms. Some individuals will have subtle cognitive changes, while others may develop more severe cognitive problems that impact how they live their daily lives.

A significant cognitive concern for many people living with Parkinson's is dementia. Most recent figures suggest that up to one-third of people living with Parkinson's will develop dementia. Dementia is the development of significant cognitive changes that considerably affect how you live your daily life and even your ability to live independently. Parkinson's dementia may also include new symptoms, such as hallucinations and long-term memory loss. Dementia may be challenging to detect because many of its cognitive symptoms can be related to other Parkinson's symptoms. For example, depression, low energy or motivation, hallucinations, or memory loss may be side effects of some medications used to treat Parkinson's. For these reasons, it is essential to talk openly to your Parkinson's physician about all your cognitive symptoms and concerns.

Let's now turn to how to face these cognitive challenges head-on.

Many people living with Parkinson's wonder what they can do to stay mentally healthy. First, it's important to realize that you are an active agent in your own health, and you can have a very real impact on your cognitive abilities. However, it is also important to have realistic expectations. Many of the cognitive symptoms of Parkinson's are the result of structural changes in the brain, and there are limits to how much they can be modified. But in most cases, cognitive abilities can be maintained and even improved to some degree.

For most people living with Parkinson's, this starts with maintaining physical health. Your brain receives all its nutrients and oxygen from the blood supply, so things that are good for cardiovascular health are good for brain health. Maintaining an active lifestyle with good nutrition and sleep can be a challenge for people with Parkinson's, but these things are vitally important to your physical and brain health.

Another key element in maintaining brain health is engaging in mental stimulation. Keep mentally active! Have conversations with people around you. Read new books. Teach someone to fly fish. Learn Italian. By encouraging your brain to engage actively and do something it's not used to, you strengthen connections in different brain networks, which may help them work more efficiently and ultimately improve the behavior they produce. Note: watching television is not a mental activity and doesn't count.

Finally, make things easier on yourself if you are experiencing cognitive symptoms. Carry a small notepad with you so you can take notes to help remember items at the store. Store commonly used objects like car keys, your purse, or your cell phone in the same place every time, so you will know where they are when you need them. Use your phone to take a picture of where your car is parked to help you find it later.

It's important to be aware that cognitive changes can be confusing, frustrating, and just as disruptive as motor changes. Just remember to be patient with yourself and remember that you're doing the best you can.

About Mark Mapstone

Mark Mapstone is professor of neurology at the University of California, Irvine School of Medicine, where he is also a member of the Institute for Memory Impairments and Neurological Disorders (IMIND).
He holds an adjunct appointment at the University of Rochester. His research focuses on early detection of neurological disease, especially Alzheimer's and Parkinson's, using cognitive tests and biomarkers obtained from blood. He has a special interest in developing strategies to maintain successful cognitive aging. In the clinic, he specializes in cognitive assessment of older adults with suspected brain disease.

»

Dr. Mapstone earned a PhD in clinical psychology at Northwestern University and completed fellowship training in neuropsychology and experimental therapeutics at the University of Rochester. He has authored more than 100 manuscripts and abstracts and is the recipient of a Career Development Award from the National Institute on Aging. His research has been funded by the National Institutes of Health, the Michael J. Fox Foundation, and the Department of Defense.

"What Is Parkinson's Disease Psychosis?"

By Cherian Karunapuzha, MD

Psychosis is a non-motor symptom of Parkinson's. It manifests in different ways, such as hallucinations, where you might see, hear, or feel something that is not there, and delusions, irrational beliefs or convictions. People living with Parkinson's have a 50% risk of developing psychosis at some point, and it can occur at all stages of Parkinson's. In the later stages, psychosis can be an integral feature of Parkinson's dementia. When psychosis occurs earlier in Parkinson's, it is usually related to starting certain medication classes or pushing to higher doses. However, it can also happen without any provoking factors in the middle stages of Parkinson's.

CAUSES OF PARKINSON'S PSYCHOSIS

The exact mechanism is not understood, but the circuits involved in psychosis seem to have an imbalance of dopamine and serotonin neurotransmitters. Some of the factors which would predispose one to get psychosis include:

- Older age of onset of Parkinson's
- Longer duration living with Parkinson's
- Presence of mood disorders like depression and anxiety

SYMPTOMS OF PARKINSON'S PSYCHOSIS

The term psychosis encompasses several features, including a false sense of presence, illusions, hallucinations, and delusions. A false sense of presence is the feeling that someone is standing beside you or is in the room with you, but when you turn around, no one is there. An illusion is a distortion or misinterpretation of something real that was sensed, like mistaking a belt for a snake. On the other hand, a hallucination is an imaginary sensation perceived without anything in the environment to provoke it. It's like seeing a dog in the corner of your room when there isn't one there. A delusion is a false, irrational belief you can't shake despite evidence to the contrary.

Typically, psychotic symptoms are subtle when they first start. In the evenings, you may begin to see shadows fleeting by or hovering at the edge of your vision, or you may have a feeling that someone is standing behind you. Gradually, objects at the corner of your vision start to look like something else, and the illusion goes away when you look straight towards it. Afterward, the images at the edge of your vision may start to become vivid and distinct. For the most part, you have insight or the ability to distinguish these symptoms from reality in the beginning.

These subtle symptoms can persist for months or even a few years, and it is often unclear when these early symptoms worsen. Sometimes, an infection or anesthesia from a surgical procedure can make them worse. As psychosis begins to worsen, it can occur more often during the day, and you can lose your ability to distinguish between reality and hallucinations. When this happens, the visions start to become intrusive and, at times, scary. At this stage, more patterns of hallucinations can begin, such as feeling things crawling on your skin, odd smells, and hearing music, along with delusions. Possible delusions include unshakeable feelings of being unduly persecuted by others or that your spouse is cheating on you. Nights can become disruptive with paranoid thoughts of strangers in the house or backyard. Frightening hallucinations and delusions are often stressful not only for the person with Parkinson's but also for care partners, and they may lead to ER visits, admissions to psychiatry units, or even nursing home placements.

PROACTIVELY ADDRESSING PARKINSON'S PSYCHOSIS

Hallucinations, along with infections and physical complications like falls, are some of the most common reasons people living with Parkinson's go to the hospital. But because even a few days of hospitalization can make Parkinson's symptoms worse (because medication regimens can be interrupted, as well as other reasons that will be explained later in Chapter 14), physicians strive to proactively prevent hospitalizations with activities like speech therapy (to prevent aspiration-related chest infections) and physical therapy (to prevent or reduce severe falls).

In the same way, Parkinson's psychosis should be caught and addressed early. However, physicians rely on you to bring up these symptoms, and only a small percentage of people experiencing Parkinson's psychosis report it to their physicians. Psychotic symptoms have a negative connotation, and many people are fearful that they could be perceived as being crazy or be placed in a nursing home if they admit to having these symptoms. Sometimes, subtle early symptoms are misjudged or wrongly attributed to something else, like poor vision, cataracts, or hearing loss. Other times, there is not enough time to discuss or screen for symptoms of psychosis during a regular appointment, as most of the time is spent discussing motor symptoms or other more obvious non-motor symptoms, like depression and apathy.

The first step towards addressing Parkinson's psychosis is to understand and accept that it is a common non-motor symptom of Parkinson's and to report these symptoms early so your wellness team can keep track of them over time and offer treatment strategies.

TREATMENTS FOR PARKINSON'S PSYCHOSIS

There are several approaches to treating Parkinson's psychosis effectively. First, ensure that there is not a provoking factor, like a brewing infection or dehydration. Then, talk with your physician about removing anticholinergic medications or reducing dopaminergic medications from your routine, especially in the evening. This may appear counterintuitive, as you might think you need more dopaminergic medications as Parkinson's progresses; however, while dopamine is good for physical symptoms, it almost inevitably worsens confusion and psychosis, especially in the later stages of Parkinson's.

If there is also a cognitive issue, starting dementia medications can help (to an extent) improve thinking and the features of psychosis. Finally, starting antipsychotic medications to treat the symptoms can also help. In the past, to treat Parkinson's psychosis, physicians had to use off-label antipsychotics that were typically used in schizophrenia. These medications often caused various side effects, including worsening the existing physical symptoms, drops in blood pressure, excessive sedation, and even deteriorating confusion. Understandably, these medications were used only when symptoms were significantly interfering with quality of life. In 2016, the first FDA-approved antipsychotic for Parkinson's psychosis was released. It has fewer side effects, meaning it can be used much earlier in the course of Parkinson's. Learn more about Parkinson's medications in Chapter 7, and for an in-depth, continually updated Parkinson's medication guide, be sure to check out the *Every Victory Counts* website.

Parkinson's psychosis can often feel like the figurative (or even literal) elephant in the room, but it is essential to bring this aspect of Parkinson's to light. The earlier you can address psychotic symptoms with your care team, the better you can manage them and improve your quality of life.

About Cherian Karunapuzha

Cherian Karunapuzha is a movement disorder specialist, assistant professor of neurology at the University of Oklahoma Health Sciences Center, and director of the OU Parkinson's Disease & Movement Disorders Center.

83

»

He completed his internship in internal medicine, residency in adult neurology, and a fellowship in movement disorders at the University of Texas Southwestern Medical Center, Dallas. He is a member of the AAN and holds board certification from the American Board of Psychiatry and Neurology.

Dr. Karunapuzha is a keen clinical educator who has received several teaching awards and is a frequently invited speaker for CME programs. Focused on community medicine, he has developed clinics for the uninsured in tandem with the patient support groups so as to improve statewide access to movement disorder specialists as well as access to research studies.

■ CHAPTER 6 – NON-MOTOR (AUTONOMIC)

OVERVIEW

Some of the non-motor symptoms you may experience with Parkinson's are connected to the effects Parkinson's has on your autonomic nervous system, which regulates functions your body automatically does, like controlling blood pressure, managing sweat and temperature, managing digestion, and controlling heart rate. Parkinson's impacts on the autonomic nervous system can cause non-motor symptoms that include:

- Constipation
- Overactive bladder and incontinence
- Sexual dysfunction, especially erectile dysfunction
- Excessive salivation (drooling)
- Excessive or too little perspiration
- Pain
- Sleep
- nOH (lightheadedness, especially when getting up in the morning or rising from a chair or couch)

While most popular Parkinson's medications do not treat non-motor symptoms, some people find certain medications effective for specific non-motor symptoms. Also, several lifestyle changes can help manage and reduce non-motor symptoms, such as exercising regularly, minimizing stress, and getting more sleep.

CONSTIPATION

Studies show that as many as 80% of people with Parkinson's experience constipation, and it can appear years before an official Parkinson's diagnosis.

As you have learned, Parkinson's lowers the level of dopamine in your body. When dopamine levels drop, the smooth muscle contractions throughout your digestive system slow down. When this happens in your colon, the stool moves very slowly, becomes dry and hard, and is more challenging to eliminate.

If constipation becomes severe constipation, the colon can become impacted and cause a medical emergency. If you do not have a bowel movement every three days or experience fullness, discomfort, or abdominal pain, no matter how much you eat, talk with your physician. Certain medications, such as pain relievers, antacids, cold medications, antidepressants, high blood pressure medications, high cholesterol medications, and cardiovascular disease medications, can make constipation worse. If you take any of these medications and experience constipation, discuss medication options with your physician.

One important reason you should minimize constipation is because it can play a significant role in ON-OFF times. Why? It centers around carbidopa/levodopa and its pathway to your brain, where it's converted to dopamine. To make its way there, carbidopa/levodopa must travel from your mouth to your stomach to your small intestine, where it is absorbed by an amino acid active carrier system and makes its way to your brain. There, it is metabolized to produce the dopamine that makes you feel your best. The more quickly the carbidopa/levodopa reaches the small intestine, the faster it passes through the intestinal walls and the brain's carrier system, and the faster you feel ON. Constipation slows the process of food through your gastrointestinal tract, meaning the process by which your carbidopa/levodopa is converted to dopamine is also delayed.

Movement disorder specialist Cherian Karunapuzha, MD, says that people with Parkinson's will have good days and bad days based on whether they empty their bowels. "When they do, they notice an immediate difference without us even having to increase the dose of the medicine," he says.

Nutritional choices play a role in constipation, and people living with Parkinson's who experience this symptom should pay close attention to how their food choices impact their digestion. One standard piece of nutritional advice for relieving constipation is to eat more fiber. Dietary fiber—non-digestible carbohydrates found in all plant foods, including fruits, vegetables, grains, nuts, and seeds—is critical for gut health. It consists of insoluble and soluble fiber, which work together to make your stools larger, softer, and capable of passing smoothly through your bowels. Though it may seem counterintuitive, a bulkier stool is easier to pass than a small and watery one.

Seek out a wide variety of high-fiber foods to help you manage constipation. Many high-fiber foods, such as beans, lentils, avocados, flax seeds, celery, broccoli, turnips, pears, peas, carrots, most nuts, oats, barley, and lettuce, contain both soluble and insoluble fiber. In general, fruits tend to be higher in soluble fiber; try adding apples, oranges, dates, dried figs, and prunes to your diet. Eating these in addition to foods high in insoluble fiber, such as whole-grain bread, bran, cauliflower, artichokes, and potatoes, will ensure you meet your daily fiber goals.

Although there are plenty of fiber supplements on the market, Parkinson's dietitians typically recommend that you get your fiber from whole foods instead. Fiber supplements usually do not provide various vitamins, minerals, and other beneficial nutrients that foods do.

Drinking enough water can also help minimize constipation. Soluble fiber absorbs water, which helps bulk up your stool while also transforming the soluble fiber into a gel-like substance. This softens the stool and allows it to move more smoothly through your bowels. However, if your body isn't adequately hydrated, it will soak up the water it needs from your food waste in the large intestine. This, in turn, creates hard stools that are difficult to pass. In general, you should aim to drink at least 64 ounces of water each day. Talk to your physician about whether those recommendations are suitable for you.

Coffee and some teas such as senna tea can also improve constipation, although too much caffeine may end up making it harder to fall and stay asleep, and it can also make a tremor worse. Some supplements such as aloe vera and magnesium can help relieve constipation. Sugar-free hard candy in moderation can also ease constipation. Your physician may also recommend an over-the-counter laxative medication or stool softener you can use to ease bowel movements.

A daily routine of 30 minutes of exercise is an essential part of keeping your gastrointestinal tract healthy and improving constipation. Different forms of exercise help in different ways. Aerobic exercise increases your heart rate and gets your blood pumping quickly, stimulating the intestinal muscles. This can help the muscles contract, which in turn helps move stools more quickly. Many yoga poses can help manage constipation, increase blood flow to the digestive tract, and stimulate intestinal contractions.

Constipation may be common in Parkinson's, but as you can see, there are many ways you can take action to manage and minimize it. Talk to your physician about treatment strategies and make daily choices to stay regular, healthy, and well. For more tips about minimizing constipation, see the 📄**Constipation Worksheet** on our ↻ *Every Victory Counts* **website**.

OVERACTIVE BLADDER AND INCONTINENCE

In Parkinson's, the brain's control of the urinary sphincter can become disrupted, leading to difficulty holding urine. As a result, people with Parkinson's may experience incontinence, accidental or involuntary loss of urine control or bowel movements. This can range from occasional minor leakage to complete loss of control of urine or bowel movements.

> *As I enter the mid-stages of Parkinson's, the most problematic non-motor issue I have is with urinary urgency. I have to plan ahead and be constantly vigilant about locations of restrooms. I am less likely now to participate in adventurous activities in the outdoors."*

— CAROL CLUPNY

There are different types of incontinence that people with Parkinson's may experience, such as:

- Urge incontinence: a frequent and urgent need to use the toilet

- Stress incontinence: an urge that usually occurs in the presence of a physical stressor, such as coughing

- Nocturia: the need to get up multiple times at night to use the toilet

There are several strategies you can try to help manage these symptoms.

1. **Avoid bladder irritants.** Various fluids and foods can irritate the lining inside the bladder, causing the bladder to contract and release urine. Avoiding these irritants can help reduce symptoms of urinary incontinence, urgency, and frequency. Examples of bladder irritants are coffee, tea, carbonated beverages, tomatoes and tomato juice, artificial sweeteners, and spicy foods, as well as acidic foods or drinks.

2. **Minimize fluids before bed.** About two hours before bed, aim to minimize fluid intake to reduce the frequency of getting up at night to use the toilet. During the day, however, be sure to drink plenty of fluids. Not consuming enough water can irritate the bladder, as well.

3. **Practice your Kegels.** Urinary incontinence can be due to weakened pelvic floor muscles. These muscles lie deep within the pelvis and help close the urethra to prevent urine from releasing when we don't want it to. Kegels are an excellent exercise to strengthen pelvic floor muscles. Consider working with a physical therapist who can help you learn how to perform this exercise and track your progress correctly.

4. **Review your current medications.** Certain medications can lead to urinary retention, urgency, frequency, or incontinence. Diuretics for high blood pressure or vascular conditions, alpha-blockers for hypertension, antidepressants, pain medications, and sleeping pills can all play a role. If you are taking any of these medications and are experiencing urinary dysfunction, discuss medication options with your physician.

87

5. **Consider urodynamic testing.** By seeing a urologist or other urinary specialist, you can use this diagnostic tool to assess how your bladder and urethra are functioning and identify the origin of your urinary symptoms. The results of your urodynamic test will help determine which medications will best alleviate your symptoms, which your physician can then prescribe.

For more resources, check out the 📄**Bladder Worksheet** on our ↗*Every Victory Counts* **website** to learn about more changes you can make to your nutritional choices and lifestyle to help manage an overactive bladder, as well as treatments to discuss with your physician and other healthcare professionals.

SEXUAL DYSFUNCTION, ESPECIALLY ERECTILE DYSFUNCTION

Sexual dysfunction, a common Parkinson's non-motor symptom, can significantly impact your quality of life. Because many people living with Parkinson's are reluctant to bring up this issue, it often goes unmentioned and untreated. The good news is that through open communication, counseling, and (if needed) adjustments to your medication regimen, you can have a healthy and enjoyable sex life while living with Parkinson's.

Parkinson's motor symptoms, including tremor, stiffness, rigidity, and dyskinesia, can interfere with sexual activity. So too can non-motor symptoms such as fatigue, excessive salivation, sweating, anxiety, apathy, depression, and cognitive changes. And while some Parkinson's medications, such as dopamine agonists, can increase sexual interest and activity, others, such as certain antidepressants, can do just the opposite.

The most common sexual problem for men living with Parkinson's is erectile dysfunction (ED). ED often goes hand-in-hand with depression, so for some people, taking an antidepressant can help. Some antidepressants, however, can decrease sex drive and cause ED; so, work closely with your physician to discuss medications that are less likely to contribute to ED. Other ED treatments include different medications, physical and/or talk therapy, and surgical implants.

Many men with Parkinson's also report concerns about hypersexuality and compulsive sexual behavior. As we discussed earlier in Chapter 5, this behavior is typically a side effect of dopaminergic therapy. Talk with your physician if you experience these symptoms since they may be treated by reducing the dose of your dopamine agonist.

Women living with Parkinson's often report that a loss of lubrication and involuntary urination during sex are their biggest concerns in this area. Because many women with Parkinson's experience decreased lubrication, sexual activity can be painful. Other symptoms women report include reduced sex drives and problems with orgasm. As with men who experience ED, women who feel concerned with losing their sexual desire can work with their physicians to see if medication changes help. Other treatment options include adding lubrication, timing sex for ON periods when your symptoms are well controlled, and working with a sex counselor or other therapist for personalized strategies.

Counseling, especially with a licensed sexologist, can help you overcome many of the sexual intimacy barriers you may feel. It's also important to remember that intimacy means many things. Physical touch, such as holding your partner's hand or hugging them, is an expression of intimacy. Redefining what intimacy means to you can be a meaningful and freeing conversation to have with your partner.

EXCESSIVE SALIVATION (DROOLING)

As we highlighted earlier, Parkinson's causes a reduction in automatic actions, including swallowing. This can impact your ability to manage the flow of saliva in and around your mouth.

Saliva is essential for many reasons. It assists in chewing and swallowing, lubricates oral tissues, provides immunity to infection, and neutralizes acid, preventing tooth demineralization. Although people living with Parkinson's typically produce an average amount of saliva, swallowing difficulties, common in Parkinson's, can cause saliva to pool in your mouth.

Excessive drooling is another common symptom of Parkinson's and can range from mild to severe. Severe drooling, which can appear as an embarrassing outpouring of saliva when your mouth is involuntarily open or when you're distracted from the need to swallow automatically, can be an indicator of more serious difficulty with swallowing (dysphagia), which can cause you to choke on food and liquids and can even lead to aspiration pneumonia.

Drooling can also lead to irritation or infection at the corners of the mouth; so, if you have swallowing problems, consult a speech-language pathologist or therapist who can assess your swallowing technique and recommend strategies that will help you swallow more effectively.

Lack of saliva or dry mouth (xerostomia) is common in people with Parkinson's, too, and may be more troublesome for people with Parkinson's than excessive salivation. It increases the risk of both dental decay and gum disease. Dry mouth can be caused by medications, Parkinson's itself, or even by aging. To treat this symptom, your dentist may suggest artificial saliva substitutes. Sugar-free hard candy (especially citrus) can help to stimulate the salivary glands. If you lack saliva or experience dry mouth, avoid irritating products such as alcohol, tobacco, and spicy and acidic foods.

EXCESSIVE SWEATING

In addition to regulating blood pressure, digestion, and heart rate, your autonomic nervous system regulates your body's temperature. If this regulation is negatively impacted by Parkinson's, you may experience excessive sweating regardless of the level of physical activity or room temperature. This can occur at any time and, when it happens at night, it may impact sleep.

To minimize and cope with excessive sweating:

- Stay hydrated
- Wear lightweight, loose-fitting clothing made from cotton or other natural fibers
- Choose clothing that doesn't show sweat
- Identify and reduce consumption of foods that may trigger sweating (spicy foods, caffeine, or alcohol)
- Identify and reduce stressors that cause sweating (public speaking, crowded rooms, etc.)

While less frequently reported, some people with Parkinson's may experience too little sweating, or hypohidrosis, which could be a side effect of an anticholinergic Parkinson's medication. Too little sweating can negatively impact your ability to control your body's temperature and can put you at risk of overheating.

If you experience excessive sweating or hypohidrosis, talk to your physician about adjusting your medication or other treatments, such as botulism toxin (Botox) injections, that may help.

PAIN

Studies show that between 60 and 83% of people with Parkinson's report experiencing pain, and chronic pain is twice as common in people living with Parkinson's than those without Parkinson's. Several different types of pain are associated with Parkinson's, and effective management requires coordination with your care team and implementation of pharma- and non-pharmacological treatments. This section addresses common questions about Parkinson's-related pain, including types of pain, treatments, the pain ladder, and which specialists to see. Although many types of Parkinson's pain are chronic, you can improve your quality of life and live well with Parkinson's by taking control of your pain management plan.

WHAT ARE THE DIFFERENT TYPES OF PAIN EXPERIENCED BY PEOPLE WITH PARKINSON'S?

Five main types of pain are common for people with Parkinson's. Multiple types may be present simultaneously or occur at different points throughout a person's path with Parkinson's. Recognizing which kind of pain you have can help you optimize treatment.

Musculoskeletal Pain. Musculoskeletal pain is pain that affects muscles, bones, tendons, ligaments, and nerves. The pain can be localized or generalized and can fade or intensify at different times. Existing musculoskeletal pain can be exacerbated by Parkinson's.

Neuropathic Pain. Rather than being caused by a physical injury, this type of pain is caused by damage to the somatosensory nervous system or a disease affecting the somatosensory nervous system, which responds to external stimuli like touch, temperature, and vibration. It tends to be consistent throughout the day and is present no matter what activity you're doing. Unlike the aching you may feel when you're doing a strenuous physical activity, neuropathic pain feels more like a tingly, crawly, uncomfortable sensation.

Dystonic Pain. Dystonia, the movement disorder in which involuntary muscle contractions cause repetitive or twisting motions, is often very painful. Many people with Parkinson's experience dystonia as a motor symptom, whether it's localized (focal dystonia), in multiple nearby body parts (segmental dystonia), or all over (generalized dystonia).

Akathisia. This movement disorder is characterized by the inability to be still. Many people who experience it feel restless or uneasy and exhibit motions like pacing, rocking back and forth, or fidgeting. Often, if it affects a particular body part, it can cause burning or pain sensations that can sometimes be relieved by moving that body part.

Central Pain. When there's damage to or dysfunction of the central nervous system from causes such as a stroke, tumor, epilepsy, or Parkinson's, central pain syndrome can result. The pain is usually chronic and constant and can affect a specific or generalized portion of the body.

HOW IS PAIN TREATED FOR PEOPLE WITH PARKINSON'S?

No matter the cause, pain is complex. When a person with Parkinson's experiences intense pain, especially in combination with other symptoms, managing it can be challenging. There are, however, several ways you can adjust your medication regimen, exercise schedule, and lifestyle to reduce your pain and improve your quality of life.

MEDICATIONS

There are various kinds of medications used to treat pain, especially for people with Parkinson's. Dr. Janis Miyasaki, MD, professor in the division of neurology at the University of Alberta's Department of Medicine, describes how physicians approach pharmacological treatment of pain for people with Parkinson's:

> *"The principle is to start with what is called the pain ladder. You always start with the least intensive, least side-effect-giving treatment."*

— JANIS MIYASAKI, MD

Step One

The first step of the pain ladder is hot and cold treatments, along with stretching and flexibility exercises. People who experience rigidity and stiffness can sometimes alleviate pain using heating pads to loosen their muscles, improve mobility by stretching, and address any residual pain with ice packs. (And remember, especially if you're new to daily exercise and have been more sedentary for a while, build your momentum and fitness levels slowly to avoid pain from overworking your muscles. Exercise is a cornerstone of living well with Parkinson's, but stretching and improving your flexibility before you begin a more intense regimen can help you stay active without getting hurt.)

Step Two

The next step on the pain ladder is low-dose, over-the-counter medications like acetaminophen and ibuprofen. Because these pharmacological interventions are relatively inexpensive, don't require a prescription, and can be managed by the person with Parkinson's, they are a great next step in treating pain. If acetaminophen and ibuprofen aren't doing the trick, transitioning to more potent non-steroidal anti-inflammatory drugs (NSAIDs) like Naproxen or Aleve may help. Remember, let your care provider know if you're taking any medications, even those available over the counter, in addition to those they have prescribed.

Step Three

The next step on the pain ladder is antidepressants. Although using antidepressants for pain relief may seem strange, medications like tramadol, tramacet, duloxetine, and many tricyclic antidepressants are often used to treat pain in people with Parkinson's when options on the lower steps of the pain ladder haven't worked. However, these medications require more careful balancing with other medications. (For example, you should not take MAO-B inhibitors with tramadol.) And because anxiety and depression are common non-motor symptoms of Parkinson's, you may need to adjust your existing antidepressants before starting new ones to manage your pain.

Step Four

The next step includes anti-epileptic medications like gabapentin and pregabalin (the former is used off-label to treat pain while the latter is often prescribed to treat neuropathic pain specifically). Though there is limited research about these medications' effectiveness in treating Parkinson's-specific pain, they have helped treat fibromyalgia pain, diabetic pain, and nerve pain; so, they may be appropriate medications if less intensive treatments have failed. However, be aware that doses high enough to treat pain effectively can also cause sedation, instability, and increased fall risk. Discuss in depth their use with your care team.

Step Five

The final step on the pain ladder is opioids. Many physicians refrain from prescribing opioids due to their addictive qualities and the potential for abuse. Still, if no other options on the pain ladder have been effective, you and your physician may consider them. Studies have shown varied results about the efficacy of opioids to treat Parkinson's-related pain, so talk to your physician about the best treatment course.

OTHER MEDICAL INTERVENTIONS

Other medications used to treat Parkinson's pain include carbidopa/levodopa or dopamine agonists. Because carbidopa/levodopa lessens dystonia and rigidity (both of which can cause pain), your physician may address your pain by increasing your dosage or the frequency at which you take carbidopa/levodopa. Other common interventions to address pain include Botox injections, surgery, or deep brain stimulation (DBS). Be sure to work with your care team members to explore all your options and decide what might work best for you.

NON-PHARMACOLOGICAL INTERVENTIONS

You can take many steps to manage your pain that are not medication-based, and lifestyle changes are often very effective. Complementary therapies and interventions like massage, stretching, yoga, increased amounts of exercise, heat and cold treatments, and physical and/or occupational therapy can help lessen your pain and improve your quality of life. It's also important to eliminate (or at least minimize) activities and behaviors that can increase your pain. Consider making changes to your environment that will make your life more enjoyable, such as investing in more comfortable furniture or sitting rather than standing on public transport. These small lifestyle changes can have positive effects on experiences with pain.

WHO SHOULD I SEE TO DISCUSS MY PARKINSON'S PAIN?

Your first point of contact should be your primary care physician. Whether that means your family physician, neurologist, or movement disorder specialist (MDS), start by asking them how to manage your pain. They may prescribe you one of the medications we listed above, offer suggestions about altering your lifestyle, and/or refer you to a pain specialist.

Pain management specialists are physicians with specialized training in evaluating, diagnosing, and treating pain; so, speaking to one of these specialists might be helpful for you. Be sure to get a referral from your primary care physician, though, to ensure you are visiting a physician who understands the complexity of treating Parkinson's-specific pain.

Health and wellness providers like physical therapists, acupuncturists, and massage therapists can also be valuable members of your care team. Be willing to try new things and approach alternative therapies with an open mind, as no one's path with Parkinson's pain is the same. What works for someone else may not work for you and vice versa. Consider visiting different specialists to find a treatment plan that works best for you.

WHAT CAN I DO DAILY TO MANAGE MY PAIN?

Remember, you're your best advocate, as only you understand how your pain feels. Understanding and communicating the kind of pain you're experiencing can significantly inform your treatment plan and allow your physicians to address your specific pain type and severity. Keep your care team informed about activities that cause pain or the times of day your pain is worse so they can help fine-tune your care plan. Do you notice the pain starting to creep in at a certain point after you take your medication? Do you feel fine when you bike but experience pain when you jog? Did you start experiencing this pain before or after your Parkinson's diagnosis? Taking stock of these sorts of questions can be helpful as you work with your care team to treat your pain effectively.

SLEEP

Many people with Parkinson's talk about sleep (lack of, interrupted, or restless) as their most troublesome non-motor symptom. Unfortunately, getting quality sleep regularly is critical to living well with Parkinson's, not just because sleep in and of itself is restorative, but because if you don't sleep well, you can't manage your other symptoms effectively.

> *Sleep? What is that? I have tried melatonin, quiet time before bedtime, going to bed at the same time each night, and tracking my sleep with a Fitbit, all in the hope of sleeping better and longer. I may not have a perfect solution, but overall, these steps help, and I save the Fitbit sleep analysis to share with my doctor."*
> — LORRAINE WILSON

For many years, the benefits and causes of sleep remained a mystery. However, in the past few years, sleep science has grown significantly. We now have a deeper understanding of the importance of sleep, why it is so essential to sleep consistently and properly, the effects of sleep medicine, and how people with Parkinson's are specifically affected.

Matthew Walker, PhD, is one of the foremost experts on sleep science. He is a professor of psychology and neuroscience at the University of California, Berkeley. In 2017, he published the *New York Times* bestselling book *Why We Sleep: Unlocking the Power of Sleep and Dreams*. While his research is not Parkinson's-specific, his coverage of the function and importance of sleep is applicable across the board.

To understand the faulty sleep mechanisms associated with Parkinson's, we first need to delve into why we sleep. Sleeping enriches our learning capacities and helps us make logical choices. It improves our psychological function and balances our emotions, allowing us to make level-headed decisions the next day. Sleep also strengthens our immune systems, prevents infection, balances metabolism, regulates appetite, encourages gut microbiomes, and lowers blood pressure, among other benefits. The bottom line is that sleep is the ultimate system reset, and every part of you benefits from it.

> **" *Every major system, tissue, and organ of your body suffers when sleep becomes short. No aspect of your health can retreat at the sign of sleep loss and escape unharmed. Like water from a burst pipe in your home, the effects of sleep deprivation will seep into every nook and cranny of biology, down into your cells, even altering your most fundamental self – your DNA."* **
>
> **— MATTHEW WALKER, PHD**

SLEEP AND WAKE CYCLES

Humans have a two-factor, built-in sleep/wake cycle. Your circadian rhythm is an internal clock that regularly makes you feel awake or tired, while adenosine is a chemical compound that builds up in your brain while you are awake and makes you feel pressure to sleep. The carefully controlled balance between these two factors—your circadian rhythm and adenosine levels—determines your sleep/wake cycle. Another critical component of regulating this cycle is melatonin, a hormone that makes you feel less awake. Melatonin is closely tied to light, so your brain produces more of it when it gets darker out. However, melatonin doesn't cause sleep; it just prompts your body that it's time to go to bed.

> **" *I find sleep to be the primary driver for what my day is going to be like. Without adequate sleep, everything is more difficult – my energy level, ability to exercise, mental sharpness, the effectiveness of my meds, etc. On nights that I do not sleep well, I must find time during the day to take a good nap."* **
>
> **— STEVE HOVEY**

THE DIFFERENCES IN REM AND NREM SLEEP

In 1952, researchers discovered that people cycle through two different kinds of sleep. The first is called REM (rapid eye movement) sleep, during which we dream, and the second is called NREM (non-rapid eye movement) sleep. You go through cycles of different lengths every night. Depending on whether you're staying awake too late, getting up in the middle of the night, or waking up too early, you might be missing out primarily on REM or primarily on NREM sleep, each of which has different consequences. For example, in an experiment from the 1960s, researchers found that depriving people of REM sleep made them moody, paranoid, anxious, and psychotic, demonstrating the importance of plentiful REM sleep.

Even with all this research on the importance and function of sleep, many people are still unaware of the various effects of poor sleep. Especially for seniors, Walker notes that "elderly individuals fail to connect their deterioration in health with their deterioration in sleep, despite causal links between the two having been known to scientists for many decades. Far more of our age-related physical and mental health ailments are related to sleep impairment than either we or many physicians truly realize or treat seriously."

While improved sleep is not a cure-all, it can certainly help with many different ailments, especially those that affect us as we age. Another meaningful change that occurs as we get older is that our sleep becomes more fragmented, meaning that we wake up during the night more often. Later, we'll take a closer look at this topic as it relates to Parkinson's.

Now that you are armed with more information about how sleep works, let's take some time to delve into why sleep is so important. We've already touched on the fact that a good night's sleep has beneficial effects on the entire mind and body, but the effects are far more multifaceted than just making you feel better rested.

EMOTIONAL IMPACTS

As mentioned earlier, sleep is essential for emotional regulation. Without a good night's sleep, your capacity to make level-headed decisions is diminished. In his research, Walker compared emotional responses for people who were awake versus asleep all night. He found that in the amygdala, a part of the brain involved in strong emotional reactions and the fight-or-flight effect, there was a 60% increase in emotional response for sleep-deprived people. He also found that sleep-deprived people had overactive striatum, which is associated with emotion, impulsivity, and reward. Therefore, when you don't get enough sleep, you are more prone to extreme positive and negative emotional swings.

The number of reported cases of sleep issues has increased dramatically in recent years. There are a variety of underlying causes, as Walker describes:

> *To date, we have discovered numerous triggers that cause sleep difficulties, including psychological, physical, medical, and environmental factors (with aging being another, as we have previously discussed). External factors that cause poor sleep, such as too much bright light at night, the wrong ambient room temperature, caffeine, tobacco, and alcohol consumption can masquerade as insomnia."*

— MATTHEW WALKER, PHD

Addressing external causes of sleep troubles can often be done using sleep hygiene techniques (as we will discuss later), while dealing with true insomnia often causes people to turn to medications. However, Walker cautions strongly against using sleeping pills as the first form of defense.

THE PROBLEM WITH SLEEP MEDICATIONS

Daniel Kripke, MD, of the University of California, San Diego, researched connections between sleeping pills and disease/mortality risk. He found that people who took sleeping pills were 4.6 times more likely to die in 2.5 years than those not taking sleeping pills. In the same period, he found that people taking more than 132 pills per year were 5.3 times more likely to die in 2.5 years, and people taking just 18 pills per year were still 3.6 times more likely to die in 2.5 years. Further, sleeping pills cause higher infection rates, increased risk of car accidents (caused by the groggy feeling the following day), high fall rates, and higher heart disease and stroke rates. These statistics are not meant to tell you to stop taking your prescribed medication. Instead, they should encourage you to consider whether a pharmacological solution is best for you and to discuss their possible use carefully with your physician.

MELATONIN

Unlike prescribed sleep medications, melatonin is available as an over-the-counter supplement and may provide some short-term benefits for sleep. Naturally occurring melatonin is a hormone that helps regulate your circadian rhythms and makes you feel sleepy when darkness falls. Melatonin is closely linked to light; when your body experiences less light, like after sunset, your brain produces more melatonin, and you feel less awake. The less melatonin your brain produces, the higher your risk of insomnia and other sleep problems. (This risk is why sleep experts recommend avoiding bright lights, especially from screens, at night. The lights interfere with serotonin's conversion into melatonin, and melatonin is essential for a good night's sleep.)

Melatonin as a supplement does not have any sleep-inducing qualities. Instead, it supplements the natural neurotransmitters associated with sleep, signaling to your body that it's time to go to bed.

Although melatonin is not considered a controlled substance and is not associated with any dependence, it may not be effective for everyone, and its effects may be short-lived. It may also be associated with some residual sleepiness and fatigue the following day. Melatonin is typically not recommended for people living with depression. As with all supplements, be sure to talk to your physician about their possible use and what dose they recommend for you.

REM SLEEP BEHAVIOR DISORDER

One widespread sleep disturbance among people living with Parkinson's is REM Sleep Behavior Disorder, otherwise known as RBD. RBD is characterized by people acting out vivid dreams, including talking, jumping out of bed, kicking, biting, etc., even though the person is often unaware of it. About 50% of people with Parkinson's report RBD as one of their symptoms, but even more strikingly, 80% of people with RBD will develop a neurodegenerative disorder within 10 years, making it a highly effective predictor. Several studies of prodromal Parkinson's indicate that sleep issues, especially RBD, are strong measures of conversion to movement disorders.

Occasionally, medications used for Parkinson's, including dopaminergic medications like carbidopa/levodopa and select antidepressants and sleep aids, can cause vivid dreams or nightmares and disrupt your sleep. As unsettling as these can be in and of themselves, this can present serious concerns when combined with RBD. If RBD causes a person to act out their dreams, they often do not feel rested in the morning. Also, bed partners of people with RBD often report violent responses by the person with RBD, which involves being punched, bitten, or kicked while the person acting out the dream is unaware of this behavior.

If you are experiencing RBD, discuss this symptom with your physician. Some medications may help, and adaptations and modifications to beds and bedrooms can enhance your safety and the safety of your partner. Some couples living with Parkinson's discover the safest and most effective way to ensure both partners sleep safely and as soundly as possible is to sleep in separate beds.

> " *I have experienced very vivid dreams for as long as I can remember, well before my Parkinson's diagnosis. One morning, my husband asked me if I was okay. He then showed me marks that appeared to have been made by my fingers around his neck. We told my movement disorder specialist who said, 'You have two choices: you can sleep in separate rooms, with the door locked from the outside for (me), or you can take a medication. You have REM sleep behavior disorder.' That was eight years ago. I chose to take medications. I still have vivid dreams, but the nights of acting out my dreams are over."*
>
> — MARTY ACEVEDO

OTHER COMMON SLEEP ISSUES

RBD is not the only sleep issue that people with Parkinson's may face. Other common symptoms include:

- **Insomnia.** Insomnia is a sleep disorder characterized by persistent difficulty falling or staying asleep. Insomnia is caused by your own body rather than by an outside force

(such as caffeine, alcohol, the wrong ambient temperature, lighting, and other factors that can impact sleep quality)

- **Sleep fragmentation.** Frequent awakenings or arousals during the night, known as fragmented sleep, interfere with your sleep cycles and can result in less time spent in deep sleep and REM sleep, the most physically and mentally restorative stages of the sleep cycle

- **Excessive Daytime Sleepiness (EDS).** EDS can be caused by the various effects of Parkinson's that interrupt sleep at night. It can also be a side effect of some Parkinson's medications

- **Nighttime sweating.** As we explained earlier, Parkinson's impacts on your autonomic nervous system can impair your body's ability to regulate temperature effectively. Ideally, chemicals and hormones in your body would begin lowering your body temperature by a few degrees as night falls to help prepare your body for sleep. If this process is interrupted, as it can be with Parkinson's, your body may release sweat instead to keep your body cool. This night sweating can lead to poor sleep quality

- **Trouble moving in bed.** Symptoms including tremor, stiffness, and rigidity can make it difficult to turn over and move in bed, as can pain caused by muscle cramping (known as dystonia) or stiffness

- **Sleep apnea.** This condition, characterized by pauses in breathing or shallow breaths during sleep, can worsen sleep problems. While sleep apnea is not caused by Parkinson's, it does occur more frequently in adults as they age

- **Fatigue.** Fatigue can feel like an overwhelming sense of tiredness, low energy, sleepiness, weakness, or stamina loss. It may appear alongside sleep problems or mood issues like depression and anxiety. Fatigue can come with non-Parkinson's-related problems like diabetes, heart and lung disease, and hypothyroidism. Poor nutrition habits, malnutrition, and dehydration can worsen fatigue, as can certain Parkinson's medications, including dopamine agonists and anticholinergic medications. We'll take a closer look at fatigue and Parkinson's later in this chapter

- **Restless Leg Syndrome (RLS).** RLS is characterized by unpleasant feelings in the legs when they are at rest that is usually relieved with movement. RLS can result from medications and medical conditions other than Parkinson's, so definitely discuss with your physician if you are experiencing RLS

HOW CAN I IMPROVE MY SLEEP?

Unfortunately, while sleep disturbances are common symptoms of Parkinson's and can severely impact quality of life, insufficient studies exist about treatments. Though many medications exist, they are not applicable across the board and often can have unfortunate side effects. More research is necessary to find better solutions.

It can feel daunting to find ways to improve your sleep, and it may be tempting to turn to pharmaceuticals to manage your sleep difficulties. However, as explained earlier, this option has the potential for adverse side effects and is often less effective than lifestyle changes in the long run. Always discuss changes that you're considering with your healthcare professional, but don't be afraid to try different techniques to find what works for you. Sleep is an essential part of living well, so make sure to prioritize it as much as possible.

> " *Rest, absolutely rest. I now regularly take a short nap without fail, and I had to get to the point where I gave myself permission to do that.*"
>
> — TIM

"Sleep hygiene" is the set of habits and behaviors that help you sleep well regularly. Below, we offer some general and Parkinson's-specific sleep hygiene tips to help you improve your sleep.

1. **Protect your bedroom.** Avoid blue light (including screen technology) to preserve your circadian rhythm and allow natural melatonin production. If you get anxious about not being able to sleep and you find yourself watching the clock, remove any visible clock faces from view in the bedroom.

2. **Prepare your sleeping area.** Reduce light and noise, lower your room temperature (around 65 degrees Fahrenheit is considered ideal), and consider using a white noise machine or app to lull you to sleep.

3. **Set a sleep schedule and develop a routine based on what's optimal for you.** Make sure to follow a regular bedtime and wake-up time, even on the weekends, because consistent sleep patterns will help you in the long run.

4. **Experiment with daytime naps.** Some people living with Parkinson's benefit from daily naps, while for some, naps can negatively affect their sleep at night. If you feel yourself needing to nap, experiment with naps of different lengths (as brief as 10 minutes and as long as two hours) and at different times of day to see what works best for you.

5. **Watch when and what you eat.** Many people with Parkinson's have constipation or acid reflux; so, tailoring your nutritional choices to avoid exacerbating those problems can also help you sleep. Avoid spicy or acidic foods, avoid too much protein (high protein levels can make it harder to absorb your medicine), and avoid sugary snacks or caffeine (which stimulate the nervous system).

6. **Limit your liquids.** Be extra careful about consuming caffeine and alcohol, especially close to your bedtime. Caffeine competes with adenosine and therefore keeps you awake rather than letting you fall asleep. Though it may help you fall asleep faster, alcohol lowers sleep quality and can make you wake up more often throughout the night.

7. **Get daily exposure to the sun.** Sunlight helps sleep partly because of its role in serotonin production, which is triggered when your skin and the retinas in your eyes absorb sunlight. Serotonin is the precursor for melatonin, the hormone that makes you feel sleepy when darkness falls. To use sunlight to boost your sleep quality, sleep experts suggest exposing your eyes to natural light early in the day. Even just two to 10 minutes of sunlight can ensure photons get through, even if there is cloud cover. Seeking out the sun in the evening is important as well. Exposure to sunlight as the sun is setting helps set the appropriate timing of secretion of the hormone cortisol, making you alert at the right times of day and sleepy at the right times.

8. **Exercise regularly.** As we have mentioned (and focus on in Chapter 9), exercise is beneficial for many systems and functions, including sleep. A study found that after four months of physical activity, adult insomniacs got an average of one extra hour of sleep per night. Exercise improves sleep quality, quantity, number of nighttime waking incidents, and the time it takes to fall asleep. Because quality sleep gives you more energy, it contributes to a positive feedback loop where you feel energized to exercise, so you exercise, so you sleep better (and, the next day, this beneficial cycle continues). Exercising in the morning can help you stay energized throughout the rest of the day. If you can exercise outside in the morning, you'll get the added benefit of better sleep: exposure to natural light early in the day may increase melatonin levels at night.

9. **Clear a path to the bathroom.** Be careful to avoid trip hazards at night. If you are particularly concerned about falls, consider including a low brightness or red-bulb lighting system from your bedroom to the bathroom to help you make your way without falling and without disrupting your circadian rhythm.

FATIGUE

Now that you know the science behind sleep and some strategies to sleep well, let's take a closer look at fatigue and Parkinson's.

Fatigue, one of the most common (and frequently, most disabling) Parkinson's non-motor symptoms, is a physical or psychological feeling of weariness, exhaustion, and lack of energy. Fatigue can affect one's quality of life in many ways. It can:

- Prevent you from being physically active
- Get worse over time, as Parkinson's progresses
- Make depression worse (it doesn't cause it, but it can add a level of intensity to it)
- Make it difficult to focus and concentrate on important tasks
- Make everything feel like an intense effort
- Get in the way of connecting with others

- Undermine countless daily activities
- Make it much more difficult and exhausting to cope with Parkinson's and non-Parkinson's-related challenges

Fatigue can be caused or worsened by several different factors, including poor sleep, depression, specific motor symptoms, and certain medications. It can also be unrelated to Parkinson's, caused by anemia or other health factors.

STRATEGIES TO MANAGE FATIGUE

- **Exercise.** It may seem counterintuitive to get moving if you're feeling fatigued; however, the right kind and the right amount of activity can significantly reduce fatigue. Experiment. Sometimes just getting out the door for a walk in the fresh air can reduce fatigue

- **Talk to your physician if you think you may be depressed.** It's possible that an antidepressant could reduce fatigue

- **Plan your time.** Identify when you tend to have the most energy throughout the day and plan to get your most important jobs done then

- **Be realistic, but still do something.** If you're feeling extra exhausted on a particular day, don't pressure yourself to accomplish everything you planned. Do something—because completing something will give you an energy boost—but be realistic about what you're capable of doing

- **Delegate.** It's not easy. You may have concerns about being a burden to others, but most people will be thrilled to help. Let them

- **Organize and declutter.** Opening up space—physically, emotionally, mentally, and logistically—can help you reduce stress and, as a result, reduce feelings of fatigue

- **Connect with others.** We know that when you feel wiped out, the last thing you want to do is attend a support group meeting or event, but positively connecting with others has the potential to not only make you feel supported and encouraged and loved, but it may very well give you the exact bump in energy that you need

NEUROGENIC ORTHOSTATIC HYPOTENSION (nOH)

Parkinson's can lower your blood pressure, as can the medications used to treat the motor symptoms of Parkinson's. Neurogenic orthostatic hypotension (nOH) is characterized by lightheadedness that occurs when a person moves from a seated/low position to standing and their blood pressure drops significantly. This rapid change in blood pressure and the resulting lightheadedness and dizziness can be one of the causes of falls in people with Parkinson's. Because injuries from falls and subsequent fear of falling can hamper your quality of life, nOH is a vital symptom to address.

While nOH is becoming more widely recognized as a common condition among people with Parkinson's, there are several other causes of dizziness not related to Parkinson's, such as dehydration and anemia. Ask your healthcare provider to help you identify root causes and potential solutions. For more, see our 📄**Low Blood Pressure and Dizziness Worksheet** on our ⟳ *Every Victory Counts* **website**.

"What Is Neurogenic Orthostatic Hypotension (nOH) in Parkinson's?"

By Jose-Alberto Palma, MD, PhD, and Horacio Kaufmann, MD

Neurogenic orthostatic hypotension (nOH) is a type of orthostatic hypotension (OH), formerly known as postural hypotension. nOH is caused by dysfunction in the autonomic nervous system and causes people to feel faint when they stand up.

WHAT IS ORTHOSTATIC HYPOTENSION (OH)?

OH is a sustained fall in blood pressure that happens within three minutes of standing. OH can reduce blood flow to organs above the heart, most notably the brain, and its symptoms can profoundly impact your quality of life. OH is more common in the elderly, and certain medications, dehydration, varicose veins, severe anemia, and conditions such as heart disease can lead to OH.

OH can be caused by the body not releasing enough of the neurotransmitter norepinephrine. When your body doesn't release enough norepinephrine, your blood vessels don't constrict when they need to, lowering your blood pressure and causing you to feel faint when you stand or sit up. When problems in the release of norepinephrine cause OH, it is referred to as neurogenic orthostatic hypotension (nOH). nOH can be seen in disorders affecting the nervous system, such as Parkinson's, dementia with Lewy bodies, pure autonomic failure, and multiple system atrophy.

HOW COMMON IS nOH IN PEOPLE WITH PARKINSON'S?

The prevalence of nOH increases with both age and number of years of living with Parkinson's. Although nOH in Parkinson's is relatively common, not everyone will experience symptoms. For that reason, people with Parkinson's should be screened for nOH, even if they have no symptoms.

nOH can be one of the earliest symptoms of Parkinson's and can appear several years—even decades—before the onset of motor problems like tremor or stiffness. Therefore, people who have nOH but do not have any significant motor or cognitive symptoms should also be monitored closely to watch for early signs or symptoms of Parkinson's.

103

WHAT ARE THE SYMPTOMS OF nOH?

nOH can appear with or without symptoms. The typical symptoms of nOH are lightheadedness, dizziness, blurry vision, and, when there's a significant drop in blood pressure upon standing up, fainting. Symptoms almost always occur when standing up, less frequently when moving from standing to sitting, and go away when lying down. People with nOH may also experience weakness, fatigue, leg buckling, headaches, neck and shoulder discomfort, and shortness of breath. The severity of symptoms varies from day to day and fluctuates throughout the day. Often, mornings tend to be most difficult, as nOH symptoms are aggravated by overnight urination, which is common in people with Parkinson's. Meals, particularly those rich in carbohydrates and sugars, also cause drops in blood pressure.

Not all people with nOH have symptoms. Symptoms emerge only when the blood pressure upon standing falls below a certain limit. In people living with Parkinson's, this usually occurs when your mean blood pressure upon standing falls below approximately 90/60 mmHg (systolic/diastolic) as measured with a blood pressure cuff on the arm. Symptoms of nOH typically disappear upon sitting or lying down, because gravity restores blood flow to the brain. Indeed, people with nOH are frequently able to tolerate wide swings in blood pressure and often remain conscious at pressures that would otherwise induce fainting in healthy people. However, fainting can still occur, especially after a large meal or alcohol consumption, in hot weather if you get dehydrated, or if you're taking medications to lower blood pressure.

In people with Parkinson's, symptoms of nOH can also be non-specific, including fatigue and difficulty concentrating, and may sometimes mimic a carbidopa/levodopa OFF state. It's easy to miss nOH unless your physician measures your blood pressure while you are in a standing position. Conversely, it is important to realize people with Parkinson's can experience lightheadedness that mimics nOH but may instead be caused by balance problems or other issues. For this reason, careful evaluation of your symptoms by a movement disorder specialist is strongly advised.

HOW IS nOH DIAGNOSED?

Diagnosis of nOH requires blood pressure readings taken while lying flat as well as while standing up. At least a 20 mmHg drop in your systolic blood pressure and a 10 mmHg drop in your diastolic blood pressure within three minutes of standing up are required to make the diagnosis.

Some people with Parkinson's don't experience a drop in blood pressure every time they stand up. In these cases, a physician may use a monitor to measure the person's blood pressure every 30 minutes for an entire day to assist in diagnosis and subsequent management of nOH.

HOW IS nOH TREATED?

The good news is that nOH is treatable. The goal of treatment is not to achieve normal blood pressure but to reduce symptoms of nOH and improve your quality of life. Management of nOH includes three components: correcting aggravating factors, lifestyle changes, and medication.

Correct Aggravating Factors

Stopping medications that can lower blood pressure, such as diuretics, anti-hypertensives, some medications used for prostate and urinary symptoms, medications for erectile dysfunction, medications for angina, and some antidepressants, is the first step. Carbidopa/levodopa can lower blood pressure and adjusting dosage may be necessary in people with Parkinson's and nOH. Anemia (a condition where you have low levels of hemoglobin, iron, in your blood) can aggravate nOH and should be investigated and treated accordingly.

Lifestyle Changes

Symptoms of nOH can improve with time, patience, and non-pharmacological changes. It is tempting to try to control nOH only with medications; however, this approach is less effective and may have adverse side effects. Treatment of nOH is more successful if lifestyle changes are also made.

Below are lifestyle steps you can take to improve symptoms of nOH. You can adopt all of them at the same time. If performed properly, these actions can lead to a dramatic improvement, even without medication.

1. **Increase water intake.** People with nOH need more water than the average person and, in general, should be drinking three quarts per day (~2.5 liters). Ideally, the best approach is to drink water together with increasing salt in your diet (see Tip #2). Tea and coffee increase urine output, so they may worsen your symptoms. Sports drinks, juices, and many carbonated beverages are not recommended due to their high sugar content (see Tip #8).

2. **Increase salt intake.** Be sure to discuss adding salt to your food with your physician, but if approved, increasing salt in your meals will help to increase your blood pressure. Although some like them, most people do not need to take salt tablets, and they cause abdominal discomfort in some people.

3. **Wear compression stockings (also known as TED stockings).** You can find compression stockings in medical supply stores. Wearing them will reduce the venous pooling that occurs when standing up and, therefore, will increase your blood pressure when standing. There are several strengths or levels of compression stockings. First, you can try medium strength (i.e., 20-30 mmHg). To be useful, compression stockings should be worn up to the abdomen. Knee-high stockings are not effective. You do not need to wear stockings while you sleep.

4. **Wear an abdominal binder (i.e., a Velcro belt around your belly).** You can find this item in medical supply stores. It functions in a similar way to compression stockings. Some people find abdominal binders more tolerable than compression stockings. You do not need to wear this while you sleep.

5. **Sleep with the head of your bed raised by at least 30° (ideally 45-50°).** Elevating the head of your bed is useful because people with nOH frequently have supine hypertension (high blood pressure when lying down), too. To avoid supine hypertension, you should not lay flat. Sleeping with the head of the bed raised will also reduce urine output, causing fewer nighttime urinations and improved blood pressure in the morning. The best way to raise the head of the bed is to get an electric bed or an electric mattress. These are commercially available in several sizes. Other less effective ways to increase the head of the bed are to use a wedge or put some books/bricks under the upper feet of the bed.

6. **Drink 16 oz. of *cold* water 30 minutes before getting out of bed in the morning.** This will increase your blood pressure when you get up. Drinking 16 oz. of cold water at any time of day will also increase your blood pressure. You can do this on an as-needed basis, ensuring that you drink the recommended total (see #1) of about three quarts per day of liquids.

7. **Start a physical therapy program.** In people with nOH, physical exercise will decrease blood pressure; however, exercise is crucial to keep muscles active and for overall well-being. To avoid low blood pressure when exercising, your physical therapist can recommend recumbent exercises (e.g., recumbent bicycle, elastic bands, rowing machine, etc.). The best exercises that are safe for people with nOH are those performed in a swimming pool. The hydrostatic pressure of the water will prevent your blood pressure from falling dramatically, even if you are standing, if most of your body is underwater (with your head out, of course, so that you continue to breathe). While you are in the water, you likely will feel much better and will be able to exercise with no significant nOH symptoms. The better your baseline fitness, the less intense your symptoms of nOH will be. Therapies such as yoga and tai chi are also highly advisable.

8. **Avoid factors that decrease blood pressure and worsen nOH.** These include hot and humid temperatures; physical exercises in the standing position that can cause blood pressure drop (see Tip #7); dehydration (see Tip #1); alcohol; and high-glycemic-index carbohydrates. Try to reduce high-glycemic carbohydrates in your meals. Try eating several small meals (five or six) instead of the three traditional meals.

9. **Be aware of your symptoms.** If you experience symptoms of nOH, you can find relief by performing physical counter-maneuvers, such as making a fist, crossing your legs, or clenching your buttocks, which increase your blood pressure when you

106

are standing. If these counter-maneuvers are not enough, sit or lie down quickly to avoid fainting and injury.

MEDICATION

While lifestyle changes can be very effective for nOH when performed properly, many people still require medication to manage symptoms. Be sure to check out the in-depth medication guide on the ⬀ *Every Victory Counts* **website** for information about medicines that may work for you.

All available drugs that raise blood pressure in the standing position also raise blood pressure while lying down, increasing the risk or worsening hypertension while lying flat with your face up. Although there is no specific data on cardio- and cerebrovascular events induced by hypertension in a flat position, physicians treating people with nOH should be aware of this potential side effect. Before beginning treatment with any of the above medications, your physician should carefully review your other medications.

About Jose-Alberto Palma

Jose-Alberto Palma is assistant professor of neurology and assistant director of the Dysautonomia Center at New York University. His work has been focused on the diagnosis, management, and understanding of autonomic disorders in patients with autonomic synucleinopathies, such as Parkinson's and multiple system atrophy, and the search for biomarkers for early diagnosis of these disorders.

Dr. Palma has been involved in several studies and clinical trials to develop new treatments for autonomic dysfunction and to describe the premotor phase of Parkinson's.

About Horacio Kaufmann

Horacio Kaufmann is a professor of neurology and medicine and the director of the Dysautonomia Center at New York University. He is one of the world's leading experts in diagnosing and managing patients with autonomic synucleinopathies (Parkinson's and multiple system atrophy), a subject that has been the focus of his research academic career for more than 25 years.

»

He has extensive experience as the principal investigator of national and international studies on autonomic dysfunction, including clinical trials for orthostatic hypotension, and identification and development of a biomarker for early diagnosis and progression of Parkinson's and related disorders.

As you can see, there is a wide variety of possible non-motor symptoms of Parkinson's, ranging from physiological effects like trouble swallowing, pain, and fatigue, to mental and emotional impacts, such as mood changes, cognitive challenges, and anxiety. Just as Parkinson's affects everyone differently, the type, frequency, and severity of non-motor symptoms each person experiences vary. Remember, just because something is listed as a non-motor symptom of Parkinson's does not mean you will experience it. Recognizing and discovering how you can best manage the non-motor symptoms you do experience are critical for learning to live well with Parkinson's.

Parkinson's Treatments and Therapies

▌ CHAPTER 7 – MEDICATION

OVERVIEW

Medications are an important part of your overall care. This chapter will review medications that can be used for the motor and nonmotor symptoms of Parkinson's. Motor symptoms particularly include stiffness, slowness, and tremor. Nonmotor symptoms are also known as "the Parkinson's you can't see," and include symptoms such as constipation, blood pressure fluctuations, and depression.

Medication management strategies are will vary, as no two people with Parkinson's will experience the same symptoms with the same severity. It is important to establish good communication with your medical provider, as not everyone will have all symptoms, and only those symptoms that are bothersome to you need to be treated. The goal of medication management is to maximize quality of life while minimizing side effects. Which medications are right for you will depend on many factors, including your age, how long you have had Parkinson's, and other health conditions you may have.

THE BEST MEDICATIONS FOR YOU

Which medication is best for you depends on many factors, including your symptoms, age, time living with Parkinson's, and risk for side effects. Any of the available medications can be used early in the progression of Parkinson's, depending on these factors.

Parkinson's symptoms may be mild for several years, requiring small doses of medication. During the first few years of treatment, controlling motor symptoms is also generally smooth, and missing a dose or two of medication may not even be noticeable. However, as the number of years with Parkinson's increases, fluctuations in the benefits of medication may emerge, and symptoms may begin to breakthrough before the next dose is due. During these OFF times, some or all of the motor and nonmotor symptoms you would have without medication can recur. You may start to feel like you are on a roller coaster when you feel good (ON) at times and worse (OFF) at others.

If these symptoms occur, you and your physician can adjust your medications to reduce your OFF periods. These adjustments may include taking medication doses closer together, using longer-acting medications, such as dopamine agonists, or using carbidopa/levodopa boosters, such as MAO-B inhibitors or COMT inhibitors.

As is the case with any medication, different people tolerate the same Parkinson's medications very differently. Some people respond well to low dosages of medication, while others may require a higher dose. Some people experience medication side effects severe enough to warrant a change of course, while others experience few or no side effects. If you experience side effects with your medication, especially if the side effects interfere with your ability to go about your normal activities, discuss this with your physician as soon as possible. Your dosage might need to be adjusted, or your physician might choose a different medication or combination of drugs.

Treatment for Parkinson's is focused on achieving the most ON time and limiting OFF time as much as possible to give you the highest quality of life. However, as medications are increased, dyskinesias—involuntary, irregular jerking or wiggling movements—can become a problem. To treat dyskinesias, medication dosages may be reduced or changed completely. Later in this chapter, we'll take a closer look at dyskinesia.

MEDICATION MANAGEMENT STRATEGIES

Medications are tailored to the individual and will vary from person to person, as no two people with Parkinson's will experience the same symptoms with the same severity. The following section reviews common strategies used as Parkinson's changes over time, primarily focused on the medication strategies to manage motor symptoms.

MILD MOTOR SYMPTOMS

Parkinson's symptoms may initially be mild for several years and not require medication. The strategy of not using medications is referred to as expectant management. During this time, it is important to focus on vigorous exercise, overall good health habits, and reducing stressors.

A good rule of thumb is to start medication when your Parkinson's symptoms become disruptive or restrictive to your life in some way, such as if tremor or slowness are interfering with daily activities at home or at work. Likewise, if you are giving up activities you've previously enjoyed due to symptoms, it may be time to start medication. Moreover, if your provider notes significant rigidity and slowness that you may not be aware of, medication treatment may be recommended even before you find your symptoms bothersome. Some people do not learn they have Parkinson's until their symptoms are already affecting their function or quality of life in some way, so medications may be recommended at the time of diagnosis or shortly thereafter.

Carbidopa/levodopa is the most effective medication for the motor symptoms of Parkinson's and is often used as initial treatment. Some people with Parkinson's and some medical providers may prefer a carbidopa/levodopa-sparing strategy. One way to use this strategy is to use carbidopa/levodopa as the initial medication, but then use other medications as add-ons to keep the dose of carbidopa-levodopa low. Another way to use this strategy would be to start an MAO-B inhibitor, dopamine agonist, or amantadine as initial medication, and carbidopa/levodopa can then be added at a later time. You will see more about each of these medications in the following pages.

MODERATE MOTOR SYMPTOMS

During the first few years of treatment, controlling motor symptoms is generally smooth, and missing a dose or two of medication may not even be noticeable. However, as the number of years with Parkinson's increases, fluctuations in the benefits of medication may emerge, and symptoms may begin to break through toward the end of dosing intervals. This recurrence of symptoms between doses is known as OFF time. As OFF times become more frequent, you may start to feel like you are on a roller coaster, feeling good control of your symptoms at some times (ON) and loss of control of your symptoms at other times (OFF).

If you experience OFF time, you and your medical provider may choose to adjust your medications. One approach is to increase the amount of medication taken at each dose. Another approach is to increase the number of times per day that medications are taken. A third strategy is to change to longer-acting medications. A fourth strategy is to add a Parkinson's medication from a different category. In the case of someone taking carbidopa/levodopa, this could mean adding a booster such as an MAO-B inhibitor or COMT inhibitor, or adding amantadine or a dopamine agonist. Working with a neurologist familiar with Parkinson's becomes increasingly important at this stage to help choose among these approaches.

Another complication that becomes more common as the number of years with Parkinson's increases is dyskinesias. Dyskinesias are involuntary, irregular wiggling or jerking movements. To treat dyskinesias, medication dosages may be reduced; medications may be divided into more frequent smaller doses; amantadine may be added; or your regimen may be adjusted to less of one medication category and more of another. Later in this chapter, we'll take a closer look at dyskinesia.

ADVANCING MOTOR SYMPTOMS

The same medications that are used for mild and moderate symptoms are also used as Parkinson's advances. However, over time there can be more Parkinson's symptoms that are less responsive to medication. Issues with speech, posture, and balance become increasingly common. The brief inability to move, called freezing, can become very problematic. The importance of integrative care; rehabilitation therapies such as speech therapy, swallowing therapy, physical therapy, and occupational therapy; targeted exercise; and mind-body therapy become increasingly important to enhance safety and quality of life in advanced stages. We'll explain the many benefits of these and other therapies in Chapter 10.

MANAGING PARKINSON'S MEDICATION FOR MORE ON TIMES

As we've discussed, carbidopa/levodopa helps minimize Parkinson's symptoms because it is converted to dopamine in the brain. OFF times take place when carbidopa/levodopa is no longer working well enough to suppress your symptoms. What, though, causes carbidopa/levodopa to stop working optimally, and what can you do to get the most from your medicine? Here, we explore some of the science behind OFF and strategies that will help you maximize your ON times to live your best life with Parkinson's.

WATER AND MEDICATIONS

To make its way from your mouth to your brain, carbidopa/levodopa must travel from your stomach to your small intestine, where it is absorbed by an extensive neutral amino acid active carrier system. A similar transport system transfers carbidopa/levodopa across the blood-brain barrier to the brain, where it is metabolized to produce dopamine. The more quickly the carbidopa/levodopa reaches the small intestine, the faster it passes through the intestinal walls and the brain's carrier system. The quicker it converts to dopamine, the more quickly you will feel ON.

The key to minimizing delayed and partial ON times is to take your carbidopa/levodopa on an empty stomach with a full glass of water. The water "flushes" the medicine quickly to the small intestine, and the absence of food in your stomach means nothing can slow its emptying. (Crushing or chewing carbidopa/levodopa can also help speed the process, as can choosing a carbonated water beverage such as club soda or sparkling water.) Ideally, you would take each dose of your carbidopa/levodopa one hour before a meal (to give it time to move from the stomach to the small intestine) or two hours after (the amount of time it takes for food to empty the stomach). Because this is not always possible, especially as your Parkinson's progresses and you take carbidopa/levodopa more often, aim to take each dose at least 30 minutes before or 30 minutes after a meal—and, again, always with a tall glass of water.

PROTEIN AND MEDICATIONS

The system that transports carbidopa/levodopa from the small intestine to the brain is the same system that transports amino acids. Both carbidopa/levodopa and amino acids must enter the bloodstream through the intestinal wall and then cross the blood-brain barrier to enter the brain. If too many amino acids are present along with carbidopa/levodopa, the medicine competes with the amino acids for absorption, and it won't enter the carrier system quickly. Similarly, some amino acids compete with carbidopa/levodopa for absorption in the brain. Their presence at the time when carbidopa/levodopa makes its way to the blood-brain barrier will delay the time it takes for the brain to transform the medication to dopamine and, therefore, decrease or delay the medication's efficacy. This, too, can lead to delayed or only partial ON times.

In your stomach, protein is broken down into amino acids, which then travel to your small intestine. For your carbidopa/levodopa to work most effectively, it should enter your small intestine when few amino acids are present; this gives it easy access to the carrier system and fewer obstacles to crossing the blood-brain barrier. To maximize your ON times, avoid protein when you take your carbidopa/levodopa and talk to your physician about how dietary changes can help you get the most from your medications.

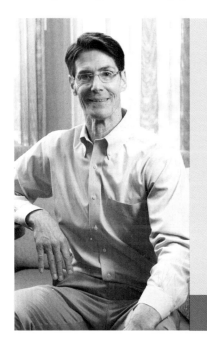

" As time goes on and my reliance on medications to address my Parkinson's symptoms increases, I have needed to be much more deliberate of what I eat and when. It's extremely important for me to make sure my medicine is fully digested before I have a meal, especially if what I am going to eat involves protein. Medication and protein are both so important, yet as my Parkinson's has progressed, so has my sensitivity to timing my consumption of the two. It's a balancing act, but it is doable!"

— STEVE HOVEY

CONSTIPATION AND MEDICATIONS

Constipation can also play a significant role in carbidopa/levodopa absorption and ON-OFF fluctuations. In the digestive system, food makes its way from the mouth to the large intestine through the alimentary canal (esophagus, stomach, and small and large intestines). Suppose your intestines aren't being emptied regularly. In that case, the carbidopa/levodopa you take won't make its way through the digestive system as it should, and, therefore, it cannot control your symptoms most effectively. Staying regular means your carbidopa/levodopa will work most effectively, and you will experience less OFF time. For more on constipation and Parkinson's, see Chapter 6.

MEDICATION-INDUCED PARKINSON'S DYSKINESIA

Literally meaning "abnormal movement," dyskinesia is an uncontrolled, involuntary muscle movement that is irregular in motion. Although it can be a stand-alone condition, in people with Parkinson's it is most often associated with long-term use of carbidopa/levodopa or other Parkinson's medications that increase levels of dopamine in the brain. This type of carbidopa/levodopa-induced dyskinesia involves symptoms ranging from writhing or wriggling to dramatic rocking and head bobbing. Severe dyskinesia, also referred to as troublesome dyskinesia, can significantly interfere with daily life and compromise gait and balance, limiting the person's engagement in activities such as running errands, participating in hobbies, meeting with family and friends, and eating in public.

As we mentioned earlier in this chapter, if a person with Parkinson's is having dyskinesias that are bothersome or present most of the time, one option is to reduce the carbidopa/levodopa dose or other related Parkinson's medications. However, if doing so would adversely affect the control of your primary Parkinson's symptoms, your physician may prescribe treatment to specifically target the dyskinesia. An extended-release formulation of amantadine has been approved by the FDA specifically for the treatment of carbidopa/levodopa-induced dyskinesia in people with Parkinson's and has been demonstrated to also reduce OFF time. Another option is to consider other forms of amantadine, which are approved to treat Parkinson's—and may be prescribed off-label to treat dyskinesia. For people with Parkinson's who are good candidates and willing to undergo surgery, deep brain stimulation (DBS) can be a successful treatment option for controlling Parkinson's dyskinesia. See Chapter 8 for an in-depth look at DBS.

MEDICATIONS AND HOSPITAL STAYS

Hospital stays for people with Parkinson's require special consideration, especially when it comes to medication. Before your hospital visit, make sure you have a complete, updated list of your medications, dosages, and the times of day that you take them. Keeping an accurate, up-to-date list decreases the likelihood of an unwanted medication interaction. As we mentioned earlier, studies have found that one in three people with Parkinson's have been prescribed contraindicated drugs while they were hospitalized, which highlights the importance of always having an up-to-date list of medications available. To help you stay organized, you can find numerous medication checklists and worksheets on our *Every Victory Counts* website.

Be sure your hospital care team understands that all Parkinson's medications must be given on time. You and/or your care partner should strongly advocate on your behalf for this important point.

In addition to your list of medications, bring with you a list of your current symptoms. This will help your hospital care team recognize these symptoms, as they may not be familiar with such problems as dyskinesia, ON-OFF fluctuations, and freezing of gait. Be sure to let them know how your movement and abilities change during ON and OFF times. This also helps the hospital care team understand why it is so important for you to get your medications on time every time.

MEDICATION PREPAREDNESS FOR HOSPITAL STAYS

Some medications can worsen motor symptoms of Parkinson's. These drugs, listed below, are often used to treat psychiatric problems such as hallucinations, confusion, or gastrointestinal problems such as nausea. It's important that your hospital team is aware that many common anti-hallucination medications must be avoided in people with Parkinson's, since they might otherwise prescribe these medications if, as is common, the stress of your illness, hospital stay, or new medications causes hallucinations or delirium while you are hospitalized. New onset delusions, paranoia, and agitation signal to the medical team that a longer hospital stay or skilled nursing is required before going home.

ANTI-HALLUCINATION MEDICATIONS TO AVOID

The anti-hallucination medications quetiapine (Seroquel), clozapine (Clozaril), and pimavanserin (Nuplazid) can be used with Parkinson's. Of these, Nuplazid is the only anti-hallucination medication approved for Parkinson's.

The following should be avoided:

- Aripiprazole (Abilify)
- Chlorpromazine (Thorazine)
- Flufenazine (Prolixin)
- Haloperidol (Haldol)
- Molindone (Moban)
- Perphenazine (Trilafon)
- Perphenazine and amitriptyline (Triavil)
- Risperidone (Risperdol)
- Thioridazine (Mellaril)
- Thiothixene (Navane)

ANTI-NAUSEA MEDICATIONS TO AVOID

Serotonin (5-HT3) antagonists work to block the effects of serotonin in order to reduce nausea and vomiting and do not worsen symptoms of Parkinson's. Ondansetron (Zofran), dolaseton (Anzemet), and granisetron (Granisol) are acceptable alternatives to the list below. Older and cheaper anti-nausea medications block dopamine, therefore worsening Parkinson's symptoms.

The following should be avoided:

- Metoclopramide (Reglan)
- Phenothiazine (Compazine)
- Promethazine (Phenergan)

MEDICATIONS TO AVOID IF YOU TAKE RASAGILINE (AZILECT) OR SELEGILINE (ELDEPRYL)

- Pain medications meperidine (Demerol), tramadol (Ultram), and methadone
- Antispasmodic medication (Flexeril)
- Dextromethorphan (cold medication) and ciprofloxacin (antibiotic)

Note: This is not a complete list of medications to avoid. If you have questions about other medications, ask your pharmacist.

For more about hospital stays and Parkinson's, see Chapter 14.

Remember, everyone living with Parkinson's experiences symptoms differently, and your medication regimen should be tailored to your unique needs and goals. Talk with your care team about how you can maximize your medications to live well with Parkinson's.

"I've Heard that I Should Wait to Begin Parkinson's Medications Because They Only Work for So Long. What Is Your Advice about That?"

By Aaron Haug, MD

This is such an important question. The purpose of medications in Parkinson's is to improve quality of life. This might mean enabling a person to continue working longer, complete daily activities more easily, or continue to enjoy a hobby. Most movement disorder specialists, myself included, recommend treating motor symptoms—tremor, stiffness, and slowness—to the point that they're no longer interfering with quality of life.

The concern that people with Parkinson's often have is that they don't want to "use up" their medication options. This is an important point, and I would say it's a misconception that medications "only work for five years" or some other time frame. There are two things going on, which can be difficult to separate because they can overlap.

The first thing is how long a person has had Parkinson's, and the other thing is how long that person has been on medications for Parkinson's. It is true that medications work best in the early years of living with Parkinson's, with greater benefit and lower likelihood of motor fluctuations and dyskinesias. However, this has as much to do with how many years a person has had Parkinson's as it does with how many years they have been on medications. When a person has lived with Parkinson's for more years, they usually need more treatment. The medicine doesn't stop working, but progression of Parkinson's leads to more symptoms. There are multiple ways to address this, including increasing the dose of one medicine or using multiple medicines together. The guiding principle is to start medication if symptoms are negatively impacting quality of life and adjust medications over time to maximize quality of life.

About Aaron Haug

Aaron Haug is a neurologist and movement disorder specialist with HealthONE Neurology Specialists in Colorado. He attended undergraduate at Creighton University and then earned his medical degree at the University of Kansas. He completed a neurology residency and a fellowship in movement disorders at the University of Colorado, including a year as Chief Resident. His medical interests include Parkinson's, tremor, other movement disorders, deep brain stimulation (DBS), and botulinum toxin injections to treat neurological conditions. Outside the office, he likes spending time with his wife and kids, running, skiing, and following Colorado Rockies baseball.

MEDICATIONS FOR MOTOR SYMPTOMS

DOPAMINERGIC MEDICATION

Carbidopa/Levodopa

Levodopa is the gold standard treatment for Parkinson's. It was one of the first Parkinson's drugs, and it is still the main drug prescribed to treat Parkinson's for many people. It acts to help with slowness, stiffness, and tremor. Carbidopa is now almost always combined with levodopa to enable more levodopa to reach the brain rather than the bloodstream. Carbidopa/levodopa can be used in conjunction with other medications to address the same symptoms. Common side effects of carbidopa/levodopa include nausea and light-headedness.

GENERIC NAME	TRADE NAME	NOTES
Carbidopa/Levodopa immediate release (IR) tablets	Sinemet	Available in three strengths: 10/100 mg, 25/100 mg, and 25/250 mg. The most commonly used strength is 25/100 mg tablets. Note that 10/100 mg tablets have less carbidopa, which is there to reduce side effects, so 10/100 mg tablets will sometimes cause more side effects such as nausea and light-headedness. Note that 25/250 mg tablets have 2.5 times as much levodopa, the active ingredient. This can help to reduce pill burden in people requiring higher doses, but can cause side effects if inadvertently taken in place of the 25/100 mg strength.

GENERIC NAME	TRADE NAME	NOTES
Carbidopa/Levodopa orally disintegrating tablets	Parcopa	Available in the same strengths as IR. Dissolvable tablets that can be helpful for people with swallowing problems.
Carbidopa/Levodopa extended release (ER) tablets	Sinemet CR	Available in two strengths: 25/100 mg and 50/200 mg. Extended-release formulation is sometimes helpful in reducing side effects. Sometimes dosed at night to help control symptoms through the night-time hours. Sometimes also dosed during the day, but absorption can be less predictable than with immediate release tablets. Brand name Sinemet CR was discontinued in 2019 but generic formulations remain available.
Carbidopa/Levodopa/ Entacapone	Stalevo	An alternative to just carbidopa/levodopa that is combined with entacapone to help with motor fluctuations. Available in six strengths. Entacapone can cause diarrhea, discolored urine.
Carbidopa/Levodopa extended-release capsules	Rytary	Each capsule contains both immediate-release and extended-release beads, with the goal of increasing ON time with fewer dosages. Note that Rytary dosing is not interchangeable with other formulations of carbidopa-levodopa. Available only as a branded product.
Carbidopa/Levodopa enteral solution	Duopa (US)	Administered through a small tube that is surgically inserted into the small intestine rather than delivered in pill form. This can be a helpful alternative for people requiring very frequent dosing or with swallowing issues. Available only as a branded product.
Carbidopa/Levodopa inhalation powder	INBRIJA	Inhaled powder used as add-on to regular regimen of carbidopa/ levodopa as rescue therapy for OFF episodes. Available only as a branded product.
Fractionable Carbidopa/ Levodopa tablets	Dhivy	25/100 mg specially-designed tablets that are intended to be split more precisely and easily into 1/4, 1/2, or 3/4 tablets. Can be helpful for people that require a very specific dose. Available only as a branded product.

Dopamine Agonists

Dopamine agonists address the same symptoms as carbidopa/levodopa, namely slowness, stiffness, and tremor. This category is generally considered the second-most effective category of medications for motor symptoms, behind levodopa. Dopamine agonists can be used alone or in conjunction with other medications to address symptoms. Over years of use, dopamine agonists are somewhat less likely than carbidopa/levodopa to cause dyskinesias or fluctuations with OFF time. Common side effects include nausea and light-headedness, and other possible side effects include leg swelling, sleep attacks, and compulsive behaviors (see Chapter 5).

GENERIC NAME	TRADE NAME	NOTES
Ropinirole	Requip	Typically dosed three times per day.
Ropinirole XL	Requip XL	Typically dosed once or twice per day.
Pramipexole	Mirapex	Typically dosed three times per day.
Pramipexole ER	Mirapex ER	Typically dosed once or twice per day.
Rotigotine	Neupro	This medication is a patch applied once a day. It provides a continuous release of medication that can be helpful for people with fluctuations or with swallowing problems.
Apomorphine	Apokyn	Subcutaneous injection used as add-on rescue therapy for OFF episodes. Subcutaneous administration may improve speed and predictability of rescue benefit over oral medications and may be helpful for people with swallowing problems. May cause significant nausea. Available only as a branded product.

> " *When I get stressed, my medications don't work right. I've found the rescue drug Apokyn to really help when my medications are wearing off. I average about one shot of Apokyn a day.*"
>
> — LINDA

MAO-B Inhibitors

Monoamine Oxidase Type B (MAO-B) inhibitors act to block the MAO-B enzyme that breaks down dopamine, which allows more dopamine to be available to the brain. Like carbidopa/levodopa and dopamine agonists, MAO-B inhibitors are used to treat slowness, stiffness, and tremor. They can be used on their own, though they typically have a milder benefit than carbidopa/levodopa and dopamine agonists. MAO-B inhibitors are often used as supplemental medications to reduce OFF time. Common side effects include nausea, light-headedness, and insomnia. Because MAO-B inhibitors increase and prolong the effects of dopamine, the side effects of dopamine may also be enhanced, including dyskinesia. There are multiple medications that are contraindicated with MAO-B inhibitors (see table).

GENERIC NAME	TRADE NAME	NOTES
Selegiline	Eldepryl	Typically dosed twice a day. Has a metabolite that can cause side effects of anxiety, irritability, or insomnia in some people.
Selegiline orally disintegrating tablet	Zelapar	Dissolvable tablets can be an advantage for people with swallowing problems. Available only as a branded product.
Rasagiline	Azilect	Dosed once a day. May be better tolerated than selegiline.
Safinamide	XADAGO	Approved 2017 as an add-on to carbidopa/levodopa to address OFF time. Available only as a branded product.

120

> " *My neurologist started my medication plan with a small dose of rasagiline, which was increased several months later, but my visible motor symptoms continued. Ropinirole was added and helped more than rasagiline alone. I met with a movement disorder specialist who added carbidopa/levodopa. I knew within days that it would be highly unlikely anyone could pick me out of a crowd as a person with Parkinson's. I ask questions and am happy my doctors make me feel like my opinion matters when it comes to medications.*"
>
> — LORRAINE WILSON

COMT Inhibitors

Catechol-o-methyl transferase (COMT) inhibitors block the COMT enzyme, thereby increasing and prolonging carbidopa/levodopa's effects. COMT inhibitors have no effect on their own and are always used in conjunction with carbidopa/levodopa. COMT inhibitors are used primarily to treat motor fluctuations and reduce OFF time. Because COMT inhibitors increase and prolong the effects of carbidopa/levodopa, the side effects of carbidopa/levodopa may also be enhanced, including dyskinesia.

GENERIC NAME	TRADE NAME	NOTES
Entacapone	Comtan	Taken with each dose of carbidopa/levodopa. Can cause diarrhea, discolored urine.
Tolcapone	Tasmar	Dosed three times per day. Rare but possible serious side effects can occur on the liver, so typically only used if other Parkinson's medications have failed.
Carbidopa/levodopa/ Entacapone	Stalevo	An alternative to just carbidopa/levodopa that is combined with entacapone to help with motor fluctuations. Available in six strengths. Entacapone can cause diarrhea, discolored urine.
Opicapone	Ongentys	Once-daily capsule. Available only as a branded product.

Amantadine Hydrochloride

Amantadine can be used alone or in conjunction with other medications to treat slowness, stiffness, and tremor. Amantadine has a unique role in the treatment of Parkinson's because it is the only medication that treats motor symptoms while potentially reducing dyskinesias. People with kidney problems need a decreased dosage. Common side effects include nausea and light-headedness. Possible anti-cholinergic side effects include confusion and constipation. Other possible side effects include leg swelling and a reddish rash known as livedo reticularis.

GENERIC NAME	TRADE NAME	NOTES
Amantadine	Symmetrel	100-mg pill strength. Maximum dose of 400 mg per day. Typically dosed twice a day—morning and mid-day—as can cause insomnia if taken late in the day.

GENERIC NAME	TRADE NAME	NOTES
Amantadine extended-release (ER) capsules	GOCOVRI	Approved by the FDA specifically for carbidopa/levodopa-induced dyskinesia. Dosed once a day at bedtime. Available only as a branded product.
Amantadine extended-release (ER) tablets	Osmolex ER	Dosed once a day in the morning. Available only as a branded product.

Anticholinergic Medication

Anticholinergic medications are used to treat tremor and dystonia in people with Parkinson's. They do this by reducing the amount of acetylcholine, a neurotransmitter that is in balance with dopamine in the body. Anticholinergic medications are also sometimes prescribed to help with drooling. Anticholinergic medications are best tolerated by younger people and should be avoided by elderly people with Parkinson's because they can increase confusion, cognitive slowing, and hallucinations. Other possible side effects include dry mouth, worsening of glaucoma, blurry vision, and urinary retention.

GENERIC NAME	TRADE NAME	NOTES
Trihexyphenidyl	Artane	Typically dosed three times per day.
Benztropine	Cogentin	Typically dosed once or twice a day.
Biperiden	Akineton	Not available in the United States.
Ethopropazine	Parsitan	Not available in the United States.

Adenosine Receptor Antagonist

Adenosine receptor antagonists block the receptors for the neurotransmitter adenosine, which acts as a central nervous system depressant. This medication is approved for use in conjunction with carbidopa/levodopa to help reduce OFF time. These medications can increase ON time without troublesome dyskinesias for many people, but dyskinesias are the most common side effect.

GENERIC NAME	TRADE NAME	NOTES
Istradefylline	Nourianz	Dosed once a day. Available in 20-mg and 40-mg strengths. Available only as a branded product.

MEDICATIONS FOR NON-MOTOR SYMPTOMS

PARKINSON'S-RELATED DEPRESSION

Selective Serotonin Reuptake Inhibitors (SSRIs)

SSRIs are the most-prescribed antidepressants for Parkinson's-related depression because of their tolerability. These medications can also be used to treat anxiety and obsessive-compulsive disorder (OCD). It often takes four to six weeks of a therapeutic dose for full effect. SSRIs are sometimes combined with other medications such as SNRIs and TCAs (see tables below), but such combinations should be used with caution due to a potential for serotonin syndrome. Possible side effects include headaches, nausea, insomnia, jitteriness, sexual dysfunction, and weight gain.

GENERIC NAME	TRADE NAME	NOTES
Escitalopram	Lexapro	Once-daily dosing.
Citalopram	Celexa	Once-daily dosing.
Fluoxetine	Prozac	Once-daily dosing.
Fluvoxamine and Fluvoxamine ER	Luvox and Luvox CR	Twice per day dosing for immediate-release fluvoxamine. Once-daily dosing for extended-release fluvoxamine.
Paroxetine	Paxil, Paxil CR, Pexeva	Typically dosed once daily. Possibly more anxiety benefit than other SSRIs. Possibly more anticholinergic side effects (e.g. dry mouth, constipation).
Sertraline	Zoloft	Once-daily dosing.

Serotonin-Norepinephrine Reuptake Inhibitors (SNRIs)

SNRIs are another class of antidepressants that can treat depression, anxiety, and OCD. Like SSRIs, it often takes four to six weeks of a therapeutic dose for them to take effect. SNRIs can raise blood pressure, and other possible side effects include headache, nausea, sexual dysfunction, and dizziness. Like SSRIs, SNRIs should be used with caution in conjunction with other serotonergic medications due to a potential for serotonin syndrome.

GENERIC NAME	TRADE NAME	NOTES
Duloxetine	Cymbalta	May have benefit for pain. May reduce OFF time.

GENERIC NAME	TRADE NAME	NOTES
Venlafaxine and Venlafaxine ER	Effexor or Effexor XR	May have benefit for pain at higher doses. Twice per day dosing for immediate-release venlafaxine. Once-daily dosing for extended-release venlafaxine.
Desvenlafaxine	Pristiq	Once-daily dosing.
Milnacipran	Savella	Specifically approved to treat chronic pain from fibromyalgia Sometimes used off-label to treat depression and anxiety. Available only as a branded product.
Nefazodone	Serzone	Requires periodic monitoring of liver function.

Tricyclic Antidepressants (TCAs)

TCAs are another class of medications used to treat depression, anxiety, and OCD. Like some SNRIs, they can also be helpful for treating pain. They are prescribed less frequently than SSRIs and SNRIs due to higher likelihood of side effects. Like SSRIs and SNRIs, it often takes four to six weeks of a therapeutic dose for them to take effect. Possible side effects include dry mouth, constipation, orthostatic hypotension, urinary retention, and confusion. People with heart conditions (such as arrhythmia or QTc prolongation) should exercise caution when using TCAs. These medications should be used with caution in conjunction with other serotonergic medications due to the potential for serotonin syndrome.

GENERIC NAME	TRADE NAME	NOTES
Amitriptyline	Elavil	Often used at bedtime due to possible sedation.
Nortriptyline	Pamelor	May have fewer side effects than other TCAs.
Imipramine	Tofranil, Tofranil PM	Can be dosed up to three times per day.

Other Antidepressants

These medications can also have benefits for depression, anxiety, and OCD. Like SSRIs, SNRIs, and TCAs, it often takes four to six weeks of a therapeutic dose for these drugs to take effect. Some of these medications should be used with caution in conjunction with serotonergic medications due to the potential for serotonin syndrome.

GENERIC NAME	TRADE NAME	NOTES
Bupropion	Wellbutrin, Wellbutrin XL	Less likely than other antidepressants to cause weight gain or have sexual side effects. More likely to have tremor as a side effect. Should be avoided if there is a history of seizures.
Mirtazapine	Remeron	May cause sedation, so also used to help with insomnia. May cause increased appetite, so also used to help with weight gain. Also available as a dissolvable tablet, which can be helpful for people with swallowing problems.
Trazodone	Desyrel, Oleptro	May cause sedation, so also used to help with insomnia.
Vilazodone	Viibryd	Once-daily dosing.
Vortioxetine	Trintellix	Once-daily dosing. Available only as a branded product.

OTHER NON-MOTOR SYMPTOMS

Constipation

One of the most common non-motor symptoms of Parkinson's, constipation can severely affect quality of life. Lifestyle changes like increasing water, increasing dietary fiber, and increasing exercise are the cornerstones of treatment. Lowering medications that may have anticholinergic side effects may be necessary. Specific pharmacological interventions are also available. Common side effects include bloating, gas, upset stomach, and dizziness. For more on constipation and Parkinson's, see Chapter 6.

125

GENERIC NAME	TRADE NAME	NOTES
Polyethylene glycol 3350	MiraLAX	OTC. Osmotic laxative. Can be used daily.
Senna	Senokot	OTC. Stimulant laxative. Best reserved for rescue use rather than daily use.
Bisacodyl	Dulcolax	OTC. Stimulant laxative. Best reserved for rescue use rather than daily use.
Lubiprostone	Amitiza	Can be considered if regular use of OTC options like polyethylene glycol are not effective.

Drooling

Sialorrhea, or excessive drooling, is another common non-motor symptom of Parkinson's. The medications listed below are used either on- or off-label to address drooling. Side effects vary by treatment, but the most common is dry mouth. For more on drooling, see Chapter 6.

GENERIC NAME	TRADE NAME	NOTES
Atropine drops		These are eye drops that can be used off-label under the tongue to treat excessive drooling. This is an anticholinergic medication; systemic side effects are possible but less likely with this sublingual dosing.
Glycopyrrolate (and other anticholinergics like benztropine, trihexyphenidyl, and hyoscyamine)	Robinul (and Cogentin, Artane, Levsin)	These are anticholinergic medications, and dry mouth is often a side effect. Possible side effects include confusion, cognitive slowing, hallucinations, worsening of glaucoma, blurry vision, and urinary retention.
Scopolamine patch	Transderm-scop	This is a patch, typically applied behind the ear every 2-3 days. Patch formulation can be helpful for people with swallowing problems. This is an anticholinergic medication. Possible side effects include confusion, cognitive slowing, hallucinations, worsening of glaucoma, blurry vision, and urinary retention.
Botulinum toxins (onabotulinumtoxinA, rimabotulinumtoxinB, incobutulinumtoxinA)	Botox, Myobloc, Xeomin	These medications are injected into the salivary glands, typically every three months. Myobloc and Xeomin are specifically FDA-approved for sialorrhea, while Botox is used off-label. Dry mouth is the most common side effect. These injectable options are often better tolerated than the anticholinergic pills and patches above.

Fatigue

Fatigue means low energy and is a common symptom in Parkinson's. Fatigue often overlaps with sleepiness and/or depression. Because medication treatment options for fatigue may be of limited benefit, treatment of any overlapping sleepiness or depression is paramount. Lifestyle changes are also important, including budgeting energy for your most important activities, exercising regularly, eating well, drinking lots of water, getting enough sleep, and taking breaks when needed. Spending time with other people helps some people feel more engaged and energetic. Medication can have some benefits for fatigue. Possible side effects include headaches, dizziness, anxiety, nervousness, and insomnia. For more information on fatigue, see Chapter 6.

GENERIC NAME	TRADE NAME	NOTES
Modafinil	Provigil	Approved to treat excessive sleepiness among people with sleep apnea or narcolepsy; used off-label for Parkinson's.

GENERIC NAME	TRADE NAME	NOTES
Methylphenidate	Ritalin	Approved to treat ADHD and narcolepsy; used off-label for Parkinson's. Should not be taken with MAO-B inhibitors.

Overactive Bladder (OAB)

The bladder is a muscle, and spasms of the bladder muscle can cause urinary urgency and/or frequency among people with Parkinson's. Lifestyle changes can be of some benefit in reducing OAB: weight loss, reducing consumption of alcohol and caffeine, and reducing fluid intake at night. Pelvic floor strengthening with Kegel exercises can be helpful. Medications can also reduce the bladder spasms of OAB. Possible side effects include headaches, constipation, dry mouth, blurry vision, and urinary retention. Most OAB medications work via anticholinergic effects, and they can have the side effects of anticholinergic medications (see Anticholinergic Medication). For more on OAB, see Chapter 6.

GENERIC NAME	TRADE NAME	NOTES
Trospium	Sanctura	Anticholinergic medication.
Darifenacin	Enablex	Anticholinergic medication.
Tolterodine	Detrol	Anticholinergic medication.
Fesoterodine	Toviaz	Anticholinergic medication.
Solifenacin	Vesicare	Anticholinergic medication.
Oxybutynin	Ditropan	Anticholinergic medication. Crosses into the brain more than other OAB medications, may be more likely to worsen confusion.
Mirabegron	Myrbetriq	This medication is a beta-3 agonist. Less likely than other OAB medications to cause cognitive side effects. Should not be used by people with uncontrolled hypertension. Available only as a branded product.
Vibregron	Gemtesa	This medication is a beta-3 agonist. Less likely than other OAB medications to cause cognitive side effects. Should not be used by people with uncontrolled hypertension. Available only as a branded product.

127

Pain

Pain is a frequent and often under-recognized symptom of Parkinson's. Pain can be compounded by other factors including age, arthritis, spinal stenosis, and neuropathy. Lifestyle changes, especially exercising and making your home safer, are important steps for pain reduction and management. Other specialists can be helpful, such as a massage therapist, physical therapist, or acupuncturist. Treatments for motor symptoms in Parkinson's (like dopamine medications and deep brain stimulation surgery) can also reduce pain. For more on pain and Parkinson's, see Chapter 6.

GENERIC NAME	TRADE NAME	NOTES
Acetaminophen	Tylenol	Used to treat pain, fever, and inflammation. Typically does not cause any neurological side effects. Sustained use of high doses can cause liver problems.
NSAIDs (Ibuprofen, Naproxen, Aspirin)	Advil or Motrin, Aleve, Aspirin	Used to treat pain, fever, and inflammation. Typically do not cause any neurological side effects. May cause stomach pain or ulcers, increased risk of bleeding, high blood pressure. Sustained use can cause kidney problems. Aspirin can cause tinnitus.
Certain antidepressants (duloxetine, TCAs)	See chart for antidepressants.	See chart for antidepressants.
Certain anti-seizure medication (gabapentin, pregabalin)	Neurontin, Lyrica	These medications are widely used for treating other painful conditions such as neuropathy and fibromyalgia. They may be of benefit for people with Parkinson's. May cause sleepiness, unsteadiness, edema, and weight gain.

Neurogenic Orthostatic Hypotension (nOH)

Neurogenic orthostatic hypotension (nOH) is a common symptom of Parkinson's. nOH refers to a drop in blood pressure when changing positions, especially when standing up. Non-pharmacological changes can be very effective. These include increasing fluid intake, increasing salt and caffeine intake, wearing compression stockings or an abdominal binder, and raising the head of the bed during sleep. Medications can also improve nOH in people with Parkinson's. Possible side effects include high blood pressure when lying down (supine hypertension). For more on nOH, see Chapter 6.

GENERIC NAME	TRADE NAME	NOTES
Midodrine	ProAmatine	Mechanism is blood vessel constriction. Possible side effects include tingling, itchiness, and hair standing up.
Fludrocortisone	Florinef	Mechanism is increased fluid retention. Should not be used by people with heart failure. Possible side effects include leg swelling. Requires intermittent testing for blood potassium levels.
Droxidopa	Northera	Mechanism is increase of circulating norepinephrine. Only medication specifically indicated for symptomatic nOH. Available as a generic but more expensive than other nOH medications.

Parkinson's-Related Dementia

Dementia refers to difficulty with thinking and memory that impairs day-to-day function and the ability to live independently. Dementia often develops in people with advanced Parkinson's. Most medications used for Parkinson's-related dementia are cholinesterase inhibitors. This means they increase the amount of acetylcholine, which is involved in thinking and memory. These medications often have a modest benefit. They can also sometimes help with reducing freezing of gait. Note that anticholinergic medications have the opposite effect (they lower acetylcholine), so the above anticholinergic medications should usually be avoided by a person with Parkinson's-related dementia. The medications below are also approved for Alzheimer's, which is a different type of dementia. Possible side effects include nausea, vomiting, diarrhea, dizziness, and tremor. For more on dementia and Parkinson's, see Chapter 5.

GENERIC NAME	TRADE NAME	NOTES
Rivastigmine	Exelon	Only medication specifically approved for Parkinson's-related dementia. Available as capsules or as a patch. Capsules are dosed two times per day. Patch often causes less nausea and can also be helpful for people with swallowing problems.
Donepezil	Aricept pill or dissolvable pill	Once-daily dosing. Dissolvable pill can be an advantage for people with swallowing problems.
Galantamine, Galantamine ER	Razadyne, Razadyne ER	Dosed two times per day for immediate-release galantamine. Once-daily for extended-release galantamine.

GENERIC NAME	TRADE NAME	NOTES
Memantine, Memantine ER	Namenda or Namenda XR	Different mechanism of action, acting on NMDA receptors. Can be combined with any of the three above cholinesterase inhibitors.

Hallucinations/Delusions (Psychosis)

Hallucinations refer to seeing or hearing things that aren't there. Delusions refer to believing things that are not true. The presence of hallucinations or delusions is technically known as psychosis. These symptoms may range from mild to severe. Possible side effects of medications to treat psychosis include drowsiness, low blood pressure, and constipation. For more on hallucinations and delusions, see Chapter 5.

GENERIC NAME	TRADE NAME	NOTES
Rivastigmine, Donepezil, Galantamine	Exelon, Aricept, Razadyne	See above for information about dementia.
Pimavanserin	Nuplazid	Only medication specifically approved by the FDA for Parkinson's psychosis. Less sedating than quetiapine. May cause edema.
Quetiapine	Seroquel, Seroquel SR	Off-label for Parkinson's psychosis. Can be sedating, so often dosed at bedtime. May cause sleepiness, dizziness, dry mouth, orthostatic hypotension, and weight gain.
Clozapine	Clozaril	Off-label for Parkinson's psychosis. More evidence of benefit than quetiapine but used less frequently due to requirement for weekly blood tests to check for low white blood cell counts. May have some benefit for tremor. May cause sleepiness, dizziness, drooling, tachycardia, and rarely seizures.

Sexual Problems

Changes in sexual function and drive can occur as part of Parkinson's, and also possibly as side effects of certain medications, particularly antidepressants. Medications for erectile dysfunction (ED) and lubrication for pain with sex (especially for women experiencing vaginal dryness) can be useful, but often lifestyle changes and alternative therapies are especially effective. Hypersexuality and compulsive sexual behavior can be side effects of dopamine agonists and can often be treated by reducing dosage. For more on sexual problems and Parkinson's, see Chapters 6 and 13.

GENERIC NAME	TRADE NAME	NOTES
Sildenafil, tadalafil, vardenafil	Viagra, Cialis, Levitra	Used to treat erectile dysfunction (ED). Can worsen orthostatic hypotension. Other possible side effects include headache, stuffy nose, and nausea.
Apomorphine	Apokyn	See above for information about dopamine agonists. Some evidence of benefit for erectile dysfunction.

Sleep

Sleep problems are prevalent among people with Parkinson's. Sleep problems may include insomnia, restless leg syndrome (RLS), periodic limb movements disorder (PLMD), excessive daytime sleepiness (EDS), and REM-sleep behavior disorder (RBD). Medication may also have a role to play in the treatment of sleep problems for people with Parkinson's, but a combined behavioral and medication treatment plan is often best. For more on sleep, see Chapter 6.

GENERIC NAME	TRADE NAME	NOTES
Carbidopa/levodopa or dopamine agonist	See charts about carbidopa/levodopa and dopamine agonists.	See previous charts for more information about carbidopa/levodopa and dopamine agonists. An extra nighttime dose of carbidopa/levodopa (especially CR) or a dopamine agonist can be used to treat RLS and PLMD.
Clonazepam	Klonopin	Most effective treatment for RBD. Can also be used to treat insomnia and RLS. Possible side effects include excessive sleepiness, dizziness, and confusion.
Gabapentin	Neurontin	Can be used to treat RLS and PLMD. Sedating side effects can be helpful for insomnia. See previous table regarding pain.
Melatonin		OTC dietary supplement. Can be used to treat insomnia and RBD. May cause headaches, dizziness, and nausea.
Sedating antidepressants (trazodone, mirtazapine)	Desyrel, Remerol	See previous table of other antidepressants. Can be used to treat insomnia.

MEDICATIONS TO AVOID OR USE WITH CAUTION

It can be challenging to keep track of all your medications, especially if you're taking medications for both motor and non-motor symptoms. However, keeping an accurate, up-to-date list of your medications decreases the likelihood of an unwanted medication interaction. Studies have found that one in three people with Parkinson's have been prescribed contraindicated drugs while they were hospitalized, which highlights the importance of always having an up-to-date list of medications available. The below medications should be avoided.

> *I was taking 28 pills a day and had really bad reactions to a couple of the drugs. I started seeing the world in a very manic way. When I stopped sleeping and my previous doctor's solution was to add a sleeping pill to the mix, I found a new doctor. Medication helps, but I wanted a more integrated approach to managing the disease, not just adding more and more pills."*
>
> — JILL ATER

CLASS	GENERIC NAME	TRADE NAME	NOTES
First generation antipsychotics	Loxapine Pimozide Fluphenazine Trifluoperazine Haloperidol Chlorpromazine Thiothixine Perphenazine Thioridizine	Loxitane Orap Prolixin Stelazine Haldol Thorazine Navane Trilafon Mellaril	These medications block dopamine receptors in the brain, thus countering the desired effects of Parkinson's medications and likely worsening Parkinson's motor symptoms.
Second generation antipsychotics	Lurasidone Asenapine Olanzapine Aripiprazole Iloperidone Cariprazine Risperidone Brexpiprazole Ziprasidone Paliperidone	Latuda Saphris Zyprexa Abilify Fanapt Vraylar Risperdal Rexulti Geodon Invega	These medications block dopamine receptors in the brain, thus countering the desired effects of Parkinson's medications and likely worsening Parkinson's motor symptoms. These medications block less dopamine than first generation antipsychotics, but they should nonetheless be avoided.
Antiemetics	Prochlorperazine Chlorpromazine Promethazine Metoclopramide Droperidol	Compazine Thorazine Phenergan Reglan Inapsine	These medications treat nausea by blocking dopamine receptors in the brain, thus countering the desired effects of Parkinson's medications and possibly worsening Parkinson's motor symptoms.
Treatments for hyperkinetic movements	Tetrabenazine Valbenazine Deutetrabenazine	Xenazine Ingrezza Austedo	These medications are used for a condition called tardive dyskinesia, which is different than carbidopa/levodopa-induced dyskinesia. These medications lower dopamine, possibly worsening Parkinson's motor symptoms.

CLASS	GENERIC NAME	TRADE NAME	NOTES
Antihypertensives	Reserpine Methyldopa	Serpalan Aldomet	These medications reduce dopamine, possibly worsening Parkinson's motor symptoms..
Antidepressants	Amoxapine Phenelzine Isocarboxazid Tranylcypromine	Asendin Nardil Parnate Marplan	Amoxapine is a TCA but unlike other TCAs also blocks dopamine receptors. Phenelzine, isocarboxazid, and tranylcypromine are nonselective MAO inhibitors and cannot be taken in conjunction with MAO-B inhibitors.

■ CHAPTER 8 – SURGICAL THERAPIES

OVERVIEW

As Parkinson's symptoms progress, increasing medications to address them can bring significant side effects, such as dyskinesia. Surgical therapies can be explored after medications are optimized, and the side effects of adding more medications start to outweigh the benefits the medications provide.

Current surgical therapies include deep brain stimulation (DBS) and enteral suspension of carbidopa/levodopa. Focused ultrasound therapy (FUS) is a non-invasive image-guided therapy that's an alternative to surgical interventions. In this chapter, we highlight these three procedures and why you may choose to get one at some point down the road.

133

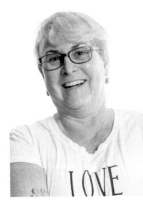

> " *I don't understand why people say they want to keep waiting to start medications or treatment or consider deep brain stimulation until they 'get bad enough.' Bad enough for what? I see that you're struggling. How bad do you have to be to want to get better?"*
>
> **— JILL ATER**

DEEP BRAIN STIMULATION

Deep brain stimulation, a highly effective treatment for Parkinson's, is a neurosurgical procedure in which electrodes are implanted into certain regions of the brain. These electrodes produce electrical impulses that regulate abnormal brain activity. The amount of stimulation is controlled by a pacemaker-like device located under the skin in your upper chest. A wire placed under your skin connects the device, called a stimulator, to the electrodes in your brain.

Here, we'll break down the what, why, how and more of DBS so that you have the information you need to determine if your path may lead you to this treatment.

> *Imagine our surprise in October 2015, when my movement disorder specialist said he had run out of medication options and recommended deep brain stimulation. My Parkinson's symptoms were reasonably well controlled with only low doses of a handful of medications. But I was constantly moving; he described my movement as wriggling dyskinesia. We then made yet another great decision and initiated the consults required prior for approval of DBS by the entire MDS clinic team. Unanimous approval received, my surgery followed on January 7, 2016. That was the day I got my life back. I'm very fortunate — DBS isn't for everyone, and results differ for each of us, but I had an immediate positive response that continues to this day. I take fewer medications, can exercise more because my symptoms are better controlled with no dyskinesia, and at present, I feel as well as I've ever felt. While DBS does not cure Parkinson's, the procedure has certainly enabled me to live my life well. We continue to travel, and I exercise more than I ever have with improved stamina, strength, balance, gait, and absolutely no falls in five years. Dystonia symptoms on my affected side are reasonably well managed with programming adjustments. Best of all, my new primary care physician noted that, if he didn't know my history, he would never have guessed that I have Parkinson's."*

— MARTY ACEVEDO

WHAT?

Deep brain stimulation to treat tremors in people with Parkinson's was approved by the FDA in 1997. Then in 2002, it was approved to treat advanced symptoms of Parkinson's. For many years, DBS was held as a last resort treatment. That's not the case anymore, as it has been approved for those in earlier stages of Parkinson's.

The procedure involves placing small electrodes into regions of the brain that control movement and are impacted during the progression of Parkinson's. The electrodes emit continuous electrical impulses (stimulation) from a stimulator device, similar to a cardiac pacemaker implanted in the chest.

As you know, in Parkinson's, dopamine-producing neurons die, thereby affecting the nerve cells in the brain responsible for body movement. Unfortunately, DBS does not affect dopamine levels in the brain. Instead, it compensates for the secondary effects of dopamine loss. So, while it's not a cure, ideally (and typically), this treatment leads to improvements in many motor symptoms such as tremor, stiffness, and slowness. As a result, this treatment may also make activities of daily living like getting in and out of chairs, walking, dressing, and bathing easier.

WHEN?

Due to some of the challenges people experience during the diagnostic process, many physicians require you to have had Parkinson's for at least three to four years before DBS becomes an option. This period—which can feel like forever—gives your physician time to make sure you have idiopathic Parkinson's and not a related condition like parkinsonism or Parkinson's plus. They also want to ensure you experience symptom relief from your Parkinson's medication(s), typically carbidopa/levodopa. That can take some trial and error to get the timing and dosing right. If your medications don't provide relief, DBS is unlikely to help.

WHY?

One of the most challenging aspects of living with Parkinson's is that it impacts your quality of life. While not everyone experiences debilitating motor symptoms, many people do, and these symptoms may get the way of you exercising, driving, communicating, working, and more. Since DBS can often result in a significant decrease in motor symptoms, many people living with Parkinson's seek it out as soon as possible.

> " *The best thing deep brain stimulation gave me is the ability to sleep through the night. For that reason alone, I'd do it again without hesitation."*
>
> — JILL ATER

Also, while DBS was not designed to decrease non-motor symptoms, evidence shows that many people experience a reduction in depression, anxiety, pain, fatigue, and more following the surgery. The reduction in those non-motor symptoms is often a downstream impact of exercising and socializing more because your more debilitating motor symptoms are reduced because of DBS.

Finally, one of the other main reasons people with Parkinson's choose to undergo DBS is that it may reduce the amount of medication you take and reduce and sometimes eliminate OFF times.

HOW?

Getting approved for DBS surgery is a process, and it involves input and expertise from a team of people. While there doesn't seem to be one path to surgery, there are some common steps you can expect to navigate on your way to the operating room.

> *It was comfortable, and I could hear them talking and what they were doing. You feel pressure and hear the drilling, but there's no sensation; they use the anesthetics. Once the surgeon implants the wires, then the neurologist tests the wires and creates this ethereal feeling while they run these sounds for them to assess if they had placed the leads exactly correctly to impact my symptoms."*

— JOHN ALEXANDER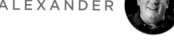

Step #1 – Meet with Your Movement Disorder Specialist or Neurologist

During this appointment, your physician will review your medical history and perform a neurological exam. Based on that, you'll discuss whether or not you're a good candidate for DBS.

Step #2 – Meet with the DBS Team

If the information discovered in Step One indicates you're a good candidate, the next step is to meet others who will assess your readiness. This team will usually include a physical therapist, neuropsychologist, speech-language pathologist, neurosurgeon, and movement disorder specialist or neurologist.

Step #3 – Discuss Your Insurance Options

This may come earlier in the process, or it may be something you address at this point. Your team will guide you on matters related to timing and how to best move through the process of getting the surgery approved.

Step #4 – Complete Your Pre-surgery Appointments

Once you've been identified as a good candidate, accessed for readiness, and made aware of the financial costs, you will get an MRI, ask your neurosurgeon questions, and complete a comprehensive physical exam to make sure you're healthy enough to have the procedure.

Step #5 – Have Surgery

DBS is a two-step surgery. During the first surgery, the physician will make the incisions and implant the electrodes. During the second surgery, which may happen anywhere from one week to one month after the first, your surgeon will implant the pulse generator under your skin on your chest.

Step #6 – Get Programmed

During this appointment, typically in your physician's office and typically two to four weeks post-surgery, someone trained in DBS programming will work with you to program the device to get the best symptom control possible. Sometimes this happens the first time the device is programmed; however, sometimes, it takes multiple tries to get it right.

Again, your physicians may do things slightly differently, but most include the steps outlined above in their DBS process.

Deciding whether to get DBS takes a great deal of research, thought, and reflection. You must discuss all your options with your care partners and physicians to make the best decision for you.

Later in this chapter, we'll discuss more about DBS. To hear stories of the "before and after DBS" and more personal accounts, be sure to check out our ⟳ *Every Victory Counts* website.

> " *Programming requires a give-and-take, and I need to clearly describe the feelings I have so my programmer can help optimize my settings.*"
>
> — JILL ATER

ENTERAL SUSPENSION MEDICATION DELIVERY: THE CARBIDOPA/LEVODOPA PUMP

Carbidopa/levodopa enteral suspension (branded under the name Duopa in the US and known as Duodopa outside of the US) is a Parkinson's medication delivery system for people experiencing persistent ON-OFF fluctuations, especially those with advanced Parkinson's. A carbidopa/levodopa gel suspension is delivered through a surgically implanted tube directly into the small intestine, where the medication is absorbed. This medication delivery directly into the small intestine has the added benefit of bypassing the stomach, the emptying of which can become unpredictable or delayed for people with Parkinson's. The small pump, which you carry or wear, allows infusion of a constant medication dose over 16 hours each day, with your physician's ability to prescribe additional doses at certain times.

Research shows that carbidopa/levodopa enteral suspension reduces OFF time and increases ON time by almost two hours a day compared to carbidopa/levodopa pills. This effect was especially noted after four weeks of therapy and persisted over 12 weeks in a study of 71 people with Parkinson's.

Carbidopa/levodopa enteral suspension can improve motor fluctuations by delivering continuous doses of carbidopa/levodopa. Dyskinesia can still occur, although it may be reduced in many cases as medication delivery levels out. The total daily dose of carbidopa/levodopa needed using carbidopa/levodopa enteral suspension may be less than that for pills.

FOCUSED ULTRASOUND THERAPY

Focused ultrasound therapy (FUS) is an early-stage, single-procedure, non-invasive technology to manage tremor and dyskinesia. It is FDA-approved and is approved to treat tremor outside the US as well. It treats Parkinson's symptoms through focused beams of ultrasonic energy that target specific areas deep in the brain, interrupting circuits involved with tremor and dyskinesia. Using a mechanism called ablation, the focused beams can disrupt targeted brain tissue to treat motor symptoms. Because focused ultrasound allows for precise targeting of areas of the brain, there is no damage to healthy tissue.

Other FUS mechanisms can temporarily disrupt the blood-brain barrier (BBB), allowing desired therapeutics access into the brain. This disruption of the BBB is also beneficial because it enables undesirable substances to leave the brain more easily.

Because FUS involves no incisions, holes in the skull, or electrodes in the brain, it can provide a powerful alternative to DBS with less risk of complications, as well as a lower cost. It does not require subsequent procedures, office visits for battery replacement, broken wire repair, or appointments to adjust simulator settings.

Researchers are currently exploring whether focused ultrasound can treat Parkinson's underlying pathology and prevent progression and restore function. Preclinical studies suggest that FUS may restore function given its ability to temporarily open the BBB to improve the delivery of therapies such as anti-alpha synuclein antibodies, neuroprotective and neurorestorative drugs, and other therapies.

Transcranial magnetic stimulation (TMS), stem cell therapy, and gene therapy are additional procedures you may hear about. As the jury is still out on their safety and efficacy, we have not included them in this manual. If you would like to learn more about them, visit the *Every Victory Counts* website.

"What Will Happen if I Get DBS?"

By Kara Beasley, DO, MBA, FACOS

Deep brain stimulation is the surgical implantation of an electric wire deep in the brain connected to a battery in the chest wall to treat Parkinson's and other movement and psychiatric disorders. The FDA first approved DBS for essential tremor in 1997 and Parkinson's in 2002. Since that time, more than 200,000 people have been implanted with these devices worldwide.

Essentially, DBS functions to provide electrical stimulation to the brain's circuit that is malfunctioning in Parkinson's and brings it back into a more normal state. DBS effectively treats the cardinal motor symptoms of Parkinson's, including tremor, stiffness (rigidity), and slowness (bradykinesia). DBS does not treat the non-motor symptoms of Parkinson's, such as drooling, constipation, or softening of the voice.

While DBS is not a cure for Parkinson's, there is overwhelming scientific evidence that proves for those who are good candidates for the procedure that DBS is safe and that it is often better than the best medical therapy alone in treating Parkinson's.

Some studies reveal DBS improves quality of life. It can make you feel comfortable in your body again, reduce social isolation, allow you to reduce your medications and eliminate side effects, and, most exciting, improve mortality. As a DBS surgeon, I have seen that DBS helps people with Parkinson's live better and longer than medication alone. DBS is effective long-term. While your Parkinson's symptoms will continue to progress, you will continue to see benefit from stimulation, and the stimulator can be adjusted repeatedly, as needed, to maximize benefit.

That said, DBS is not for everyone.

> *I had to take a lot of medication for a while before I had DBS. I had visual, auditory, and olfactory hallucinations. I smelled things that weren't there. I was aware that what I was seeing and experiencing was not real, but it's still disturbing to be sitting alone at 3 am, seeing animals scurrying around on the floor, and hearing whispering in the shadows. I felt like I was living in my own private version of* The Shining."
>
> — COREY KING

139

There is a window for DBS. The ideal candidate is healthy enough to undergo surgery (regardless of age), still has a good effect from medications (even if medications are less predictable, less effective, or cause too many side effects), and has not experienced too much cognitive decline. To determine whether you are a candidate, your neurologist will require an evaluation that includes ON-OFF testing.

It is vitally important that you and your physicians discuss your DBS goals and establish reasonable expectations for what might or might not improve for you before you opt for DBS. Remember, YOU are a critical part of your treatment team!

While I admit that performing these procedures every day means I'm more accustomed to brain surgery than most, DBS is a minimally invasive surgical procedure. It involves a pre-operative MRI scan, usually performed under sedation, which is then used by your treatment team to plan precisely how to get from the outside to the target deep in the brain while avoiding crucial brain structures. Then, on the day of surgery, the wire or "lead" is implanted through a hole in the skull the size of your thumb. When the lead is in the correct spot (target), it is locked into place and coiled under the skin. This procedure requires a night in the hospital, and Parkinson's symptoms will usually improve for a short period. This is called the "lesional effect" or "honeymoon effect" and is temporary. Then, one week to one month later, the lead is connected to a battery or "generator" implanted in the chest wall like a pacemaker. Once this is complete, the device is fully implanted. The last step is an ongoing process called programming, in which your neurologist will use a magnetic device to "turn on" the electricity and "turn off" your symptoms.

There are currently two types of DBS leads on the market. The traditional lead delivers a circumferential ball of electricity. The steerable lead allows the programmer to direct the electricity in a certain direction to minimize side effects. There are several techniques for placing DBS leads. The choice of technique depends on the surgeon's discretion, their comfort level with various techniques, and a discussion about your own goals and concerns.

The most common surgical technique is awake DBS surgery, in which you are sedated for the placement of a rigid frame or a tower known as frameless DBS. Both devices are affixed to the skull, but the frameless device allows your head to move, whereas the frame secures your skull to the surgical table. Whether frame or frameless, you continue under sedation until after the surgeon drills the thumb-sized hole in the skull. The sedation is then turned off, and the surgeon places a "microelectrode" in the brain while you are awake but comfortable, "listening" to single brain cells on the way down to the target. The brain itself has no pain receptors, so this part of the surgery is very well tolerated; in fact, you might even find it interesting to hear your brain "talk." Each part of the brain has a different electrical sound, and the surgeon will use these sounds, along with your movement, to ensure the target has been reached. Once the target has been reached, the actual lead is implanted in the same place and tested for how effectively it improves your symptoms.

Also, the team will closely watch for any side effects from the stimulation that might occur from electricity "overflowing" into other structures in the brain. Once the lead is in the perfect spot, it is secured and coiled under the skin. The frame or frameless tower is removed, and a small dressing is placed on the scalp. Most people spend one night in the hospital and go home the next day. The advantage to this awake DBS technique is that the surgeon and treatment team can ensure that the lead is in the exact right spot, thanks to your brain's responses while awake.

The alternative technique for placing the lead is to place it while asleep, known as "asleep DBS" surgery. This is performed under general anesthesia. The frame or frameless tower is placed in the same fashion as the awake DBS surgery, but the microelectrode recordings and testing are not conducted because the brain is "asleep." Some surgeons use a robot to place the lead more precisely in this technique. To ensure that the lead is in the perfect spot, the surgeon will then use a CT scan or MRI in the operating room to see where the lead is placed and compare it to the precise pre-operative plan. The advantage of this technique is that you are asleep during the entire surgery. The disadvantage is that the surgeon can't test for efficacy or side effects in the operating room.

Regardless of the technique used to place the lead, the generator (battery) placement is the same and is performed one week to one month after the lead implantation. During this procedure, you are placed under general anesthesia. An extension wire is tunneled under the skin to connect the lead, which was implanted in your brain, to the surgically-placed battery in your chest wall.

There are several battery options available. The traditional option is called a primary cell battery and requires no charging. These primary cell batteries typically last three to five years. A second option is a rechargeable battery that requires recharging every few days to few weeks, similar to a cell phone battery. Finally, a third option allows the battery to sense electrical activity in your brain and turn on and off only when the brain waves fall outside the set parameters. This allows for more personalized stimulation. You will discuss the choice of device and battery options with your surgeon before implantation.

Once the battery is in place, you will return to your neurologist, who will optimize your device's stimulation settings.

While risks and complications with DBS implantation are rare, every surgery has them. Risks include:

- Bleeding or stroke
- Infection
- Lead breakage
- Lead movement
- Failure to improve
- The lead ending up in the wrong place
- Adverse side effects of stimulation

You and your care partner must talk to your surgeon about these risks and understand them fully, including which are correctable, before undergoing DBS.

If you have read this article and are excited about the possibilities of DBS, be your own advocate. Talk to your neurologist about whether DBS is suitable for you. Do your research, prepare your questions, and seek a neurosurgeon specializing in DBS to get your additional questions answered.

About Kara Beasley

Kara Beasley is a neurosurgeon with Boulder Community Health. Dr. Beasley completed a dual degree in medicine and biomedical ethics at Midwestern University in Glendale, AZ, and is one of only a few dually credentialed neurosurgeon bioethicists worldwide. She completed a general neurosurgery residency at Philadelphia College of Osteopathic Medicine in Philadelphia, PA, and an MBA at the University of North Carolina's Kenan-Flagler Business school.

Before joining Boulder Community Health, Dr. Beasley obtained fellowships in stereotactic radiosurgery at Cooper University Hospital in Camden, NJ, and functional and restorative neurosurgery at the Cleveland Clinic Foundation in Cleveland, OH. In part, Dr. Beasley chose to dedicate her career to the surgical treatment of Parkinson's after meeting people living with Parkinson's and learning about deep brain stimulation during her training. She is a member of the Davis Phinney Foundation's Board of Directors.

"Why Is Enterally Administered Carbidopa/Levodopa a Good Choice for Managing Motor Fluctuations in Advanced Parkinson's?"

By Martin J. McKeown, BEng, MD, FRCP(C)

Effective therapy in Parkinson's requires learning about all the potential alternatives, weighing each potential risk and benefit, and then choosing the best one for you. In early Parkinson's, the response to medications is robust and can be dramatic. However, as Parkinson's progresses, the therapeutic window (the difference between medication levels in the brain that are too little or too much) diminishes, making it challenging to maintain the correct dose.

ENTERALLY ADMINISTERED CARBIDOPA/LEVODOPA: ANOTHER THERAPEUTIC OPTION

What other options are available if you experience fluctuations with medications but you're not a candidate for deep brain stimulation? Enterally administered carbidopa/levodopa gel is an excellent alternative in some circumstances. Often referred to by the brand-name product, Duopa (referred to as Duodopa outside of the US), enterally administered carbidopa/levodopa is a gel formulation of standard carbidopa/levodopa medication typically given in pill form but is administered with a pump via a tube that passes through the abdominal wall into the gut. The medication itself is contained in a reservoir bag inside a stiff, plastic cassette that fits into a portable, battery-powered pump worn around the waist.

Meta-analyses have suggested that enterally administered carbidopa/levodopa results in significantly improved motor scores and, perhaps more importantly, improved quality of life measures in people with Parkinson's.

POTENTIAL RISKS OF ENTERALLY ADMINISTERED CARBIDOPA/LEVODOPA

Like all therapies, there are potential downsides to enterally administered carbidopa/levodopa. The majority of these are seen within the first two weeks following the surgical procedure. The tube may become clogged or kinked, and there may be an infection around the insertion site. Once the tube is in place and the insertion site is suitably healed (typically after a couple of weeks), a careful titration process ensures that the medication levels are just right for you. This procedure varies but typically relies on frequent (at least hourly) observations by trained personnel to ensure that the medication infusion rate is optimal. This sometimes requires staying overnight in the hospital or near a hospital for a couple of days.

After the tube has been inserted, there are no complications, and the appropriate dispensing of medication has been achieved, side effects may emerge, like what many people experience when taking the pill form of carbidopa/levodopa: upset stomach, dyskinesia, or dizziness upon standing. However, a couple of issues appear more commonly with enterally administered carbidopa/levodopa: decreased weight and increased risk of peripheral neuropathy. The reasons for the weight loss are unclear. Often people with severe, disabling dyskinesia can lose weight because of their continual movements. Once the dyskinesia is reduced with enterally administered carbidopa/levodopa, they may regain some weight back. However, some people continue to lose weight for unknown reasons. Peripheral neuropathy, often also seen with the pill form of carbidopa/levodopa, may result from vitamin deficiencies, which you can prevent with oral supplementation.

WHO SHOULDN'T BE CONSIDERED FOR ENTERALLY ADMINISTERED CARBIDOPA/LEVODOPA THERAPY?

People with mild Parkinson's symptoms who respond well to oral medication don't need to proceed with enterally administered carbidopa/levodopa. Additionally, anyone who is unmotivated, non-compliant, or has poor care partner support may have difficulty managing the logistics of storage, delivery of the cassettes, and the pump's operation. Finally, the medication is expensive, and health insurance coverage may be an issue.

While not a solution for everyone, enterally administered carbidopa/levodopa can be transformative for someone who experiences frustrating ON-OFF fluctuations but is not a candidate for DBS. People who have suffered from severe motor fluctuations may find this therapy allows them to maintain independence and substantially improve their quality of life. Therefore, enterally administered carbidopa/levodopa is an excellent option for advanced Parkinson's.

About Martin McKeown

Martin McKeown is the PPRI/UBC Chair in Parkinson's Research, Director of the Pacific Parkinson's Research Centre, and Full Professor in the Department of Medicine and Electrical and Computer Engineering (adjunct) at the University of British Columbia, Canada. He did his Engineering Physics, Medicine, and Neurology training at McMaster, University of Toronto, and University of Western Ontario. He completed a three-year research fellowship at the Computational Neurobiology Laboratory at the Salk Institute for Biological Studies in San Diego before being hired as an Assistant Professor of Medicine and Biomedical Engineering at Duke University. He has been responsible for a variety of peer-reviewed research projects funded through the National Institute of Health, the National Parkinson's Foundation, the Canadian Foundation for Innovation, the Natural Sciences and Engineering Research Council of Canada, the Canadian Institutes of Health Research, the International Association of Translational Neuroscience, and the (US) Whitaker Foundation. He is a member of the Neuroscience A (NSA) Canadian CIHR Scientific peer review committee and a member of Parkinson Canada's Research Policy Committee.

CHAPTER 9 – EXERCISE

OVERVIEW

" *Exercise needs to move from a recommendation to a prescription for people with Parkinson's.*"

— JAY ALBERTS, PhD, DEPARTMENT OF BIOMEDICAL ENGINEERING, CLEVELAND CLINIC

Again and again, research and personal experience highlight the critical importance of exercise for people with Parkinson's. Regular physical exercise can improve mobility and coordination, boost your mood, reduce stiffness, and minimize soreness and fatigue. And each year, more studies prove that exercise may slow the progression of Parkinson's itself.

Exercise, beneficial for everyone, is essential for people with Parkinson's because research has shown that it may be neuroprotective. Multiple studies explore the possibility that exercise helps protect nerve cells at risk of damage, degeneration, or cell death. In other words, the most vulnerable cells are strengthened before they experience damage— thanks to exercise. This process, called neuroprotection, may occur with high-intensity aerobic exercise.

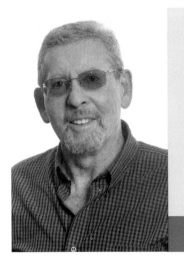

" *I have always thrived on a daily dose of fresh air and sunshine. Living in Colorado has made outdoor exercise more feasible than when I grew up in Cleveland. My wife and I have been cycling together for many years, so noticing I was losing ground was a hard reality to accept. A couple of years ago, I was introduced to the benefits of an electric bike. I haven't looked back since.*"

— RICH WILDAU

The idea that exercise can protect nerve cells is not unique to Parkinson's. Exercise has been shown to mitigate depression, limit memory problems associated with normal aging, and reduce the risk of developing Alzheimer's. It is unknown what specific type of exercise has the most significant potential for neuroprotection, but intensive, high-energy aerobic exercise has shown the most promise and is actively under study in people with Parkinson's.

Exercise and movement may also help your body and brain find new ways to move.

Parkinson's damages parts of the brain, and exercise aids your brain in discovering new nerve cell connections. This process is called neuroplasticity, which can be thought of as disconnecting the old wires in the brain and redirecting new wires to make different pathways. Using these alternative brain pathways may enable you to perform and gain strength in a task you otherwise have trouble performing. For instance, people with speech problems might be able to sing, or those who have difficulty walking might dance or march to music with a specific beat because these tasks engage different areas of the brain.

“ *The best evidence for slowing the progression of Parkinson's is exercise.”*

— BENZI KLUGER, MD, MS, FAAN,
UNIVERSITY OF ROCHESTER MEDICAL CENTER

EXERCISE'S IMPACT ON PARKINSON'S SYMPTOMS

In addition to possibly slowing the progression of Parkinson's, exercise can help you live well with Parkinson's right away. It helps reduce motor symptoms such as rigidity, stiffness, slowness, and postural instability, and it has also been shown to reduce tremors in people with Parkinson's. It can positively impact gait, balance, and functional mobility, as well as fine motor skills.

“ *A study of more than 2,000 people living with Parkinson's showed that those who were exercising for 150 minutes or more per week had better mobility, physical function, and cognitive performance compared to those who were not exercising. The people who were exercising regularly also experienced less disease progression over the course of a year.”*

— GAMMON EARHART, PT, PhD, FAPTA,
WASHINGTON UNIVERSITY SCHOOL OF MEDICINE

Just as importantly, exercise has been shown to reduce non-motor symptoms of Parkinson's, including sleep problems, constipation, digestion, depression, fatigue, and cognitive decline. Exercise not only minimizes daytime fatigue and sleepiness but can also help you sleep more soundly at night.

Later in this chapter, Jay Alberts, PhD, of the Cleveland Clinic will explain more about the many ways exercise is medicine for people living with Parkinson's.

CREATING YOUR EXERCISE ROUTINE

Exercise for people with Parkinson's can help at any time, and the earlier you start, the better. That said, it is never too late to add more physical activity to your daily life. Before starting or increasing the intensity of an exercise program, be sure to have a conversation with your healthcare professional about anything specific to your symptoms and health that you should be aware of as you exercise.

> *Whatever form of exercise or movement therapy you choose, you need to follow through with it. Make it a habit. Pick something you enjoy doing, and you'll be more likely to stick with it."*
>
> — DAVIS PHINNEY

It's important to incorporate several different types of exercises that specifically target your symptoms. Later in this chapter, Lee Dibble, PT, PhD, ATC, shares a proven prescription for exercise that will help you to live well (and better) with Parkinson's.

> *A growing body of work demonstrates the importance of exercise for living well today with Parkinson's. Because people with Parkinson's may have many different symptoms, the right exercise prescription for an individual may include some combination of endurance, strength, and balance training."*
>
> — MARGARET SCHENKMAN, PHD, PT, FAPTA,
> UNIVERSITY OF COLORADO SCHOOL OF MEDICINE

The way each person experiences the symptoms and challenges of Parkinson's varies with age, years since diagnosis, and level of physical activity (or inactivity). In the same vein, the way that you exercise with Parkinson's will vary. What feels good today might not be the exercise you choose tomorrow. That's okay. In addition, your routine will be different from what your neighbor does or what others in your Parkinson's community do. That, too, is okay. Ultimately, how you choose to exercise is up to you. What is most important is that you start and continue moving.

> *It is currently believed that if anything can slow the progression of Parkinson's, it's regular exercise."*
>
> — BASTIAAN BLOEM, MD, PHD,
> RADBOUD UNIVERSITY MEDICAL CENTRE

"How Is Exercise Medicine for the Brain?"

By Jay Alberts, PhD

While many great scientific discoveries are rooted in a dimly lit laboratory or clinical environment, some are not. In 2003, I pedaled a tandem bike with a close friend who'd been diagnosed with Parkinson's a few years earlier on a multi-day group bike tour through the corn and bean fields of Iowa. Little did I realize that an important discovery about the effects of exercise on Parkinson's motor function was about to be made.

A few days into the ride, my friend noticed a dramatic improvement in her handwriting as she wrote out a birthday card—effortlessly and legibly. Initially, I thought that maybe our pie and homemade ice cream diet was responsible for these motor function improvements. Who wouldn't feel better after indulging in such treats? But, it turns out it was neither the pie nor ice cream; it was riding the tandem that was making the difference.

> *I have always been moving, probably since the day I was born. Even as a little kid, I hated sleeping because of FOMO – Fear Of Missing Out. From figure skating to alpine skiing to marathon running, to backcountry skiing and skinning, to climbing 14er's – it's always been hard to tie me down. At the time that I was diagnosed, I had just had a total knee replacement and a cyst removed from my lower spine. I am convinced that having been active non-stop for years had prevented, or at least delayed, the onset of Parkinson's for me. It was only my season of immobility that allowed Parkinson's to get a foothold. I truly believe that 90% of my Parkinson's is progressing slowly because of consistent purposeful exercise. I cannot state this strongly enough. If a person is truly dedicated to living well with Parkinson's, he or she must find an exercise routine that includes: cardio, yoga, strength training, balance, and cross bodywork. There are no medications that can even come close to matching the benefits of exercise. Neuroplasticity is a wonderful thing."*

— PATTI BURNETT

FORCED EXERCISE

What is special about tandem cycling? Couples without Parkinson's jokingly call it a marriage test because of the coordination and communication required on a bicycle built for two. But for my friend with Parkinson's and me, the tandem enabled us to engage in a type of exercise called forced exercise.

Forced exercise essentially means assisting a person in exercising at a greater rate than their preferred, voluntary exercise rate. In this case, my friend with Parkinson's could pedal at a rate of approximately 50 revolutions per minute (RPM) when she was exercising by herself. When she rode tandem with me, our pedaling rate or cadence was 80–90 RPM. Thus, I was "forcing" her to pedal faster than she could by herself.

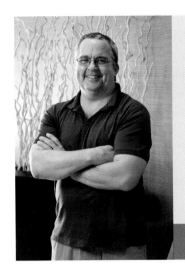

" *I've found specialists like a psychiatrist or a neuropsychologist to be necessary tools for coping and growing. I'm not afraid to reach out for help. People take their cars in for routine maintenance, and I believe we have to do that with our minds as well. Often we think we can fix something ourselves, but our mind is far more intricate than a car."*

— BRIAN

RESEARCH TIMELINE

Since this discovery, my colleagues and I have dedicated more than 17 years to studying the effects of exercise, primarily forced exercise, on motor and non-motor performance. Each project has inspired the next, and the research continually supports the belief that forced and high-intensity aerobic exercise improves motor function (and more) in people with Parkinson's. Here, I'll share more about how our research has unfolded.

2009: My team and I studied the effects of exercise on cognitive and motor functioning in a group of people newly diagnosed with Parkinson's. Results suggested that aerobic exercise has a strong potential to slow the progression of Parkinson's symptoms in individuals not yet treated with Parkinson's medications.

2012: In our clinical trial called CYCLE, we began comparing the effects of forced exercise cycling on motor and non-motor performance compared to voluntary rate cycling and a non-exercise control group. Results showed that an eight-week, high-intensity aerobic exercise program markedly enhances overall motor function, certain aspects of walking, and cognitive function in people with Parkinson's.

2015: My research team and I examined dual-tasking—the simultaneous performance of two attention-demanding tasks—and Parkinson's. This study used a virtual reality assessment to improve motor and non-motor function in people with Parkinson's.

2018: My colleague Dr. Anson Rosenfeldt and I began a two-year study on the effectiveness of Pedaling For Parkinson's—an existing, low-cost community cycling class—and how participation in the class may slow Parkinson's progression. Moving from the lab to real life was a big step toward increasing access to classes so even more people can live well with Parkinson's.

2019: A $3M National Institutes of Health (NIH) grant funded our study on the impact of exercise on Parkinson's. This project built on data recorded in the CYCLE study, measuring the long-term CYCLE protocol's effectiveness in a home-based setting. My research team and I set out to use performance data from this research to determine whether a certain exercise level can slow Parkinson's progression.

2020: Data from Dr. Rosenfeldt's and my recent study indicate that cycling may be an ideal exercise mode for people with Parkinson's because regardless of disease severity, individuals can achieve and maintain a moderate to high intensity of exercise. Additionally, the study's compliance data highlights several important points, including that people with Parkinson's regularly attend community-based cycling classes without external encouragement, and they can achieve and maintain moderate levels of exercise intensity without direct oversight.

" Every time I don't feel like exercising, my friend drags me out. When he doesn't feel like going, I do the same thing for him. It's also the social aspect, getting out of the house. We get exercise, we're participating in life, and we're counting on each other."

— COREY KING

HOW INTENSE IS INTENSE ENOUGH?

In July 2020, Dr. Rosenfeldt and I published a paper about how exercise should be a universal prescription for people living with Parkinson's. We have seen how, in the past two decades, aerobic exercise has become a mainstream recommendation for managing multiple symptoms of Parkinson's. Data from animal studies and select human trials indicate that aerobic exercise may facilitate structural and functional changes in the brain. Recently, several large human clinical trials have been completed and collectively support the use of aerobic exercise, specifically high-intensity aerobic exercise, in improving Parkinson's motor symptoms.

And we have seen that despite these findings, exercise recommendations continue to lack specificity in terms of frequency, intensity, and duration. Our goal was to determine how much exercise and intensity were the ideal prescription for people with Parkinson's.

Based on positive clinical findings and trials, here is my advice: people living with Parkinson's should perform aerobic exercise in the following dose (after, as always, consulting with their healthcare teams and getting clearance to begin an exercise regimen of this intensity):

- Three times per week
- 30–40 minutes for the main exercise set
- 5-10 minutes for a warm-up period

- 5-10 minutes for a cool-down period

- 60–80% of heart rate reserve or 70–85% of heart rate max (Instead of heart rate, individuals can achieve an intensity of 14–17 on a 20-point rate of perceived exertion RPE scale)

- You should be able to answer questions while exercising, but you should not be able to have a conversation

Data continues to show that exercise is medicine for Parkinson's. To realize its benefits, however, you must take the medicine. Get moving regularly and at high intensities. By doing so, you will, through your own experience, be able to proclaim that exercise really is medicine for Parkinson's.

About Jay Alberts

Jay Alberts is the Vice Chair of Innovations within the Neurological Institute at the Cleveland Clinic and staff in the Department of Biomedical Engineering. Dr. Alberts' research is focused on understanding the effects of exercise on the motor and non-motor symptoms associated with Parkinson's. In addition, he studies how Parkinson's impacts cognitive and motor function under dual-task conditions in order to develop rehabilitation strategies that improve these declines.

Within clinical transformation, Dr. Alberts develops technology to objectively quantify Parkinson's symptoms using consumer electronic devices and to develop subsequent models of clinical care. He serves as the principal investigator on a number of studies, including ones supported by the National Institutes of Health, Department of Defense, and the Davis Phinney Foundation. He was presented with an Alumni Achievement Award from Iowa State University in 2011 for his translational research related to Parkinson's and was awarded the prestigious Sones Award for Innovation in 2013 from the Cleveland Clinic.

"What Does the Research Say about Parkinson's and Exercise?"

By Lee Dibble, PT, PhD, ATC

Over the past two decades, substantial evidence has emerged to reveal significant and clinically meaningful benefits of exercise for persons with Parkinson's. Distinct research lines have converged to strengthen the foundation of evidence that physical activity and exercise can result in intangible benefits. These lines of evidence are:

1. Longitudinal (epidemiologic) studies
2. Physical activity interventions for diseases associated with sedentary behavior and aging
3. Exercise studies in animal models of Parkinson's
4. Synthesis of human studies of exercise and Parkinson's

Evidence from multiple longitudinal observational studies suggests that people who regularly engaged in moderate to vigorous exercise had a decreased risk of developing Parkinson's. The apparent risk reduction is substantial and present even if the regular exercise was performed in the third or fourth decades of life.

The positive effects of physical activity and exercise are present regardless of age or type of illness. There is strong evidence that regular participation in physical activity and exercise decreases the occurrence and adverse consequences of heart disease, diabetes, and obesity. Also, exercise studies consistently improve cognitive abilities even in the presence of dementia. Physical activity and exercise indirectly improve movement abilities and quality of life in persons with Parkinson's by preventing other potentially concurrent diseases.

Multiple exercise studies in animal models of Parkinson's demonstrate improvements in mobility, nerve cell function, and the potential for increased survival of nerve cells within the brain's affected area. In contrast, animal studies that impose inactivity demonstrate increased degeneration of nerve cells and loss of mobility. Proposed mechanisms for the observed positive effects include increased production of nerve cell growth factors and the growth of new blood vessels that supply oxygen and nutrients to at-risk areas of the brain. At the very least, these findings suggest that exercise has a positive impact on the brain and the rest of the body.

Research shows that those who participate in exercise programs, regardless of the type of exercise, enjoy a better quality of life, walking ability, balance, strength, flexibility, and cardiovascular fitness compared to those who do not exercise. Specific positive effects of different types of exercise are highlighted below:

152

Aerobic/Cardiovascular endurance exercise: Aerobic exercise has been found to have multiple beneficial effects, including potential disease-modifying effects. Varying modes of delivery (such as treadmill training or "forced exercise" on a tandem bicycle) have resulted in cardiovascular fitness improvements and overall motor symptom reductions. Larger scale research trials are now underway to more deeply understand the extent and mechanisms of aerobic exercise effects in individuals before starting their Parkinson's medications and in those with mild to moderate Parkinson's.

Balance Training: Research groups worldwide have demonstrated the benefits of exercises targeted at improving balance and reducing falls in people with Parkinson's. Despite differences in methods and interventions, these studies found that exercise improved functional mobility and reduced the incidence of falls, particularly in individuals with mild to moderate Parkinson's. These studies reinforce the power of exercise and specific balance task practice to improve balance and reduce fall risk. Such fall reductions may have a dramatic impact on quality of life.

" *You can lose balance, but you can get it back. Balance is a learned process."*

— EDIE ANDERSON

Flexibility Exercise: Spine and extremity flexibility exercises have shown significantly improved mobility and performance of daily activities in people with Parkinson's. Participants in one of these studies also performed aerobic exercise and improved their walking ability and efficiency of walking.

Resistance Training: In numerous studies examining resistance exercise, multiple benefits of strength training have emerged. Regular resistance exercise significantly improved muscle strength and muscle function, reduced disease severity, and improved mobility. One of these studies had participants continue with exercise after the initial intervention period, and the resistance training improvements were sustained for two years.

Upper Extremity Skill Training: Improvement of dexterity of the upper extremity has been demonstrated in numerous studies. In one such study, participants practiced handwriting tasks five days a week for six weeks on an electronic tablet. In addition to improvements handwriting size, participants improved their ability to maintain writing size in the presence of distraction and improved in writing tasks that were not practiced.

Respiratory Training: Given potential concerns about voice, swallowing, and cough in people with Parkinson's, breathing training programs have been shown to improve various functions. Training of muscles involved in expiration and inspiration may improve swallowing safety, voice strength and quality, and cough strength.

In summary, most well-controlled exercise studies suggest a vitally important role for exercise in managing Parkinson's. Since exercise improves many of the early symptoms of Parkinson's, individuals with Parkinson's, their care partners, and healthcare providers should work together to incorporate exercise and physical activity into a Parkinson's management strategy early after diagnosis to prevent disability rather than react to it. Current and future studies will provide additional clarity on the effects of individualized interventions based on specific types of symptoms (e.g., flexibility exercise to address muscular rigidity and pain). Also, these studies will expand the understanding of the effects of exercise on non-motor features such as cognition, depression, fatigue, pain, and blood pressure regulation.

About Lee Dibble

Lee Dibble is a professor in the Department of Physical Therapy and Athletic Training at the University of Utah. Dr. Dibble has also co-directed the Department of Physical Therapy's Clinical Operations at the University of Utah and has served on the Utah State Physical Therapy Association Board of Directors and the Utah State Parkinson Disease Association Executive Board.

His research focuses on exercise and motor learning countermeasures to combat postural instability and balance disorders and has conducted studies examining eccentric muscle training in mobility-limited populations. Dr. Dibble has a PhD in Exercise and Sports Science, focusing on Motor Learning and Motor Control from the University of Utah, and is a Certified Athletic Trainer, licensed Physical Therapist, and licensed Athletic trainer. He has published more than 70 research articles and has served as an associate editor for the Journal of Hand Therapy *and as an associate editor for the* Journal of Neurologic Physical Therapy.

"How Can I Stay on Track with my Exercise Routine?"

By Terry Ellis, PhD, PT, NCS and Tamara Rork DeAngelis, PT, DPT, GCS

Even knowing how powerful a tool exercise is for living well with Parkinson's every day, staying on track and making exercise part of your daily routine can be difficult. Here are three reasons why:

#1 – Maybe you haven't been a regular exerciser. It can be overwhelming to change from a non-exerciser to an exerciser at a later stage in life. While you may know that along with taking medication, exercise is one of the very best ways to feel better, minimize your symptoms, and slow the progression of Parkinson's, it may be hard for you to imagine starting an exercise routine. It would be nice if you could flip the switch and become an exerciser, but sometimes it's not that easy!

#2 – Maybe you have been dealing with pain, motor symptoms, trouble sleeping, fatigue, declining mobility, and maybe even depression for many years. Showering you with all the potential benefits of exercising is not going to be enough to get you going. You may need more support to get started.

#3 – Exercising can be challenging. And high-intensity exercise can be even more challenging. And we're human. Sure, there are those among us who love to push themselves and face the challenge and the grind of exercising every day. But not all of us do.

> *When I was first diagnosed, I stopped running and cycling because I was depressed, and I lost a year of well-being. Don't stop what you've been doing, don't let stuff go. If you sit on the couch, you'll feel worse, and it's going to get harder. Find something you love to do and do it."*
>
> — TIM HAGUE

So, now what? If you don't gravitate toward regular exercise or feel well enough to do it, here are a few ways to help you get started and stick with it.

#1 – Build confidence. If you have never considered yourself an exerciser, start to reconsider that idea. As soon as you begin to take a walk for your health, you are an exerciser. You don't need a gym membership to be an exerciser! Minor changes to your daily routines, such as doing 10 minutes of squats before breakfast or stretching your calf muscles at the kitchen sink, can slowly help build your confidence.

#2 – Identify barriers. Before you begin an exercise program, plan how you will overcome day-to-day challenges that may prevent you from sticking to your routine. Here is a list of some common barriers:

- I have a busy schedule and am not able to fit exercise into my life
- I have fatigue, so I am too tired for exercise
- I am not confident in my ability to exercise successfully
- I don't enjoy exercise and therefore find it difficult to motivate myself to participate in a long-term program
- I don't know where to begin or which exercises are best for me

 # 3 – Overcome barriers. Once you've identified the barriers that may limit your success with exercise, use the following strategies to help you get started and stay on track:

- **Schedule it.** Just as you would schedule a meeting at work or a visit with a friend, you can schedule exercise. If you put it on your calendar, you're more likely to do it. Schedule a specific time during the day when you feel your best and have good energy

- **Get guidance.** If you experience fatigue or sleepiness during the day, speak with your physician about possible ways to address these issues. Over time, exercise may increase your energy level and reduce feelings of fatigue

- **Get informed.** If you aren't sure what you should be doing for exercise or have questions about what exercises are best for you, visit a physical therapist who can help you get started. Once you've done that, you also can work with a personal trainer or another fitness professional who can help you find new ways to make your workouts challenging and fun

- **Experiment.** Add music or bring a friend to make your time exercising more pleasurable. Many people find that participating in a group exercise program adds to both their enjoyment and commitment to exercise

- **Stay accountable.** Tell friends, family, coworkers, and others that you are going to start an exercise program. When they ask you about it, you can proudly report that you have reached your goal to make exercise a part of your life. You can also stay accountable to yourself by keeping an exercise log. See our 🗎 Exercise Journal Worksheet on our ⟳ *Every Victory Counts* website

- **Focus.** For various reasons, you might stop exercising for a short period. The goal is to get back on track as soon as possible. It is important to keep in mind the reasons for your commitment to exercise and to focus on all the benefits you experience. There will be bumps in the road to becoming a lifetime exerciser, but if you keep going, you can continue to make a difference in your health and well-being

#4 – Mix up your exercise routines. By doing different routines each day, you can stay engaged and interested in your exercises. If you're feeling uninspired to go for a jog, find a dance class you can join online or in person instead. If your workout schedule says you need to do yoga but you feel like boxing instead, go for it! Cross-training keeps your muscles and brain challenged while keeping you from slipping into exercise boredom. It also helps you avoid injuries caused by strain or overuse of certain muscle groups. Remember that you don't need fancy equipment or a gym membership to cross-train effectively. Take a fast-paced walk one day; do a push-up, plank, and sit-up routine the next; jump rope or work out with a boxing video the next. Mix and match and keep exploring new exercise options.

I can be paralyzed by dystonia and then get on the treadmill and walk. I also roll on a foam roller and roller balls to help work out tight muscles."

— LINDA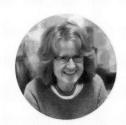

Whatever exercises you choose, start strong to stay stronger longer. Explore the many ways exercise can help you manage your symptoms and improve your quality of life.

About Terry Ellis

Terry Ellis is an associate professor and Chair of the Department of Physical Therapy & Athletic Training, College of Health & Rehabilitation Sciences, Boston University.

She is also the Director of the Center for Neurorehabilitation at Boston University and the Director of the American Parkinson Disease Association National Rehabilitation Resource Center housed at Boston University. Her research investigates the impact of exercise and rehabilitation on physical capacity and community mobility in individuals with neurological conditions, including Parkinson's and stroke. She also has expertise in using mobile health technology to help persons with Parkinson's engage in lifelong exercise to improve overall mobility, community engagement, and quality of life. Dr. Ellis has a PhD in Behavioral Neurosciences from Boston University School of Medicine and is a licensed physical therapist with board certification in Neurologic Physical Therapy. She has published numerous articles and lectures internationally on rehabilitation, exercise, and mobile health technologies in people with Parkinson's.

About Tamara Rork DeAngelis

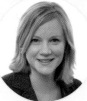

Tami Rork DeAngelis is a senior physical therapist at the Center for Neurorehabilitation at Boston University. She has been providing physical therapy services, contributing to research, and implementing educational programs to people with Parkinson's for more than a decade.

»

Dr. DeAngelis is also the coordinator for the American Parkinson Disease Association (APDA) National Rehabilitation Resource Center at Boston University, providing information and resources on exercise and rehabilitation to persons with Parkinson's, families, and healthcare providers nationwide.

She co-authored the BE ACTIVE & BEYOND booklet, an exercise program for people with Parkinson's, distributed by the APDA, Inc. She lectures in the Doctor of Physical Therapy program at Boston University, Parkinson's support groups, professional conferences, and symposia about the benefits of rehabilitation for persons with Parkinson's. Dr. DeAngelis received a bachelor's degree in biology from Lafayette College, a master of science in physical therapy from Boston University College of Health and Rehabilitation Sciences: Sargent and her Doctorate in Physical Therapy from Temple University. She is also a board-certified specialist in Geriatric Physical Therapy and a member of the American Physical Therapy Association.

"Why Do my Symptoms Sometimes Worsen after I Exercise?"

By Sarah King, PT, DPT

As a Parkinson's physical therapist, I regularly talk to people who struggle to keep up a regular exercise program because the side effects that follow exercise are frustrating and disruptive. Let's explore four reasons why your Parkinson's symptoms may be getting worse after exercise and how you can adapt your Parkinson's exercise program to minimize the side effects so you (and your brain and body) can reap the benefits.

Reason #1: Your body is stressed out.

What it looks like: Immediately after exercise, you notice symptoms like tremors, dyskinesia, or freezing are worse. This may last from a few hours to a few days.

What's going on: Do you notice your symptoms are exacerbated when you're under a lot of psychological stress? Exercise is physical stress on your system and, while beneficial in the long run, it can impact your system in the same way that mental stress does in the short term.

What to do:

1. Ease your way into exercise, starting with 5-10 minutes of fast-paced walking a few times during the day.

2. If you have a lot of stress and anxiety daily, try implementing 10-15 minutes of meditation or mindfulness to calm your nerves each morning, so exercise isn't taking your stress levels over the edge.

3. Schedule your workouts so you can relax afterward and aren't anxious about getting from the gym to your next appointment.

Reason #2: Your medication isn't optimized.

What it looks like: You start your workout feeling relatively strong but then you hit a wall. You notice wearing OFF symptoms like stiffness, difficulty walking, worsening posture, and increased slowness.

What's going on: Your symptoms may be creeping back up during exercise because your medications are wearing OFF. This occurs with carbidopa/levodopa medications when you've reached the end of the effective dose and your dopamine levels are low.

What to do:

1. Talk to your movement disorder specialist, as they can help you modify the dose, timing, or frequency of your medication schedule.

2. Keep a log of your ON and OFF times and share them along with any other important notes (like what time you eat and exercise each day). Your physician may alter your medication or encourage you to modify your dosages around exercise to keep you from wearing OFF mid-session.

3. See our 📄 Daily Medication Log on our ⟳ *Every Victory Counts* website.

Reason #3: You're fatigued.

What it looks like: You feel a general level of physical or mental exhaustion that stretches beyond normal tiredness. To even begin any workout feels like an accomplishment due to your utter lack of energy and motivation. When you do manage to exercise, you're wiped out. You may notice walking seems incredibly difficult due to heaviness in your legs or extreme freezing. Exercise is such an endeavor that you're tempted just to avoid it altogether.

What's going on: The energy-producing, stress-regulating cells in your body (called mitochondria) aren't working effectively, leaving you lacking the energy it takes to exercise regularly.

What to do: While it feels counterproductive, exercising regularly actually improves how well your mitochondria function. However, it can take a few months to improve your exercise tolerance, and you may need to take it slowly. Vow to stick with your exercise program for at least three weeks before throwing in the towel. Finally, recognize that improving fatigue takes a comprehensive approach.

> " *When I was diagnosed with Parkinson's, I was training for a marathon. While I don't do nearly the exercise I used to do, I'm still physically active. I'm not running marathons, but I walk on the treadmill. I keep moving, and I tell myself it's okay not to do everything I used to do.*"
>
> — LINDA

Reason #4: You're not exercising effectively.

What it looks like: You're working out regularly but feel you're not getting the results you want. Your symptoms continue to creep up without any real improvements in your flexibility, strength, balance, coordination, or stamina.

What's going on: When it comes to seeing results from your exercise, your program's intensity and consistency are key. While you may be getting some general exercise benefits, you may not be challenging your brain and body in a way that's effective for your Parkinson's symptoms.

What to do: According to the research on Parkinson's exercise, there are seven components to include in your Parkinson's exercise program for optimal results. Layer these elements over your current exercise program for improved results.

- BIG, POWERFUL MOVEMENTS used to combat the slow, small movements that are common in Parkinson's
- PARKINSON'S-SPECIFIC EXERCISES that target the motor and non-motor symptoms of Parkinson's
- Movements that are PHYSICALLY CHALLENGING for your body
- Movements that are MENTALLY CHALLENGING for your mind
- Exercise that's also SOCIAL to combat all-too-common feelings of isolation and loneliness
- Being ACCOUNTABLE to someone to ensure you show up regularly
- Having FUN! If you enjoy it, you're more likely to come back for more

160

About Sarah King

Sarah King is a Parkinson's physical therapist and former owner of Invigorate Physical Therapy & Wellness in Austin, TX. She earned her Doctorate in Physical Therapy from Texas State University in San Marcos and a bachelor's degree in exercise science from Truman State University. She has spent more than a decade working in the health and wellness field, first as an ACE Certified Group Fitness Instructor and then an ACSM Certified Personal Trainer.

She is a Parkinson's Wellness Recovery (PWR!) trained therapist, an extension of the LSVT Big and Loud program for people with Parkinson's. She served on the Board of Directors as Secretary for her local non-profit, Power for Parkinson's, which offers free fitness classes to people with Parkinson's and their care partners. She is also a member of the American Physical Therapy Association (APTA) as well as the Texas Physical Therapy Association (TPTA)

"How Can Dance Help Me Manage Parkinson's?"

By David Leventhal

Dance, whether experienced in a structured group class, socially with a partner, or solo in your kitchen, delivers the same Parkinson's-specific motor and non-motor attributes that other forms of exercise do while offering some unique benefits.

When you dance, you engage in a richly evolved art form, harnessing the power of music, imagery, and expression to experience movement in a fun, creative way. When you dance, you think about movement like a dancer—with intention, rhythm, and a creative, problem-solving mindset. Many people with Parkinson's comment that dance can motivate you to start moving and keep moving, no matter what stage of Parkinson's you're in.

> **"***As physicians, we stress the importance of physical activity, social interaction, and mental stimulation to our patients with Parkinson's. Dance for PD gives them all three. But it is much more than a possible therapy or treatment; the PD dancers have told us this type of dance restores their self-image and brings them joy."*
>
> — HELEN BRONTË-STEWART, MD, MS

Physically, all dance forms—be it tap, ballet, tango, salsa, hula, or flamenco—rely on a shared "DNA" of basic movement elements that are exceptionally helpful for people with Parkinson's. These elements include dynamic balance, rhythm, weight shift, coordination, dual tasking, articulation and control, large amplitude movements, and sequencing (stringing movements together). This last element is important because it invites you to practice and execute a series of different moves as a "phrase" or movement sentence. By practicing dance sequences, you can build fluidity and reliability into your movements. (This is how professional dancers prepare for seamless performances.) Also, dance styles introduce you to new and diverse ways of moving, which in turn can expand your movement vocabulary and the wide range of physical options available to you.

More than a purely physical form, dance is a cognitive activity that requires you to integrate elements of motor planning (step patterns, speed, direction) with imagination and music, all to express yourself and connect with others. Dancing, whether you're seated in a chair or traveling across the room, requires mindful intention and provides, in return, a satisfying sense of personal agency and control.

Part of that satisfaction comes from musicalizing your movements. When you think like a dancer, you infuse music into every part of your body—music becomes your coach, guide, and teacher. Music provides rhythm but also indicates quality, imagery, intent, and story. It tells you when and how to initiate a movement and suggests moving your arms sharply or softly. Music, in a dance experience, is never utilized as background or distraction—it has the power to coordinate your movements and integrate your body, mind, and spirit into a cohesive, unified iteration.

Because dance focuses on your movement's qualities, not just the steps, dance can help you detour around limitations and help you feel fully immersed in your movement experience. Dance adds Technicolor delight to movements—like walking or turning—that might otherwise feel challenging. Think about the difference between how people walk to work in the rain and how Gene Kelly dances (and sings) in the rain. The people walking to work are putting one foot in front of the other, with intention, in a steady rhythm while holding an umbrella—but Gene Kelly transforms those same basic elements into a dynamic explosion of movements and qualities that allow him to tell a story and express joy. You don't have to dance like Mr. Kelly to recognize and take advantage of how dance can transform rote, challenging, or drab movements into a dazzling palette of possibility.

More than 40 peer-reviewed studies and reports by such entities as the World Health Organization point to the physical, cognitive, social, and emotional benefits of dance. People with Parkinson's who use dance to address symptoms and live well speak to the sense of confidence, creativity, and community that dance gives them and to the value of thinking like a dancer in their daily life.

Whatever draws you to try or maintain dance as a part of your movement portfolio, these four points can help you get the most out of your experience:

- Every style of dance offers similar core benefits. Find a style you like and make dancing a habit

- Don't worry about perfection. Focus on learning and doing as much as you can, and remember that the essence of dance is joy

- There's nothing wrong with dancing safely at home (it's better with a partner), but joining a group class online or in a studio offers the additional benefits of social interaction, a sense of community, and the opportunity to work with professional dance teaching artists who can expand your movement horizons and share insights they've gleaned from years of training and performance

- Think like a dancer even when you're not technically dancing. Use music while you're walking down the street, use imagery to take that first step out of bed in the morning, move big like you're performing on stage, and stop, think, and plan your movements as a choreographed dance sequence if you ever find yourself feeling stuck or frozen.

About David Leventhal

David Leventhal is a founding teacher and Program Director for Dance for PD®, a program of the Mark Morris Dance Group that has now been used as a model for classes in more than 300 communities in 25 countries. He leads classes for people with Parkinson's around the world and trains other teachers in the Dance for PD approach. He has co-produced five volumes of a successful At Home DVD series for the program and has been instrumental in initiating and designing innovative projects involving live streaming and Moving Through Glass, a dance-based Google Glass App for people with Parkinson's. He received the 2016 World Parkinson Congress Award for Distinguished Contribution to the Parkinson's Community and was a co-recipient of the 2013 Alan Bonander Humanitarian Award from the Parkinson's Unity Walk. He graduated from Brown University with honors in English Literature. He is a member of the Davis Phinney Foundation Board of Directors and Inclusion, Diversity, Equity, and Access (IDEA) Advisory Board.

"What Are the Benefits of Boxing for People Living with Parkinson's?"

By Brett Miller, PT

Boxing, they say, is as much a match of mental agility as it is physical ability. Anyone who has ever trained and stepped into the ring knows this is true. Inner struggle and mental warfare are pervasive themes in boxing. We know boxing is a sport that forces individuals to look deep inside themselves and discover who they are and who they want to be. Some of the world's most famous and greatest boxers of all time have faced not only their relentless opponents but also themselves.

Doesn't this boxing match sound synonymous with the ongoing fight against Parkinson's? Throwing your combinations, getting backed into the corner, sticking and moving, jabbing and uppercuts—all mixed with the inner struggle, unpredictability, mental warfare, physical and mental fitness.

Research and testimonials support the science of boxing and why it's a "go-to" exercise for many people with Parkinson's. Research performed by a group of sports scientists from the US Olympic Committee came to a surprising conclusion that, pound for pound, based on ten different athletic skills, the most demanding sport in the world is boxing. Endurance, strength, power, speed, agility, flexibility, hand-eye coordination, and mental aptitude were among the tested categories.

To anyone who has ever boxed, this conclusion makes perfect sense. When I talk about boxing, I explain it as a "one-million-mile-per-hour chess game." You are planning your next five offensive and defensive moves while also carrying out and executing the present move while also maintaining the ability to reflect and change course at a second's notice. This is why boxing is so tough, whether you have Parkinson's or not—but also why it is incredibly successful at managing Parkinson's symptoms.

The intense training of boxing-specific exercise (non-contact), otherwise known as high-intensity interval training (HIIT), profoundly impacts neurological fitness and neuroplasticity. Research points to the fact that high-intensity exercise has a neurological protective response to the destruction of dopamine cells. Additionally, when we engage in high-intensity exercises like boxing, we release a protein from the central nervous system known as brain-derived neurotrophic factor (BDNF). The critical roles of BDNF are to optimize memory, sharpen our learning process, speed up the synapse of our motor neurons (synaptogenesis), and create neurogenesis, the process by which new neurons are formed in the brain. The science of boxing enables this. When done two to three days per week as prescribed by a licensed exercise professional, it can be the difference between living with Parkinson's and living your best life with Parkinson's.

There are numerous additional benefits from the high-intensity sport of boxing: improvements in eye tracking, peripheral awareness, hand-eye coordination, ability to change focus on many objects, reaction times, contrast sensitivity, dynamic visual acuity, depth perception, and hemispheric transference. Boxing to manage Parkinson's has also been shown to improve range of motion, strength, functional mobility, and confidence, and it has been shown to decrease the risk of falling.

On top of all these benefits, the camaraderie built with your fellow fighters and coaching staff is invaluable for people living with Parkinson's.

So, how can you begin to reap all of boxing's benefits?

As a physical therapist specializing in working with people with Parkinson's, my recommendation to most people would be to begin a boxing program two or three days a week. Check with your physician to get the go-ahead, then seek out a credentialed trainer experienced in proper boxing technique who also knows proper modifications for exercise programming and Parkinson's. Working with someone who understands Parkinson's and its typical motor and non-motor symptoms (and their response to high-intensity exercise) is important for preventing injury and minimizing other possible risks.

> *I fall a lot. However, physical therapy and exercise, especially working out in the pool and boxing, have all helped me understand falling and how to catch myself."*
>
> — BRIAN

Equally important is finding a place that welcomes you home. Seek out a facility or center where you will enjoy spending time two, three, even five days a week. A place where you can feel vulnerable, real. A place where you can let it all go without ego or judgment. A place where the coaches are professional, and the camaraderie shows up in the form of family gatherings and support groups outside of the facility. Where everyone knows your name and lifts you up. Find a boxing center and community with this combination, and you will be the worst enemy Parkinson's has ever seen. You will triumph.

When you doubt this, remember Muhammad Ali's words: "Impossible is not a fact. It's an opinion. Impossible is not a declaration. It's a dare. Impossible is potential. Impossible is temporary."

Brett Miller is a licensed physical therapist with 26 years of experience in sports therapy, acute and intensive care, long-term care, and wound care. He has worked in the fitness industry for 24 years with extensive experience in kickboxing, boxing, spinning, rowing, and strength and conditioning. He is the founder and owner of 110 Fitness and the Head Coach of Rock Steady Boxing South Shore. He has worked as the strength and conditioning coach for world-class boxers and Olympic athletes, focusing on injury prevention and rehabilitation.

Additionally, Brett Miller has been the owner and operator of Boston Orthotics, Inc. for the past 17 years. He was also an adaptive sports coach at New England Disabled Sports at Loon Mountain in Lincoln, NH, for 18 years. Brett is a US Army veteran, a PWR!Moves® Certified Therapist, and is certified in Concept 2 Rowing, Pedaling for Parkinson's, SCW Boxing Fitness, SCW Aquatics Exercise, Tai Ji Quan: Moving for Better Balance, CPR/AED, and is a licensed boxing second in the state of Massachusetts. Brett serves as a Davis Phinney Foundation Ambassador and is also a research consultant for innovative US research companies, prominent Boston hospitals, and the Cleveland Clinic.

166

"How Can I Stay Consistent if I Haven't Been a Lifelong Exerciser?"

By Amy Carlson, MS

I was never a dancer. A klutz? Yes. A dancer, No. And then...Parkinson's.

In the very beginning, I could ignore the fact that I was a person with Parkinson's, so I did. But somewhere along the way, my body and my brain moved into what I call the "ability margin," and I had to answer the call whether I was ready or not. It was not something I wanted; I was in the middle of a career, raising a family, loving the life I had. Parkinson's was not in the plan.

And then, to add insult to injury, I learned that I needed to exercise. No thanks! It's not that I wasn't an active person. At the time, there wasn't a double black diamond run that I wouldn't try, but I didn't think of skiing, snowboarding, waterskiing, or hiking as exercise. Those were fun things. The word "exercise" recalled images of being pelted with balls in a gym class dodgeball game. Or maybe being struck out at the plate yet again during softball in middle school.

In a fit of compliance with physician's orders, I went to a Zumba class. There was my 40-something self, looking past a bunch of spandex-clad 20-somethings to see my Parkinson's body in the mirrors of a dance studio. I watched in something akin to horror as I saw, perhaps for the first time, what Parkinson's had done to my brain and body. The right side of my body moved in time with the music. The left side of my body lurched in some sort of damp shallow echo of my right side. I left the class in tears. Exercise was evil.

Then I was coerced (bullied) by a persistent person with Parkinson's named Trish to attend a Dance for PD class in Pasadena. Begrudgingly, I walked in from the bright sunlight to the draped high ceiling dance studio. Around the room were people my age (40s) or older and a young woman with a few discrete tattoos clad in what I would come to understand is true dancer attire: her uniform included an overlarge David Bowie concert tee-shirt, well-loved turquoise leggings, and thick black socks. She welcomed us into a circle of chairs in the middle of the room. There were no mirrors. The eight dancers, all older than me except for my daughter who sat by my side, watched her reach for the ceiling. Then we did too.

> " *Not only does exercise help Edie with her Parkinson's, it has helped me a lot. We both encourage each other and get to know each other better. It's always encouraging when you see your partner working hard, no matter how far the disease has progressed.*"
>
> — SCOTT ANDERSON

In that class and the hundreds of hours I've spent studying dance since that day, I have come to learn one thing about dance:

Dance = Sound + Movement

Whether that sound is Bach or The Beatles or Beat Poetry or the beat of a single drum and whether that movement is choreographed or organic or just a body walking down the street. If sounds encourage a body to move, that body is dancing.

I believe that dance has given me access to movement in a way that eludes the damage done in my brain by Parkinson's. It feels as if there is another language at my disposal to send messages of movement to my body, a space in my brain that has a newer relationship with my muscles. At first, dance was intoxicating because I could escape Parkinson's in the dance studio. I could get so far into the dance that my Parkinson's disappeared. Later I found ways to exorcise the demon dyskinesia via dance. By letting the odd movements flow and move with my willed movements, I found that a unique and compelling choreography came to the fore. Now, I find that even in my most OFF states, I can coax my dancer muscles to life just enough to overpower my brain's conviction of immobility and initiate movement. So far, dance is agile enough to move me alongside my Parkinson's.

I know that my body is more flexible, strong, and supple than it has ever been in my adult life. Pulled muscles, sprains, and strains are a thing of the past. Now, my muscles are tuned and responsive to my needs. The stiffness and ache that used to come in the days after an overzealous physical outing are over. My body welcomes a good workout.

My state of mind is revived by the release of emotion that comes through movement. The expression of pain, anger, and frustration, or the exploration of joy, exuberance, and tranquility through my core, limbs, and extremities, gives freedom to the paradoxical feelings that Parkinson's spurs.

The cognitive challenge of dance requires my prefrontal cortex to utilize executive function. My mind plans and executes movement, organizes and remembers choreography, and translates everything into motion both purposefully and automatically.

For me, dance has been the perfect companion to take me through my journey with Parkinson's. Parkinson's permits you to rock your world. Parkinson's is an invitation to change. Flip the script. Change the way you live your life. Find a movement you like, learn to love it, and permit yourself to take time for that movement every day.

About Amy Carlson

On an ordinary Thursday in November of 2011, Amy's ring finger on her left hand began to vibrate. By February of 2012, the vibration was clearly visible, incorporated much of her left arm, and she experienced constant pain in her left shoulder. Later that year, Amy was diagnosed with Parkinson's. She says that Parkinson's has changed her life but perhaps not how most people would expect. She has come to believe that, in its own way, Parkinson's has saved her life, changing her in ways that she would have never expected. Her life has become slower, more deliberate, and more immediate. As a Davis Phinney Foundation Ambassador, Amy's goal is to help others learn about how to live well. She sees so many people with Parkinson's who are alone, confused, and frightened or have run out of hope. Amy wants to be that voice in the darkness that provides direction. She wants to pay it forward because so many people have helped her on her Parkinson's journey.

CHAPTER 10 – COMPLEMENTARY THERAPIES

OVERVIEW

Conventional medicine has come a long way when it comes to helping people with Parkinson's live well. Between the varieties and combinations of medications and surgical therapies, many people with Parkinson's have been able to find conventional treatment regimens that work well for them.

However, the options to help people with Parkinson's live well don't stop there. There are various complementary therapies that people with Parkinson's experiment with, under the care of their medical team, to reduce symptoms even more.

Complementary therapies are those that are used alongside traditional medical treatment. This is different from alternative therapies, which are used in place of traditional medical treatment.

People with Parkinson's choose to try complementary therapies for a variety of reasons:

- They aren't getting the relief they want from their Parkinson's medications
- They see it as a way to take control of their health
- They've heard from friends with Parkinson's that a specific therapy worked for them
- They like the social aspect that comes with participating in many of the complementary therapies
- Their complementary therapy(ies) of choice makes them feel more at ease, relaxed, and at peace

In this chapter, we share various complementary therapies that people in our community have tried. This is not an exhaustive list. If you're wondering why we left something off this list, it's either because

- It's not something we've had experience with and/or
- We don't feel comfortable mentioning something that is unproven, expensive, and could cause harm or worsen your Parkinson's symptoms

For example, many people promote herbal medicines and homeopathy to help those with Parkinson's. We have heard too many stories where adding these kinds of treatments can make Parkinson's worse, in addition to being very expensive; so, we've decided to leave them off our list.

As with everything we share in this manual, please discuss the use of any complementary therapies with your medical and care teams to help you make an informed decision before you jump in. Be open about what you're interested in, tell the truth about what you've tried, and stay in constant communication with your team. This might seem obvious; however, one study found that more than half of people with Parkinson's did not consult their physicians before starting a complementary therapy. We encourage you to be part of the 50% who do.

First, we'll explore the three most common complementary therapies that all people with Parkinson's would benefit from having as part of their prescription for living well: physical therapy, occupational therapy, and speech-language therapy.

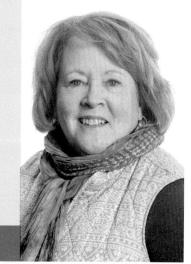

> *We are blessed to have a Parkinson's care physical therapy clinic that we collaborate with and have seen firsthand what physical therapy, speech, and occupational therapy can do for a person with Parkinson's. IT IS CHANGING LIVES by keeping patients stronger and independent longer! So many are resistant because the doctor hasn't mentioned it. ASK for it!! GO often!"*

— CAROLYN RHODES

PHYSICAL THERAPY

Physical therapy works to restore and maintain the body's functional performance. In general, a physical therapist (PT) evaluates and treats problems related to movement and musculoskeletal problems. Since balance, walking (including freezing of gait), slowness, and rigidity are primary motor symptoms of Parkinson's, and because fatigue, poor leg power, and stamina are common symptoms that limit daily activities, physical therapy is an essential part of your treatment.

> *As a physical therapist and owner of a Parkinson's wellness center, I consider the* Every Victory Counts *manual to be the 'Parkinson's bible.' It's a gift I give to every person that steps in my facility with Parkinson's."*

— BRETT MILLER

Individualized care is one of the primary reasons working with a PT is so beneficial. The best type of exercise is different for everyone; while some benefit most from high-intensity training, others need to focus more on balance and flexibility. PTs can assess your mobility, work with you to set goals that are meaningful to you and how you live your daily life, and create a personalized plan for you.

Your initial physical therapy evaluation might include testing for muscle range of motion, muscle strength, degree of rigidity, walking, balance, and posture. The evaluation may include turning, standing, sitting, lying down, rolling over, and getting up out of a chair and from a lying-down position. A PT can also measure physical endurance. Suppose a walking device, such as a cane, walker, or wheelchair, is needed to maintain safety and independence. In that case, the PT will evaluate your movements to determine the most appropriate device, and they can provide instructions for proper use.

Physical therapy can include any or all of the following:

- A home or gym exercise program tailored to you, your Parkinson's, and your current level and abilities
- Balance training and posture exercises
- Stretching and strengthening exercises
- Conditioning or endurance exercises
- Footwear assessments
- Strategies for fall prevention
- Instruction in "safe falling" to the floor and proper techniques for getting up off the floor
- Techniques to lessen freezing of gait
- Walking aid training (walkers, wheelchairs, lift belts)
- Treatment of joint, back, neck, or muscle pain and problems
- Dry needling trigger point therapy
- Care partner training for in-home therapy exercises and transfers

Find a good physical therapist but make sure that that person is able to challenge you to work beyond your current level of fitness. If you select a PT who only treats patients in later stages of Parkinson's, he or she may not be willing to move you to a higher state of fitness for fear of injuring you. Be honest with them and let them know that if they are unable to give you difficult enough exercises, you will need to look elsewhere. They need to trust that you know your body and abilities and are willing to stretch yourself to attain a better quality of life."

— PATTI BURNETT

Although all PTs will have some knowledge of movement disorders, Parkinson's physical therapists have had additional training in neurologic physical therapy and are certified in this specialty. Later in this chapter, we'll take a closer look at the many ways physical therapy and working with a Parkinson's PT can help you live well today and every day.

OCCUPATIONAL THERAPY

Occupational therapy and therapists can help you with many everyday activities at work, home, and play, from dressing and eating to overcoming freezing problems at home or in the community to installing and using adaptive equipment.

" *Occupational therapy has helped me a lot with fine motor skills, like handwriting. My fine motor skills are terrible, so I have a box I made up with things like a deck of cards, a small ball I squeeze with my hands, a medicine bottle with some money in it, scissors, an adult coloring book with colored pencils, a clothespin, a rubber band, etc. I play with all these supplies when I'm watching TV or sitting around to practice and improve my fine motor skills."*

— LINDA

Occupational therapy can include any of the following:

- Treatment for arm and shoulder strength problems, hand dexterity, and handwriting difficulty
- Motor biofeedback, stress management, and relaxation techniques
- Dressing, hygiene, performing daily chores, meal preparation
- Performing transfers (to and from a bed, tub, toilet, wheelchair)
- Improving mobility, task efficiency, and safety
- Use of adaptive equipment or aids (grab bars, commodes, tub seats)
- Work-related concerns
- Home assessments for safety
- Driving assessments
- Home exercise programs
- New methods of performing the tasks of daily living to preserve energy and reduce fatigue
- Identifying problems with movement freezing and the environment
- Medication and time management
- Cognitive therapy

- Care partner education and training
- Non-motor symptom treatment: dizziness, sleep, hygiene, bowel and bladder management
- Food preparation

Later in this chapter, we'll take a deep dive into how occupational therapy can help you live well.

SPEECH-LANGUAGE AND SWALLOWING THERAPY

Speech therapy is more than just speech; it is about communication. 70% of communication is non-verbal; people rely on facial expressions, change in tone, body language, and actual word meanings to communicate. The main goals of speech therapy are to improve someone's ability to communicate effectively, improve communication in social interactions, and increase the safety of someone's swallowing skills.

Communication is one of the most important skills in life. Speech pathologists have research-based strategies to help you maintain your voices. It's good to have an evaluation done early on for baseline information and to learn how to keep your voice healthy and strong. Speech, like learning to play an instrument, needs to be practiced regularly to maintain skills. I know as I am a speech pathologist with Parkinson's!"

— CAROL CLUPNY

A speech-language pathologist (SLP) evaluates and provides treatment for speech, voice, language, cognition, and swallowing disorders. Once you are evaluated, you and your SLP will design a plan of care that's best for you.

WHY SHOULD I SEE A SPEECH-LANGUAGE PATHOLOGIST?

The following speech and swallowing changes can occur during Parkinson's and are reasons for speech-language therapy:

- Soft voice
- Slurred or mumbled speech
- Rapid or run-on speech
- Stuttering
- Decreased facial expression (facial masking)
- Drooling
- Frequently needing to clear the throat

- Swallowing difficulties, such as difficulty swallowing pills, swallowing several times with each bite, coughing while eating, or sensing that food is stuck in the throat
- Coughing and throat clearing due to aspiration (food or saliva getting into the breathing tube or lungs) while eating and drinking

I went to speech therapy because I was getting really weak in my voice. After the initial SpeakOUT! program I did with the Parkinson Voice Project, I joined their Loud Crowd, which gives you ongoing maintenance and accountability. It forces you to do your exercises and continue practicing, which I need."

— LINDA

TREATMENTS AND STRATEGIES FOR IMPROVING SPEECH AND SWALLOWING

- Speech exercises to improve speech volume and intelligibility
- Cognitive strategies to improve speaking and language function
- Understanding the impact of facial expression and speech changes on communication and relationships
- Counseling about communication and the impact of body and facial expression
- Instruction on proper neck and body positioning while swallowing
- Recommendations for dietary changes based on swallowing abilities
- Improvements to eating habits for safer eating and weight control
- Care partner instruction on the Heimlich maneuver and more

Sometimes a modified barium swallow is needed to diagnose swallowing problems. This radiology procedure can visualize the passage of food or fluids from your mouth to your stomach. This test can determine whether food or fluids are entering the lungs, called aspiration. Aspiration occurs when material goes past the vocal cords, goes down toward the airway, and then filters down into the lungs. Parkinson's can increase your risk for aspiration, leading to more serious problems such as aspiration pneumonia and pulmonary edema; so, it's important to ensure you have a healthy swallow. Be sure to look on our *Every Victory Counts* **website** for a **video** that describes aspiration and what it looks like.

We'll look more in-depth at physical, occupational, and speech-language therapy later in this chapter.

14 ADDITIONAL COMPLEMENTARY THERAPIES

In addition to these three vital therapies, many others can help you live well with Parkinson's. Here, we highlight 14 other complementary therapies that many in our Parkinson's community have found valuable and have no evidence of being dangerous for someone with Parkinson's.

" *Working at a chiropractic clinic when diagnosed with Parkinson's I was immediately aware of the varying therapies that could be available to people with Parkinson's. I loved massage and acupuncture the most and found value in yoga, adjustments, and supplements. I searched out a functional or holistic movement disorders PA. After I shared with her my enthusiasm for complementary and alternative treatments, here is what she told me, 'You realize, don't you, that Parkinson's is a progressive neurological disorder that will increasingly affect every system of your body, and there is little you can do to slow down this process? Your prescription meds will not cure it but merely treat your symptoms.' Well, was I ever disillusioned and determined in my mind and heart to prove this woman wrong."*

— PATTI BURNETT

ACUPUNCTURE

Acupuncture involves inserting thin needles through the skin to stimulate certain points in the body and improve the flow and distribution of energy in the body. Several studies have shown that acupuncture and conventional treatment were more effective in reducing pain and relieving symptoms than conventional medicine alone. While it is considered generally safe, talk to your physician about possible side effects such as fatigue, lightheadedness, soreness at the needle site, and worsening of your symptoms before you try it.

AROMATHERAPY

Aromatherapy is the practice of inhaling or applying to the skin aromatic essential oils derived from a wide variety of healing plants. Aromatherapy has been shown, anecdotally, to help people reduce pain and stress, improve sleep, soothe sore joints, improve digestion, decrease anxiety and depression, promote relaxation, and more.

ART THERAPY

Art therapy is a type of psychotherapy that allows you to use art to express your feelings and communicate issues that may be difficult to talk about. Art therapy can help you explore feelings, reconcile emotional conflicts, foster self-awareness, manage behavior and addictions, develop social skills, reduce anxiety, and more. Many people who live with Parkinson's say that being creative helps them focus, relax, and live more in the moment.

Look on our ⤴ **website for articles written by people** who use art therapy every day to live well with Parkinson's.

> *I am a nature photographer and was concerned that my tremor would take photography away from me. Five years with Parkinson's, and I'm still enjoying my daily photo walks. Yes, the mechanics of photography are more challenging, but the joy it continues to give me far outweighs any diminishment of my skills!"*
>
> — KERRY HOWARD

AYURVEDA

Ayurveda is based on the belief that the mind and body are connected and that each person has a mind-body type that should guide their choices about nutrition, exercise, and all other areas of life. The guiding philosophy of this therapy is to take actions that put you in the flow, rather than taking the path that will cause you to struggle and strain against your natural way of being.

DANCE THERAPY

The American Dance Therapy Association (ADTA) defines dance/movement therapy as the psychotherapeutic use of movement to promote the individual's emotional, social, cognitive, and physical integration.

> *Dancing provides an arena to feel like an integrated body working as a whole instead of feeling like a patient. In dance class, we welcome both the struggling parts and thriving parts of the body and the awareness of how things can change unexpectedly day to day. Embracing and honoring your dancer body can be liberating and fortifying—it is something gained among so many things lost when dealing with Parkinson's. Breathing compassion into the struggling parts, breathing gratitude into the thriving parts, and the ability to see all those parts as an integrated, whole body is a practice that participants can carry with them every day."*
>
> — SARAH LEVERSEE, DANCE FOR PD® INSTRUCTOR

We've had so many people with Parkinson's share with us what a big difference dancing has made in increasing their energy and improving their quality of life. For more on the many ways dance can help you live well with Parkinson's, flip back to Chapter 9.

FELDENKRAIS METHOD

The Feldenkrais Method® is based on the idea that the brain oversees movement; so, to change your movement, you must change your mind. For a person with Parkinson's, the natural rhythm and flow of perception, feeling, and movement are disrupted, and routine behaviors such as walking, speaking, swallowing, and more can become difficult, if not completely unavailable. The Feldenkrais Method teaches people movement sequences designed to enhance their functional ability. As you learn better ways to move, you can improve your balance, breathing, cognition, coordination, facial masking, swallowing, and more. This method can be taught privately or in group classes.

LAUGHTER YOGA

Typically practiced in a group setting and led by a trained instructor, laughter yoga centers around breathing techniques, clapping, chanting, and, as the name suggests, laughter. Although there is little clinical evidence supporting its benefits, it has been said to help manage stress, anxiety, depression, and more. You can learn more about laughter yoga on our ⏚ *Every Victory Counts* website.

MASSAGE THERAPY

Many people with Parkinson's use massage therapy to improve well-being and alleviate symptoms of pain, rigidity, fatigue, depression, and even tremor. There's very little risk involved with getting a massage, so many physicians highly recommend you include this type of therapy in your treatment. The good news, too, is that many insurance providers will cover massage therapy sessions because it is considered a common treatment for Parkinson's.

MINDFULNESS

To be mindful is to be aware of what's going on around you, how you feel, and the space you're in. It sounds simple enough, but being mindful is easier said than done. That's because it's very easy to let thoughts about the future, medication schedules, to-do lists, worries, and anxiety become top of mind.

Therefore, mindfulness practices such as meditation are designed to help people practice being in the moment, suspending judgment, practicing self-compassion, and becoming detached from every possible outcome. If you're able to make this a regular practice in your life, you can gain the power to reduce stress, enhance performance, improve sleep, improve concentration, improve cardiovascular and immune health, reduce pain, increase coping skills, change your brain, and more.

❝*I can't control that I have Parkinson's, but I can control how I live with Parkinson's.***❞**

— DAVIS PHINNEY

177

MUSIC THERAPY

Music therapy is the use of music within a therapeutic relationship to address the physical, emotional, cognitive, and social needs of individuals. For some people with Parkinson's, music therapy decreases freezing, improves gait and speech, increases postural control, and improves cognition. Plus, many have reported that their music therapy classes are the most fun they have all week.

PILATES

Pilates is a non-impact form of exercise designed to improve spinal structure and alignment and strengthen the core. There's little clinical evidence for its efficacy related to people with Parkinson's; however, a regular Pilates practice for many people helps to improve balance, posture, strength, flexibility, and quality of life. While Pilates is often offered in a group class format, if you decide to give it a try—after getting the go-ahead from your physician—consider working one-on-one with a certified Pilates instructor first to learn how to use the equipment and avoid injury.

REIKI

Reiki is a Japanese technique that involves laying hands on or near different parts of a person's body. It's based on the idea that we all have a "life force energy" that flows through us, and it's what causes us to be alive. A low life force energy causes illness and stress, and a high life force energy causes greater health and happiness.

> " *I truly believe Reiki has eased my symptoms and calmed my mind. Reiki helped me to get closer to achieving my dreams, and it changed my whole perspective about illness."*
>
> — KARL ROBB

TAI CHI

Tai chi integrates balance, flexibility, and coordination (motor function) with focused mental attention and multitasking (cognitive function). Findings show that individuals who participate in these exercises experience improvements in Parkinson's related to motor symptoms, including balance and mobility, and a reduced number of falls. The research also indicates that engagement in these exercises helps to reduce depression significantly.

YOGA THERAPY

Even if you have never practiced yoga before, chances are you've heard people talk about the benefits they receive from doing it. And while traditional yoga classes may be beneficial for people with Parkinson's, when determining the path you might like to take, it's important to distinguish between a yoga teacher and yoga therapist and a yoga class and a yoga therapy session.

- **Yoga class:** a place where students practice a certain system of exercise
- **Yoga teacher:** someone who guides students through their practice and teaches various yoga methods in a correct and safe way
- **Yoga therapy session:** designed to help the student get relief from symptoms or health conditions that are troubling them. Sometimes these are group sessions; however, more often than not, they are one-on-one sessions
- **Yoga therapist:** an individual who has undergone specialized training in assessment, practice development, and a variety of different health conditions such as cancer, depression, trauma, and Parkinson's

Yoga therapy is one of the complementary therapies that has research proving its efficacy. It has been shown to reduce tremor, improve balance and gait, increase flexibility, improve posture, loosen painful muscles, and reduce stress. While yoga therapy is considered generally safe, it's still a good idea to talk to your physician about it before giving it a try. When you're ready to move forward, make sure you work with a yoga therapist who has been specifically trained to work with people living with Parkinson's.

Adding complementary therapies to your conventional treatments is a great way to empower yourself to live well with Parkinson's. By taking this holistic approach to wellness, you can experiment with a variety of ways to heal your body, mind, and spirit.

"How Can I Get the Most Out of Physical Therapy?"

By Mike Studer, PT, MHS, NCS, CEEAA, CWT, CSST

As a physical therapist with more than 30 years of experience, I have witnessed a transformation in our understanding, management, and hope when it comes to Parkinson's. Most people living with Parkinson's seek physical therapy to help with balance, fall prevention, and walking. In contrast with even 15 years ago, we now have the research-based tools to modify the effects of Parkinson's and to improve safety and mobility for daily life.

Some of the most common walking and balance challenges that I address include:

- Short steps or shuffling (festination)
- Difficulty changing directions
- Difficulty keeping balance while rising to stand or sitting down from standing
- Halting, hesitating, or freezing while walking
- Involuntary movements of the body, arms, or legs (tremor and/or dyskinesia)

Clearly, there is a purpose to walking: to move safely and efficiently from one place to another. Often, people facing walking and balance challenges choose to reduce their walking to avoid injuring themselves in a fall. While this may seem like an effective strategy, it can lead to more weakness and, therefore, a greater risk of falling due to the combination of a movement disorder plus weakness plus fear. This can limit people in moving even from a bed to a wheelchair and cause them to consider giving up walking altogether. So, what is the solution?

HOPE AND EXPECTATIONS

While there is no single physical therapy solution that suits everyone with Parkinson's, there is certainly reason to be hopeful. Research-based evidence tells us (and my personal experience supports this) that people with movement disorders at any level of ability can improve their mobility through therapy. Rehabilitation professionals working with people with Parkinson's expect to make a positive difference that lasts.

> **"***The information that's covered in this manual is critical to helping people slow the progression of Parkinson's. When my clients start implementing what they've learned, their entire world starts to change for the better, and they feel hopeful again.***"**
>
> — SARAH KING, DPT

Some of the most well-researched techniques in rehabilitation for gait and balance issues for people living with Parkinson's include these categories:

- **High-intensity exercise.** In this category, you will practice activities that require speed (treadmill or fast walking), power (strength applied quickly in time, such as a fast effort to "jump up" to standing), or excursion (often referred to as "big" movement, with an exaggerated arm swing or step length).
- **Agility training.** Tasks that involve a rapid alternation of movement—such as the efforts of a combination "right-left-right" as in boxing, or as in the footwork in dancing—will test your agility. This type of exercise could include efforts to step

around barriers or obstacles, as in hopscotch.

- **Combining auditory or music conditioning.** Adding music to your exercise routine or moving to a pace set by a particular beat can help you move more fluidly.

- **Concentration-focused.** Efforts to rebuild distraction tolerance and the automatic nature of some routine tasks is the goal of concentration-focused exercise. Research has proven that people with Parkinson's can preferentially lose, but also improve, their ability to move with distractions. Walking, dressing, getting out of bed, and brushing teeth are but some examples of life's automatic movements, thanks to years of repetition. However, Parkinson's and the absence of sufficient rehabilitative training can interrupt automatic access, putting you at risk for falling when distracted during these and other routines.

- **Compensatory.** Identifying and prescribing the right adaptive equipment/assistive devices or environmental changes to best serve your needs of remaining safe and active (walkers and canes, some of which are equipped with visual or auditory cues in the form of laser lines, metronomes, or music) is how you compensate for movements you may no longer be able to do.

- **Personalization for Success.** The best rehabilitation is personalized for you. Your symptoms, preferences, and the things you respond to best add up to the right physical therapy approach. Additionally, your therapy should be based on research specifically shown to be effective for Parkinson's. This research tells us to use more repetitions, practice daily, include general exercise, incorporate activities focused on balance, and make it fun! When movement and exercise are fun, you will work harder and receive more benefits from your efforts. Research also tells us that participating vigorously in something that is enjoyable causes the brain to release dopamine-- that's right, the very same chemical that Parkinson's limits!

There are also things you can do at home to continue to improve your walking and balance skills. Ideally, you'll first visit a physical therapist with experience and a passion for movement disorders so that you can receive a personal examination that includes measurements of your abilities. Having a personalized baseline with measurements and data that you can work to improve over time can be very inspiring. Often, tracking progress gives people more drive to work on home exercises with greater effort and regularity. Ask your physical therapist to build an individualized program so that you can re-measure your abilities at intervals and see your progress.

If you are limited in your search or access to physical therapy, consider selecting exercises from the list below, remembering to include repetition, daily practice, and activities that are fun for you.

PARKINSON'S TREATMENTS AND THERAPIES

EXERCISES* YOU CAN DO AT HOME

1. **Sitting to standing repetitions.** Practice a few repetitions of standing up FAST, then do some VERY SLOWLY, with control.

2. **Standing still with your feet together.** If this is challenging, practice this with your body near a bed or with a care partner.

3. **Big step forward, big step back.** Stand with your back on a chair or bed. Take one BIG step forward and return to the starting position. Then, switch your legs. As you become more comfortable, you could increase the speed and the length of steps.

4. **Walk short distances with weights around your ankles.** Try three-pound or five-pound weights and walk with guidance from a care partner or a cane or walker to begin. Slowly increase the time spent by a few minutes at a time. FOCUS on lifting your feet up (not shuffling).

5. **Change directions.** Walk with turns, forward-backward walking, etc. Walk in your home, preferably in a hallway. Start by moving forward. Turn around midway down the hall the first time. Then, make it more complicated and take a few steps sideways or backward. This can be challenging. Take extra caution as you begin, enlisting help from your care partner as needed.

6. **March in place with high knees.** This can be done while sitting or standing. Exaggerate your movement and extend your time as you become stronger.

7. **Full-circle turnarounds.** With assistance, stand in a hallway, and turn a full circle.

8. **Standing still, or sitting to standing, with eyes closed.** Stand in one place and practice balancing with your eyes closed. Try standing up from a seated position with your eyes closed. This is another challenging exercise. Start with assistance and use caution.

*You should choose exercises based on your individual needs, the ability to perform them safely, and the availability of care partners or other people who can assist you as needed.

SAFETY FIRST

All exercises practiced for the first few times can be challenging, if not dangerous, if misprescribed for your situation. Some tips to ensure that your efforts to improve your balance and mobility do not result in an injurious fall include:

- Asking and waiting for help EVERY time you try a new exercise

- Limiting distractions when trying a new balance exercise

- Using smaller ranges of motion to begin your first few trials each time you exercise

Finally, consider your overall activity level and general fitness. If you feel limited in your ability to walk for long periods (more than six minutes at a time), consider using a walker or walking with a care partner so you can go farther, safely, several times per week. Staying consistent and exercising regularly will allow you to increase both your stamina and balance.

About Mike Studer

Mike Studer is a physical therapist and the owner of Northwest Rehabilitation Associates in Salem, Oregon. He was awarded the "Clinical Excellence" award in 2011 by the Academy of Neurologic Physical Therapy and was awarded the same honor by the Academy of Geriatric Physical Therapy in 2014. He received his Bachelor of Science degree in physical therapy from the University of Missouri-Columbia and is a neurologic certified specialist.

"How Can Occupational Therapy Help Me Live Well with Parkinson's in my Home?"

By Amanda Craig, OTR/L, CBIS

An occupational therapist (OT) can talk for days about the assistance and support that occupational therapy can provide to people with Parkinson's. My short answer to how an OT can help you live well with Parkinson's? We can help with almost everything. All aspects of your life that you need or want to do. The end.

Now that you know that, here's the longer answer: Occupational therapists recognize that all people need to be active and occupied in order to be satisfied. Occupational therapy helps people of all ages (beginning to the end of life) with their "occupations." To an OT, "occupations" are any activities that occupy your body, mind, emotions, and time. That's right; we're not only focused on employment. Our list of occupations can include any aspect of life, from eating, showering, dressing, sleeping (yes, we consider sleeping an occupation), playing, working, volunteering, driving, parenting, pet-parenting, home care, and many more.

Occupational therapists break down tasks to determine why a person is experiencing decreased participation or efficiency within their activities. An OT investigates a person's challenges in order to create a customized treatment plan. These skill deficits may include but are not limited to gross and fine motor skills, vision, hearing, pain, fatigue, thinking skills, emotional coping skills, and communication skills.

The goal of occupational therapy is to help you be as independent as possible for as long as possible. To meet that goal, an OT can help you maintain or strengthen your ability to care for yourself, care for your house, take care of your loved ones, and get around in the community.

So, with this in mind, let's look at some ways an OT can help you live well with Parkinson's at home. Why? Because much of our lives are spent in our homes. We eat, sleep, and cultivate passions there. We create art, food, and music there. We study and educate ourselves there. And, of course, we visit others and maintain relationships there. So, home needs to be a place that supports our goals and allows us to thrive.

To set yourself up for success at home, an OT can visit your residence and learn about how you live on a day-to-day basis. They may take measurements and ask you to perform some of your daily, normal tasks, like getting around in your bathroom, preparing food in your kitchen, getting in and out of your closet, and feeding your pet. Afterward, they will provide you with recommendations and potential resources, which might be specific to your needs or might be general accessibility recommendations. The OT should also let you know what home changes are important to make right away and what can be made in the future as your Parkinson's progresses.

Ultimately, OTs want to offer home solutions that will increase a person's engagement in an activity. We want any modifications in the home to allow you to increase your overall participation. And we want to contribute to maintaining or improving your overall health and wellness.

Depending on your needs, goals, symptoms, and lifestyle, an OT may recommend modifications to your seating arrangements and furniture, kitchen organization, lighting, bathrooms, and stairs and walkways. Additions and improvements to your home such as grab bars, push-pull doorknobs, bed canes, touch-on lights and faucets, doorbell cameras, and improved lighting can make your home not only more comfortable but safer as well.

Whether you're looking for an OT who specializes in this kind of home evaluation process or any of the countless other occupations of life, seek out an OT who can help you meet your specific needs and goals. An occupational therapist is an ideal partner to have on your Parkinson's adventure.

About Amanda Craig

Amanda Craig is a licensed occupational therapist and owner of Ada Therapy Services, PLLC in Boise, ID. Amanda provides individualized outpatient treatment for adults and adolescents experiencing functional "real life" deficits caused by neurological and chronic conditions. The therapists at Ada Therapy Services subscribe to the founding principle of occupational therapy: all people need to be active and occupied to be satisfied. Amanda completed her graduate degree in occupational therapy from Idaho State University and a bachelor's degree in business from Philadelphia University/Thomas Jefferson University in her home state of Pennsylvania.

"Why Should I See a Speech-Language Pathologist?"

By Michelle Underhill, MA, CCC-SLP

Many people living with Parkinson's experience difficulties with communication, swallowing, and cognition. These challenges may show up as a quiet voice, mumbled speech, trouble finding words, avoidance of certain foods or liquids, extra saliva in the mouth, mucus in the throat, frequent coughing or throat-clearing, and difficulty organizing or remembering information. How many of the following statements relate to you?

- People often ask me to repeat what I said
- I run out of air quickly
- I speak up less often than I used to
- It's not my voice that's the problem; it's their hearing
- I start talking, then get stuck on a word. It's awkward and uncomfortable
- I cough more when I'm eating/drinking
- I have too much saliva! I can't keep up with it. Sometimes I drool a bit
- I'm losing weight; it's too much of a hassle to eat
- It's hard to keep up with the conversation
- I can't do the puzzles/games/activities I used to enjoy

WHEN SHOULD YOU SEE A SPEECH-LANGUAGE PATHOLOGIST (SLP)?

If any of the above statements ring true for you, establishing a relationship with an SLP will help you discover strategies to improve how you function in everyday life. If you have recently been diagnosed with Parkinson's, undergoing an evaluation with an SLP can establish your "baseline" status and provide you with valuable information to prepare for the future. Use this time to create a plan to maintain or improve your vocal strength and articulation, ensure safe swallowing, and build strategies to help with cognitive challenges.

When you meet with an SLP, share your specific concerns, the situations that create problems, and observations others have shared with you. The SLP will conduct an evaluation targeting your personal difficulties and complete a comprehensive speech-language pathology assessment. Your evaluation should include an interview, a review of your medical history, and assessments of your speech, language, voice, swallowing, and cognition (thinking and memory). These assessments may be informal (discussion, observation, self-reports) or formal (standardized tests). Your SLP will consider your results against normative data for your age to assist in determining which outcomes are considered "within normal age expectations" and which results fall outside of that range.

WHAT DOES SPEECH THERAPY LOOK LIKE?

There are many activities designed to help you improve your communication, swallowing, and cognition. Your SLP will determine which approaches are most appropriate for you. Your initial evaluation and subsequent visits will focus on speech, language, voice, swallowing, and cognition. For fun, you can start practicing them as soon as you get the chance.

- **Speak LOUDLY.** Place a sucker inside your cheek and practice speaking to help you to articulate more clearly. When others have difficulty understanding you, restate the information in a shorter sentence or use different words. Pretend you are using a "presentation voice" to help you exaggerate your articulation.

- **Language.** If you didn't understand what someone says, ask for repetition or more information. Express your thoughts and ideas to your loved ones and friends—they want to hear what you have to say! When you struggle to find a word, describe it in other ways (what it looks like, where you use it, etc.). Keep talking; the word you're looking for may come to you, or it may occur to your conversation partner.

- **Voice.** Be louder than you think you need to be. If you are comfortable, you are probably too quiet. Breathe! It is easier to be loud and clear when you have air in your lungs to support your voice. When you are loud, the quality of your voice tends to improve automatically.

- **Swallowing.** Whether you have too much saliva in your mouth or not enough, try sucking on lemon candy, small suckers, or chewing gum. Yes, this will create more saliva, but it will also help you to swallow more frequently. The more you practice swallowing, the more those muscles receive exercise. If you struggle with thick mucus in your throat, these strategies will help you to get it either swallowed down or cleared up and out.

- **Cognition.** Consider how you prefer to learn information. Do you need to hear it? See it? Feel it? If you need to see something to remember it, take a mental picture in your mind when you want to commit something to memory. Write a note or say it out loud. Find mental challenges that take you outside of your comfort zone but are still accessible. Look for activities that require new learning and mental effort and also bring you joy.

An annual evaluation is recommended and may or may not be followed by therapy, depending upon your needs at the time. Continue with your personal strategies and exercises each day. When you complete work outside of therapy sessions, you maximize your progress. You may find that you prefer to stay in regular contact with your SLP for maintenance therapy to stay on top of any changes you are experiencing.

Seek out a speech-language pathologist to help you live well with your Parkinson's today and in the future.

About Michelle Underhill

Michelle Underhill is a speech-language pathologist and the owner of Northern Colorado Therapy Services, a multidisciplinary private practice specializing in the care of people living with Parkinson's. She has extensive experience in evaluating and treating individuals with Parkinson's at all stages and is a certified clinician in LSVT LOUD. She is passionate about the positive impact of therapy on daily functioning and has focused her career on sharing hope and power within life's various circumstances. Ms. Underhill completed a bachelor's degree in communication disorders from Colorado State University and a master's degree in speech-language pathology from the University of Northern Colorado.

187

CHAPTER 11 – NUTRITION

OVERVIEW

One of the most common questions we're asked is this: *"What should I eat now that I've been diagnosed with Parkinson's?"*

The answer is that there is no one answer. Just as each person with Parkinson's experiences different symptoms, each person reacts differently to different types of food. In some ways, this is good news. It may require more experimentation and a little more trial and error; however, there's also more hope that there are some tweaks you can make to your nutritional choices to help you feel better and mitigate some of your symptoms. The key is knowing that the foods you eat affect how you feel, and this knowledge can be a decisive first step in finding more ways to live well.

FINDING THE BEST EATING PLAN FOR YOU

The most important fact to know about Parkinson's nutrition is that one size does not fit all. Work with your physician to find a starting point, tweak, and adjust from there based on your unique needs. One of the more critical reasons to do this is because when it comes to finding a nutritional plan that works best for you, timing will likely play a key role. That's because, as we explained in our chapter about medication, eating protein can affect the absorption of Parkinson's medications. If you don't time it right, you may think that certain foods aren't working when it's just a matter of timing.

Before making any changes to your nutrition, be aware that the suggestions outlined in the following pages are meant to serve as guidelines only. Review any nutritional changes with your physician and wellness team, especially if you have diabetes or heart or gastrointestinal problems, and ask your physician about the effects of your nutritional choices on your medications.

A RECOMMENDATION FROM PARKINSON'S EXPERTS: EAT THE MEDITERRANEAN WAY

While there is no one-size-fits-all nutritional plan for Parkinson's, there are sound guidelines that can serve anyone well. Eating well means getting the appropriate vitamins and nutrients from foods and not from a pill. Eating well means that the foods you choose will reduce your risk of diseases, such as cardiovascular disease, hypertension, diabetes, obesity, intestinal problems, stroke, and cancer.

So, what style of eating reduces these risks, boosts your energy, promotes heart and brain health, and is recommended by countless Parkinson's experts? The Mediterranean diet. (A quick note: We are not fans of the word diet because, for so many, it implies that you will eat a certain way for a certain time period and that there are good foods and bad foods. So, while we choose to focus on the term nutritional choices rather than diet, the "Mediterranean Diet" is the common label for this way of eating.) A Mediterranean diet focuses on vegetables, fruits, whole grains, beans, nuts and seeds, and olive oil. Some people also eat fish. But, because it is a plant-based way of eating, you can easily create a Mediterranean diet plan that is vegetarian, vegan, or lower in carbohydrates than standard diets. Eating the Mediterranean way is not only healthy but completely customizable, affordable, varied, and convenient.

We are not fans of the word diet because, for so many, it implies a time limit. So, while we choose to focus on the term nutritional choices rather than diet, the "Mediterranean Diet" is the common label for this way of eating.

Eating a Mediterranean diet is associated with a lower risk of Parkinson's (studies have shown this can reduce the risk of Parkinson's anywhere from 14 to 48%) and later age of disease onset. It also provides many benefits to people living with Parkinson's; consistent findings show that the Mediterranean diet is proven to reduce the risk of many diseases, such as stroke, hypertension, heart disease, diabetes, depression, dementia, and cancer, proving its global impact on health.

Recommendations based on Mediterranean diets include:

- High in fruits and vegetables: 8-10 servings daily
- High in fish: 2-3 times per week (for a total of 8-12 ounces)
- Low in meat (especially red meat): 1-2 times a week, at most
- High in plant protein: nuts, seeds, beans
- Olive oil as the primary oil
- High in whole grains
- Low in processed, refined sugar
- Foods in their whole state (rather than processed)

John Duda, MD, national director of the Parkinson's Disease Research, Education, and Clinical Center for the Department of Veteran Affairs and associate professor of neurology at the University of Pennsylvania's Perelman School of Medicine, says, "the best evidence out there suggests that a whole-food, plant-based diet—a Mediterranean diet—is best for long-term health and wellness. The evidence is clear that adopting this type of diet will reduce your risk of dementia, depression, constipation, and a whole host of other things that will help you in the long run. A diet full of fiber and full of plant-based nutrients that include a whole host of antioxidants and anti-inflammatory molecules could help protect your brain. That's the diet I recommend."

PARKINSON'S NUTRITION Q&A

Although, for the reasons we mentioned above, nutrition for Parkinson's is not an easy topic to address, here are some of the most common questions we receive about Parkinson's and nutrition.

#1 – Should I only eat organic food?

Exposure to pesticides is the strongest link between the environment and Parkinson's. Eating organic foods can reduce the ingestion of pesticides, but organic produce, dairy, and meat do cost more than conventional products. Be sure to wash all produce thoroughly in warm water, especially if organic foods are not an option. The "Dirty Dozen" and "Clean Fifteen" are lists published annually of foods with higher and lower pesticide exposure, respectively, to help you choose which foods to eat organic.

#2 – I'm constipated all the time. Is there anything I can do to help manage this symptom?

Constipation is the most common gastrointestinal problem for people with Parkinson's. Increasing the amount of water you drink and fiber intake are two things you can do to improve constipation symptoms. Most experts recommend at least 64 ounces of fluid a day, and some recommend prune juice as an excellent way to increase fluids intake and relieve constipation.

Increasing the number of high-fiber foods like apples, prunes, dates, figs, radishes, berries, nuts, beans, and whole grains can also help relieve your constipation. Remember that introducing additional fiber should be done slowly to allow your digestive system to adjust to the effects. Exercise can also help; simply walking can help promote movement in your bowels. For more about constipation and Parkinson's, head back to Chapter 6.

#3 – If I take regular doses of carbidopa/levodopa, should that impact when and what I should eat?

Yes. Proteins may influence the effect of carbidopa/levodopa in food. Proteins can compete with carbidopa/levodopa uptake both from the gut and across the blood-brain barrier and may, therefore, inhibit the effect of carbidopa/levodopa. If you take regular doses of carbidopa/levodopa, you should talk to your physician about taking your medicine one hour before eating, especially before high-protein meals. (And remember, take all medications with a full glass of water, which helps flush the medicine quickly from your stomach to your small intestines, where it is absorbed. Try sparkling water or club soda to speed delivery even more.) However, protein is still essential for your diet, so it can help to create a schedule to manage your medication and protein intake throughout the day so that you're not eating your high-protein meals simultaneously with your carbidopa/levodopa. Try concentrated protein sources (yogurt, nuts, and fish) as a snack between medication doses.

#4 – Why is it so important that I stay hydrated when I'm living with Parkinson's?

Getting the ideal amount of water each day can help you in countless ways. As we have mentioned, water can be especially beneficial when you take your Parkinson's medications. When you take your medication with a full glass of water (and nothing else), it enters your small intestines quickly, giving it a fast track to your brain. As we've mentioned, choosing carbonated water can also aid in faster uptake of your medication.

Drinking enough water is also essential to help promote general health and relieve symptoms of constipation. When someone experiences long periods of dehydration, their cells can't function properly and die, leading to degeneration and disease. Dehydration also leads to poor circulation and blood flow, resulting in high blood pressure, organ failure, and more. You may experience decreased thirst with Parkinson's, so it can be helpful to create a hydration plan, carry a water bottle, and track your daily water intake to ensure you're drinking enough.

#5 – Lately, I've been having a lot of trouble chewing and swallowing. It makes it difficult to eat. What can I do?

This is a common problem for many people with Parkinson's. One strategy is to focus on your food's consistency and consider softer food, like applesauce or broiled fish. You can also add moisture to your food, such as gravy or sauce, so that it's easier to swallow.

Another option is to blend your meal partially. You can do this by putting 75% of your meal in the blender and saving the rest to eat as solid food. Slow cookers are also great at cooking meats or vegetables, so they are tender and easy to swallow.

If you have trouble swallowing liquids, you can thicken fluid with things like applesauce. And, as we explained earlier in this manual, it can be incredibly beneficial to visit a speech-language pathologist to learn specific ways to improve your chewing and swallowing.

#6 – I keep losing weight (that I don't want to lose). What's happening, and what can I do about it?

Weight loss is a common side effect of Parkinson's. In fact, in many cases, weight loss precedes motor symptoms and is considered an index for Parkinson's progression. There are various potential causes at play, such as overall malnutrition, increased energy output, decreased energy input, nausea or vomiting, and lack of appetite. If you have unwanted weight loss, the best thing to do is to talk to your physician about creating a plan to manage your caloric intake. Creating a meal plan to gain and then maintain your weight will vary by individual, but shakes, smoothies, avocados, nuts, and seeds are all simple ways to consider adding nutritional calories to your diet. If loss of smell is a problem for you, you can also consider using more spices to make your food taste better.

#7 – No matter what I do, I keep gaining weight. What's happening, and what can I do about it?

Weight gain is another common side effect that can occur from a decreased ability to exercise or as a result of gastric emptying, in which you may feel like you're uncontrollably gaining weight despite not eating much. The discrepancy may have to do with your body going into starvation mode as it tries to recalibrate your energy input and output. Again, the best course of action is to speak with your physician about a weight loss plan that aligns with your specific issues and goals. Also, you might consider an anti-inflammatory diet if you're suffering from weight gain associated with gastric emptying. (More on that below.)

If your weight gain seems to be associated with compulsive eating, a common impulse control disorder that dopamine agonists can cause, talk with your physician about managing or changing your medications or options for managing any compulsive eating behavior. For more about impulse control disorders and Parkinson's, see Chapter 5.

#8 – I told someone at my Parkinson's support group about the pains I have in my stomach, and she mentioned gastric emptying. What is it, and if that's my issue, what can I do about it?

Gastric emptying or gastroparesis relates to a delayed movement of food from the stomach to the intestines that can cause stomach pains, bloating, nausea, and feelings of uncomfortable fullness after only a bite or two of food. It's not known whether this condition is associated with Parkinson's itself or carbidopa/levodopa treatment. Still, whether it is or isn't, there are a few things you can do to address your symptoms. Try eating smaller but more frequent meals of easy-to-eat, anti-inflammatory foods, such as berries, leafy green vegetables, fatty fish, olive oil, nuts, and tomatoes. Limit caffeine, alcohol, grains, and dairy to see if this helps. Currently, there is no medication for gastric emptying that is compatible with people with Parkinson's, but you can talk to your physician and your registered dietician about other possible strategies and treatments.

#9 – Should I take supplements?

In general, it's best to get vitamins and minerals from the food you eat rather than through supplements. And while some research shows that supplemental vitamin D and calcium may be beneficial in promoting bone health, if bone thinning is an issue for you, there's much debate about that as well. The truth is, no supplements have been proven beneficial to Parkinson's.

Supplements or alternative medication compounds are not regulated by the FDA, meaning there is no external, unified oversight of the quality or consistency of the supplements you may find on the store shelf. Just because something is an "herbal preparation" or "natural compound" does not necessarily mean it is any safer than prescription medication. If you wish to take supplements, look for products that carry USP (United States Pharmacopeia) or similar verification for your home country. This independent laboratory tests the purity, potency, and bioavailability of products. In effect, this test ensures that what is on the bottle label is, indeed, what is contained in the pill or supplement. Otherwise, the actual purity and strength of the substance might differ from what the bottle label claims. Consumer Lab (⌾ consumerlab.com) tests different brand names and can provide you with similar information.

For your safety, always discuss potential interactions between supplements and your prescribed medication with your pharmacist and physician.

#10 – I've heard a lot about the benefits of drinking coffee lately. Is it beneficial for people with Parkinson's?

It is not clear whether there are any benefits to drinking coffee for people who have already been diagnosed with Parkinson's. Most of the recent research that has come out about coffee has to do with its ability to reduce the risk of developing diseases such as Parkinson's and Alzheimer's. Once you have already developed Parkinson's, its benefits are debatable.

Provided it doesn't irritate your stomach, coffee is okay to drink, but you should talk to your physician about any symptoms associated with drinking caffeine (for some people, it can be a bladder irritant or make their tremor worse). Coffee can help if you suffer from daytime sleepiness but consider having your last cup long before bedtime as caffeine late in the day can interfere with your sleep cycle if you're especially sensitive to it.

#11 – Can I drink alcohol?

There's no definite answer as to whether alcohol has any effect on the symptoms of Parkinson's; however, alcohol can interfere with the efficacy of certain prescription medications, so talk with your physician about how it might reduce the effectiveness of the medications you take.

Like caffeine, alcohol can be a bladder irritant for some people. If this is the case for you, avoiding alcohol may help alleviate urinary discomfort. Similarly, alcohol late at night may interfere with your sleep; if that is a problem for you, avoiding it may help you sleep better through the night.

#12 – I have terrible insomnia. Are there any nutritional choices I can make that might help me fall asleep and stay asleep longer?

Sleep issues are prevalent among people with Parkinson's. In fact, changes in sleeping habits are often among the first signs of Parkinson's. Fortunately, you can make changes to improve your ability to get the rest you need, as we explained earlier in this manual. When it comes to optimal nutrition for sleep, most physicians and dieticians recommend watching what you eat and when you eat it, limiting your fluid intake in the evenings (especially alcohol and coffee), and limiting your sugar intake. Try to avoid heavy meals before bed. A light snack consisting mainly of complex carbohydrates and a small amount of protein, such as cheese or peanut butter and crackers, is thought to help your brain produce serotonin and increase tryptophan. Carbohydrates cause the pancreas to release more insulin, which in turn helps tryptophan enter the brain. Valerian root and chamomile teas are both calming and touted to help sleep. (Of course, ask your physician before taking any supplement or herb.)

If you wish to explore sleep aids, discuss their use with your physician. And, if your poor sleep is a result of REM Sleep Behavior Disorder (RBD), be sure to speak with your physician and your care partner so you can get the help you need. Learn more about sleep and Parkinson's in Chapter 6.

#13 – Is there anything I can do with my nutritional choices to manage the side effects I experience from all the medications I take?

Depending on the side effects you experience, there may be ways to help minimize them with your diet. For example, if you experience nausea, eating bland foods like saltines and cold liquids may help, as can eating slowly and in small portions. Other foods and beverages that can help manage nausea include ginger (in root, candied, crystallized, or tea form) and starchy foods such as rice, toast, cereal, or oatmeal. Papaya, pineapple, yogurt, and peppermint tea can ease bloating and gastric upset.

Ask your physician to review which medications can be taken with food to reduce nausea. Drink plenty of water. If your physician encourages you to take vitamins or supplements, take them with dinner or at the end of the day, as these can cause nausea. Try grinding or crushing your meds and mixing them with fluids if approved by your physician.

Finally, if nausea and bloating persist due to medication, your physician may prescribe supplemental medication to treat these symptoms.

#14 – There's a lot of information out there about the link between the gut, brain, and inflammation in diseases such as Parkinson's and Alzheimer's. What's essential for me to know about it, and what are some of the healthiest anti-inflammatory foods I can eat? What food should I stay away from?

There is increasing evidence that there's an association between Parkinson's and gut health, though our absolute understanding of the connection remains incomplete. Studies have found lower levels of Prevotella, a "good" gut bacterium, in people with Parkinson's, along with higher levels of inflammatory bacteria. While more research is needed to understand the connection to Parkinson's, eating a diet rich in anti-inflammatory foods is generally found to be beneficial for your overall health, and there's no harm in including anti-inflammatory foods in your diet if you can tolerate them.

Some healthy anti-inflammatory foods include coconut oil (which contains medium-chain triglycerides) and fatty fish like salmon or tuna, dark leafy vegetables, tomatoes, nuts, certain spices, and soy. Curcumin, found in turmeric, is a potent anti-inflammatory compound. While probiotics do not contain the health-promoting gut bacteria missing in people with Parkinson's, some studies suggest that probiotics can help constipation in Parkinson's.

The top foods to stay away from if gut inflammation is a problem for you include refined carbohydrates, white bread and pastries, French fries, soda, red meat, and margarine.

#15 – Are there ways to help manage my lightheadedness through nutritional choices?

Eat smaller, more frequent meals, and reduce your consumption of alcohol and caffeine. Increase the number of other fluids you drink daily but be sure to talk with your physician if you have heart or kidney disease before increasing fluids or salt. You can try increasing salty and high electrolyte fluids, such as V8 juice, broths, and non-sugary sports drinks (avoid sugary drinks, especially if you have diabetes), if your physician gives you the okay for this experimentation (see Chapter 6 for more strategies).

#16 – I feel constant fatigue and sleepiness. How can food help minimize these symptoms?

Increase your fluid intake to prevent dehydration. Eat breakfast, and then and in all meals, pay attention to the amount or ratio of carbohydrates, proteins, and fat you are consuming. Aim for a balance of each of these food groups.

You may be tempted to snack on highly processed foods for energy, yet this can deplete your energy level. Simple sugars supply faster energy but can later lead to energy drain; the boosting effect of sugar lasts only 30 minutes. Instead, eat a balance of simple and complex carbohydrates. Healthy simple sugars for energy include fruits and honey. Complex sugars are found in whole wheat and grain products and starchy vegetables like peas and corn.

Eat smaller meals rather than big, heavy, and fatty meals. Focus on eating energy-boosting foods, such as almonds, walnuts, lentils, and oats. Drink caffeine (coffee, hot chocolate, tea) in the morning but avoid it later in the day. Finally, try chocolate! A small (one ounce) amount of low-sugar, dark chocolate can be an energy booster.

#17 – Are there foods that can help me fight anxiety and depression?

Certain foods have been shown to boost brain health and improve symptoms of certain mood disorders. These foods include dark chocolate, fatty fish, fermented foods, oats, berries, bananas, nuts and seeds, coffee, avocados, beans, and lentils. Avoid foods that can cause blood sugar spikes and crashes, such as sugary drinks and simple carbohydrates.

Alcohol has been found to make mood disorders like depression more severe, so talk with your physician and other care team members about its consumption if you experience depression or are taking antidepressant medications.

HOW TO VET FAD DIETS

In the Appendix, we'll take a close look at how to evaluate various Parkinson's resources, from studies to medications to therapies. Much of that advice can be taken when evaluating claims about diets and nutrition plans. Here, we'll share some signs that a diet may not be nutritionally or scientifically sound.

1. **It guarantees fast results.** Whether you're exploring a new diet plan to lose weight, gain weight, or simply feel your best, remember that it takes time to feel the effects from dietary changes. Don't get caught up in claims about losing 10 pounds in 10 days or feeling more energized within 24 hours of switching diets. Focus on the long game, remembering that living well with Parkinson's is a marathon, not a sprint.

2. **It severely limits the food you can eat.** A balanced diet is exactly that—balanced. If an eating plan requires you to cut out too many food groups, it's unlikely you will not be able to meet your body's nutritional needs through food. Be sure to work with your physician if you wish to explore a diet that sets strict limits on any one food group.

3. **It involves purchasing a certain product.** If you need to buy brand-name packaged foods, food kits, pills, beverages, or other products to benefit from a diet plan, think twice. There's a chance the company is just trying to profit when you could buy and prepare foods that meet the plan's nutritional values for much less money.

4. **Celebrities and public figures hype it.** A star who claims that a particular diet helps them stay healthy might be telling the truth, but they are also likely profiting from their role as spokesperson.

5. **It claims to be a one-size-fits-all plan.** We've said it before, but it's worth repeating here: different diets work for different people. It's true that for some people, eating a low-carb, keto diet makes them feel their best. Some people indeed feel best when eating a vegan diet, and some people feel the same no matter what they eat. Remembering this is key. Just because a trendy diet works well for someone you know doesn't mean it's right for you.

"As a Person Living with Parkinson's and a Registered Dietician, What Advice Do You Have for Using Nutrition to Live Well with Parkinson's"?

By Marty Acevedo, RD

I grew up in the South, where my favorite meals included fried chicken or pulled pork, green beans cooked all day with a bit of fatback for seasoning, banana pudding and pecan pie, and lots of sweet tea. As I learned more about nutrition in general in pursuit of my degree and, ultimately, my career as a registered dietitian, my personal "diet" began to change. A move to California solidified my commitment to a healthier lifestyle.

My diagnosis with young onset Parkinson's came at 44; like many people, I felt several symptoms preceding this diagnosis for at least a decade. I'm convinced that the internal tremor present for as long as I could remember played a role in maintaining a healthy weight. Perhaps, my "diet," based upon the then-popular Food Pyramid, along with my commitment to exercise, delayed the onset of symptoms.

Like most of us, my knowledge of Parkinson's was limited when I learned of my diagnosis in 2004. My education had provided limited insight into nutrition for Parkinson's, other than how protein intake might require modification around the timing of carbidopa/levodopa dosing.

Naturally, my science and medical background led me to research every aspect of Parkinson's, including nutrition. I quickly concluded that a lifestyle that included intake of fresh fruits and vegetables, lean meats and more fish, whole grains, lower-fat dairy products, and moderate intake of sweets and alcohol would continue to serve me well. While my research delved into other "diets," such as keto, paleo, gluten-free, vegan, intermittent fasting, and other meal plans, I knew that a Mediterranean, plant-based diet made the most sense for me. After all, this was not a significant change for me and is consistent with my lifelong mantra that there are no "bad" foods and that we should practice moderation in all things, including our nutritional intake.

I've always felt that we should get our nutrients from food, not from a pill or supplements. While supplements are warranted when deficiencies are identified, they are usually not necessary for most of us. Like in Parkinson's, there is much that we do not know and fully understand about nutrition. There may be beneficial substances in food that we've yet to identify. Those nutrients that we have identified work synergistically to provide us with all the tools necessary for our bodies to work and thrive. For example, the Mediterranean diet provides vitamins, minerals, fiber, carbs, protein, fat, and other nutrients necessary for each of us.

I'm fortunate to have benefited from exceptional care, including appropriate medication and deep brain stimulation (DBS) five years ago. While DBS gave me my life back, the procedure also resulted in unexpected weight gain, even though my diet did not change and I had begun to exercise more than I ever had. Likely, my resting energy expenditure diminished once that internal tremor and my dyskinesia were no longer present. But because I value the benefits of better managing my symptoms through DBS, I can certainly live with a higher number on that scale.

My outlook is that we are best served by adopting a healthy lifestyle rather than following a specific "diet" or worrying about our weight. To me, this means healthy, balanced meals that provide appropriate nutrients, identification of problematic foods (for example, I am lactose intolerant, so adjust my food choices accordingly), adequate intake of water and other liquids, and daily exercise.

While there is no particular "diet" universally recommended for Parkinson's, the Mediterranean diet and lifestyle include foods that act as antioxidants and are phytochemicals. Foods with these properties may well have a positive impact on the progression of Parkinson's, along with a potential neuroprotective effect. Further, adopting the lifestyle aspect of this way of eating—more relaxed, with fewer stressors, a renewed sense of acceptance and appreciation for life in general, and regular exercise—has enhanced and improved my journey in ways I never thought possible.

198

Living well with Parkinson's is truly a journey, and that journey is different for each of us. I'm beginning my seventeenth year of living well with Parkinson's and look forward to what's yet to come. I believe that the lifestyle I've chosen, along with a strong support team of clinicians, family, and friends and an equally strong sense of purpose in my life will allow me to continue to live my life well with Parkinson's.

About Marty Acevedo

Marty Acevedo was diagnosed with essential tremor in 2004 and with Parkinson's in 2010. She says that she experienced gait disturbance, dystonia, and REM sleep behavior disorder ten years before her diagnosis. After her progression through the grieving process, Marty decided that her diagnosis would not define her life. Marty felt called to help others who share this journey and quickly became involved with the Parkinson's Association of San Diego. Serving as secretary on the board of directors, she targeted her knowledge and passion towards educating others living with Parkinson's, encouraging exercise and socialization, and helping others to find their best life.

Marty is most proud of her involvement in developing and implementing an integrated, medically evidence-based program for people with Parkinson's at a local wellness center.

Marty is an avid traveler with her husband and their travel van, having covered 35 states and multiple national parks. Exercise, enjoying the ocean and beach, maintaining and cultivating new friendships, learning new things, and sharing her positive outlook are all vital to her daily life.

Living Well with Parkinson's

■ CHAPTER 12 – EMOTIONAL HEALTH

OVERVIEW

As you continue to learn, Parkinson's impacts your whole self. Therefore, attending to your emotional health is just as important as caring for your physical and mental health. In this chapter, we'll share ways to stay present, to view obstacles as opportunities, to ask for help when it's needed, to give back, and to build self-care and compassion into your daily life.

> **"** *I have no doubt that my attitude strongly correlates to my emotional health on any given day. So, I focus on an attitude of gratitude! This foundation keeps any struggles in perspective and opens the door to a daily dose of joy."*
>
> — LORRAINE WILSON

THE MIND-BODY CONNECTION

What was once a philosophical discussion is now an emerging area of healthcare called mind-body medicine. Specialists who practice mind-body medicine share the belief that thoughts and emotions influence healing and well-being. Rather than viewing the brain and body as separate entities, this philosophy views them as linked together to form each person's unique existence.

Western medicine often focuses on the physical body and emphasizes quick treatments with pills or surgery—ignoring the impact that emotions, mind, and spirit have on the healing process. Health and wellness are optimized when equal attention is given to each of these areas.

> **"** *"Parkinson's has been a blessing for me. It made me realize my strength, courage, and confidence. Not everyone with Parkinson's will agree, but this is why each journey is unique."*
>
> — GRETCHEN WHITE

Many believe our minds have a critical role in healing. This is understood all too well by people who experience tremor. An increase in life stress is often directly tied to an increase in tremor. Relaxation, in turn, can reduce tremor.

The "power of the mind" is so important that modern-day scientific studies are designed with this mind-body connection in mind. For instance, medication studies are designed to compare a medication's effect to a placebo or sugar pill. Simply wishing, expecting, or believing that a treatment will work increases the likelihood that it will. Recent attention has been paid to the influence of the placebo effect on clinical trials related explicitly to Parkinson's.

Examples of techniques that focus on the mind-body connection include:

- Biofeedback
- Cognitive behavioral therapy
- Hypnosis
- Feldenkrais Method
- Breathing techniques
- Meditation and guided imagery
- Relaxation techniques and stress reduction
- Yoga therapy and laughter yoga
- Spiritual practice such as prayer or chanting

Later in this chapter, we'll discuss many of these techniques and how they can help you live well every day. No matter what you choose, the important thing to remember is that how you think affects how you feel, and how you feel affects how you think. Your mind, therefore, can have a positive effect on your body. Find activities that bring you joy, meaning, and a sense of calm. Do them often and pay attention to how they positively impact your whole self.

> *If I had a heart attack and didn't consult a cardiologist, people would think I was crazy. If I knew I had Parkinson's and didn't consult a neurologist, you'd think I was crazy. If I'm having mental health issues and don't consult a psychologist or psychiatrist, is that wise? No. We'll seek health for just about anything else, which tells me that we have a poor response to our own mental health because it's terrifying."*
>
> — TIM HAGUE

HOW SUNLIGHT CAN BOOST YOUR MOOD

The human body was built to work in partnership with the sun. Its light can transform our moods, focus, sleep, energy levels, immune systems, bone density, and mental health. As a result, spending time in the sun can be particularly beneficial to people living with Parkinson's who experience symptoms like depression, apathy, poor sleep, pain, and fatigue.

When the sun's ultraviolet light is absorbed through your skin, your body produces vitamin D, and vitamin D, in turn, promotes the production of serotonin. Serotonin, in turn, produces feelings of happiness and well-being. Like dopamine, the chemical messenger impacted by Parkinson's, serotonin is a neurotransmitter that helps brain cells and other nervous system cells communicate. Serotonin helps regulate mood and helps you feel emotionally stable. In other words, like dopamine, serotonin helps you feel good. And when you feel good, you are more likely to take actions that help you live well with Parkinson's, such as exercising, connecting with others, and staying involved in your community.

> " *For me, living well with Parkinson's means facing adversity with grace, gratitude, and grit. That means rising above circumstance to a greater purpose, deeper meaning, and a soulful journey along the way. And by sharing this with others, together, we make the world a little brighter!"*
>
> — KAREN FRANK

Sunlight and its impacts on serotonin can also help improve your quality of sleep. Serotonin production is triggered not only when your skin absorbs sunlight but also when sunlight hits your eyes. The sunlight sends cues to specific areas of the retina that trigger the release of serotonin. Serotonin plays a vital role in mood, focus, and sleep; it is the precursor for melatonin, the hormone that makes you feel sleepy when darkness falls. Time in the sun, therefore, helps regulate your sleep-wake cycle and can lead to better sleep.

Spending time in the sun also encourages your body to produce beta-endorphins. These hormones cause a feeling of well-being, strengthen your immune system, relieve pain, increase alertness, reduce depression, and more.

Even short periods outdoors can bring countless benefits. According to the World Health Organization, getting just 15 minutes a day of natural sunlight can reduce stress and anxiety and may help you sleep better at night. Are you looking to boost the benefits even more? While you're soaking up the sun, get moving. Bring a friend. Pick up trash. Tend a garden. Volunteer. And watch how your life, so linked with the sun, is transformed.

NOTE: People with Parkinson's are at greater risk for developing melanoma. If you plan on being outside for a while, apply sunscreen once the rays have touched your skin for at least 15-20 minutes.

GET OUTSIDE

Just as the human body was built to work in partnership with the sun, we are also meant to be outside. As Florence Williams details in her book *The Nature Fix*, being outdoors in natural spaces makes us happier, healthier, more creative, more empathetic, and more apt to engage with the world and with each other.

Furthermore, George MacKerron, an economist at the University of Sussex and developer of the Happiness study, discovered through his work that one of the most significant variables that contribute to happiness is not who you're with or what you're doing. It's where you are. On average, people are happier outdoors in green and natural habitats than outdoor urban environments. So, to the extent that it's possible to surround yourself in green, it would be worth it to do so.

> " *One of my greatest joys as an Ambassador is to help others live well today. That includes promoting physical activity and ways to strengthen one's social, emotional, and spiritual wellness.*"
>
> — LORRAINE WILSON

While spending time in the natural outdoors may be easier for some than others, there are actions all of us can take, no matter where we live, to bring more of the green outdoors into our lives.

Here are just a few of the ways:

- Spend an hour a day digging, planting, and weeding in your garden
- Take your shoes off and let your feet touch the ground, the grass, the earth
- Practice yoga barefoot in the grass
- Take a blanket to the nearest park and have a picnic with your favorite person
- Take a walk outside first thing in the morning and touch (or hug) a few trees
- Park a mile from your destination and walk the rest of the way while examining all the trees, clouds, and flowers you see
- Read a book on a park bench
- Bring the outdoors in by growing herbs on your windowsill and putting plants in every room of your house
- Walk, run, or ride a different route to work every day
- Collect items from your outdoor travels and use them to create art or bring more of the outside in
- Swim in an outdoor body of water and feel it, listen to it, and smell it with all your might
- Find a sacred outdoor space to call home and return to it each time you need a nature fix (This could be a specific bench in a park, a flower bed with your favorite smells, a tree that reminds you of home, a pond where you can hear the frogs...)
- Invite someone to your favorite outdoor spot and make a memory

- Stargaze while nestled in a blanket on your deck or on the grass
- Go on the hunt for dirt roads and the nooks and crannies they lead to
- Eat farm-to-table whenever you get the chance
- Learn a new outdoor activity
- Visit a botanical garden in your area or go to the zoo
- Or anything else you can dream up

HOW MUCH TIME OUTDOORS IS ENOUGH?

Tanya Denckla Cobb, an environmental public policy mediator, has a tool for that. She calls it the Nature Pyramid. It's like the FDA's food pyramid, but this one has a recommended daily allowance for the amount and types of outdoor experiences we need to have for a healthy life.

Beatley writes, "we are hard-wired from evolution to need and want contact with nature. To have a healthy life, emotionally and physically, requires this contact. The empirical evidence of this is overwhelming: exposure to nature lowers our blood pressure, lowers stress and alters mood in positive ways, enhances cognitive functioning, and in many ways makes us happy. Exposure to nature is one of the key foundations of a meaningful life."

Now's the time. Get on out there!

GIVING BACK TO LIVE WELL WITH PARKINSON'S

"The best way to find yourself," Gandhi said, "is to lose yourself in the services of others."

When we ask people in our community what they do to live well, the vast majority say that giving back is at the top of their list. Whether they give back by leading support groups, creating community programs, participating in clinical trials, educating themselves so they can educate others, or raising money for Parkinson's, giving back gives them a purpose and helps them connect with others.

Evidence shows that giving back can reduce stress while improving happiness and mood. In 2020, the Cleveland Clinic reported that health benefits associated with giving back include lower blood pressure, increased self-esteem, less depression, lower stress levels, longer life, and greater happiness and satisfaction. "When you look at the functional MRIs of subjects who gave to various charities, scientists have found that giving stimulates the mesolimbic pathway, which is the reward center in the brain—releasing endorphins and creating what is known as the 'helper's high,'" the report says.

You can also experience a "warm glow" when giving back. In a 2006 report from the National Institutes of Health, researchers explain how studies show that "when people give to charities, it activates regions of the brain associated with pleasure, social connection, and trust, creating a 'warm glow' effect."

> *I can honestly say that aspects of my life have changed for the better because of Parkinson's. We can dwell on the negative, but how does that make life better? Parkinson's has given me a sense of purpose to give back to the community, the Parkinson's community, and the community at large. I've been so inspired by others whose efforts have made me, my family, and the world we live in a better place. This has encouraged me to do my part for others."*

— STEVE HOVEY

Acts of kindness can help you stay active, social, and connected, three critical components to living well with Parkinson's. Social scientists and psychologists believe that giving promotes social connection—when you give, you are more likely to receive. This belief in reciprocity builds "a sense of trust and cooperation that strengthens our ties to others," according to the University of California, Berkeley's *Greater Good* magazine. "Research has shown that having positive social interactions is central to good mental and physical health."

Giving back also allows you to put your struggles and worries in perspective, which can boost your feelings of gratitude and optimism. A 2017 study from Cambridge University underscores this idea, finding that participants in a three-week study who engaged more by helping others (as opposed to sharing and receiving support for their problems) felt decreased levels of depression and increased feelings of gratitude. Marianna Pogosyan, PhD, says this is because "when helping others navigate their stressful situations, we are enhancing our emotion regulation skills, and thus, benefiting our emotional well-being."

HOW CAN YOU GIVE BACK?

Acts of kindness can be large or small, ongoing or one-time moments. Calling a friend, donating to a food bank, participating in a tree-planting project, ringing a bell for charity, cuddling puppies at a shelter—these and countless other activities can brighten someone else's day and your own as well.

> *Don't sit at home idle. Get involved and be an advocate for your condition."*

— MICHELLE LANE

Feeling inspired and want some ideas on how to give back, especially to your Parkinson's community? Here are three ideas you could get started on today:

Advocate

How does advocacy help people with Parkinson's? It not only increases awareness of Parkinson's, but it also builds community and creates the opportunity for people to solve problems together. By being involved at the local, state, and national levels, you can influence funding decisions and policy, healthcare, and the research needed to find a cure.

Lead a Support Group

Don't have a Parkinson's support group in your community, or don't have one that's an ideal fit for you? Create one! Shape it in a way that speaks to you, whether that means it's online, a come-as-you-are meeting, a "Parkinson's Happy Hour," a Parkinson's book club, a walk-and-talk meetup, or anything else that comes to mind and suits your needs and goals.

> *I am learning that when I help others, my own problems diminish in significance. This has been especially the case with leading a support group for a small number of women with Parkinson's. Each of them has her own set of challenges, and it has been rewarding to watch a bond of trust develop between the six of us. We are all so different – with different past careers, symptoms, ages, medications, and attitudes. Yet to watch the six care for each other, speaking words of life, and carrying each other's burdens bring me joy. I have come to love these women."*

— PATTI BURNETT

Educate

Getting people to understand Parkinson's isn't easy. Stereotypes, misunderstandings, healthcare, and the media have done an excellent job of misrepresenting or stigmatizing people with Parkinson's ever since it was first recognized as a disease. While it is not your job as a person with Parkinson's to teach everyone you interact with about Parkinson's (how exhausting!), finding people who are open, kind, and patient and sharing your story with them is a step toward creating a more inclusive environment. Authentic conversations about Parkinson's can create meaningful change. So, the next time you're in a situation where you feel frustrated because others don't understand you, if you have the desire and energy, go ahead and teach them a little something.

Now, what about taking care of your own mind? Some people benefit greatly from meeting with a counselor regularly or having a rich spiritual life.

COUNSELING

Counseling can be helpful even before things become overwhelming. Just as it is important to address physical health issues early, it is equally important to address the emotional and psychological impact of living with Parkinson's soon after diagnosis. Trying to manage your symptoms, avoid complications, and live with a chronic disease can drain both you and your family or care partner. Support, knowledge, understanding of available resources, and knowing where you can turn for help are some of the best defenses to avoid feeling overwhelmed and burned out.

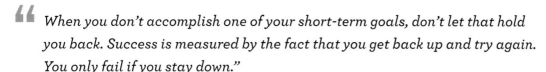

> *"When you don't accomplish one of your short-term goals, don't let that hold you back. Success is measured by the fact that you get back up and try again. You only fail if you stay down."*
>
> — EDIE ANDERSON

Counseling can help you, your family, and your relationships. Some of the types of counseling available to you include:

- **Individual Counseling.** Many people find it easiest to deal with emotional issues by working with a counselor individually. In this setting, you can discuss any concerns you have in a private, one-on-one session.

- **Group Counseling.** Group counseling can provide a social outlet for individuals who are experiencing similar problems. In this type of counseling, individuals with similar problems form a group with a counselor to discuss their problems together. This type of counseling differs from community support groups in that the counselor helps facilitate the discussion and directs proactive outcomes. It is sometimes easier to gain insights and identify positive coping strategies when learned through others' experiences.

- **Relationship and Family Counseling.** Parkinson's can be difficult for you, your care partner, and your family. Many times, when the spouse becomes the care partner, the relationship dynamics change. The goal of relationship counseling is to provide a safe place for communication and honesty. This, in turn, may help to redirect time and energy to the quality of the relationship.

SPIRITUALITY AND PERSONAL BELIEFS

Your culture, upbringing, values, and religious or spiritual beliefs directly affect your health and well-being. For some, spiritual solace is their most significant source of guidance and support. Many people with Parkinson's say that their religion or spiritual connections help keep them grounded and hopeful. Studies have proven the healing effect of prayer and the importance of religious and spiritual connections in surviving with conditions such as cancer and AIDS. Some people turn to their religious community as a source of support and guidance. Others may find spiritual connection at a different level, such as with nature or through meditation or social activism.

Your personal and cultural beliefs surrounding healing are also important parts of your well-being. Entire systems of care exist—some with a history steeped in cultural traditions, such as Native American medicine, Ayurvedic medicine, and Chinese medicine. For instance, acupuncture is used in combination with traditional medicine to treat mood disorders, tremor, pain, and gastrointestinal problems. These ancient healing systems of care can complement standard Western medical treatments. For more information about these and other complementary therapies, jump back to Chapter 10.

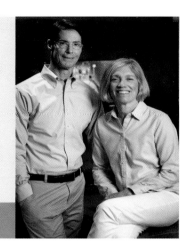

> **"** *For us, our faith is important. It gives me another aspect of community that I wouldn't have otherwise, and it's where we get our strength. You're not in control of most things that happen in life, Parkinson's being one of them. This is what we've been given. We move forward with God to lean on, and it gets us through the tough times."*

— NANCY HOVEY

"What Do I Need to Do to Live Well?"

By Davis Phinney

When I was first diagnosed with Parkinson's, my foundation for living well was exercise. As a professional athlete, that's what I knew, and it was my bedrock. More than 21 years into this journey with Parkinson's, though, the role exercise plays in my view of living well has changed. Now, it's an integral part of my day, rather than the focus of it. I do it for the physical benefits and what it facilitates—better sleep, more energy, appetite, and a positive mood.

The one thing that has remained constant for me in my approach to Parkinson's is my philosophy: celebrate the little victories. I say this with conviction—not only to you but often, to myself—because Parkinson's so frequently can dampen your enthusiasm for life. It's vital to be able to acknowledge when you've experienced something good. You've got to stop to see it, to "chalk it up." I don't always mark those occasions by raising my arms up in victory like I did when I was a cyclist, but I do make a point of pausing long enough to recognize it.

I try to be conscious of these victory moments. Even something as simple as taking joy in reading a funny essay or feeling the warmth in a hug from my wife or watching one of my kids compete in a sporting event is cause for celebration.

Before Parkinson's, I spent a good amount of my day thinking about the past or things yet to come, obscuring the present moment. Today, I'm much better at bringing myself back to the moment at hand and letting worries or fears pass by. When I do, I'm able to appreciate and celebrate my moments of victory as they unfold.

I make a conscious point of not dwelling on negative thoughts. For me, anxiety is best managed by being present in my thoughts and actions as much as possible throughout the day. Instead of lamenting what I can't do or how things have changed, this approach frees me to see and savor the joy that occurs in so many ways throughout the day. Put my socks on while standing up? That's a victory. Rode my bike for coffee with friends? Another victory. Got in a few ski runs on fresh powder? Definitely a victory. The occasions may not be momentous themselves, but I believe that *every victory counts!*

"How Can Being Mindful Help Me Live Well with Parkinson's?"

By Davis Phinney

Meditation may sound like something only for monks or mystics, but it isn't so different from other training we do for Parkinson's, like physical or speech therapy. In all instances, we're trying to gain control of our thoughts and encourage ourselves to respond in a certain way that we've predetermined. Sometimes that response is to "do nothing" or watch the thoughts pass through our mind without reacting or judging. Sometimes the response is to calm rising anxiety and slow down our breathing. Gaining control in any sense takes practice, just like it takes practice to walk in new ways or to swing your arms when they no longer want to swing naturally.

They say mindfulness—or focusing entirely on the "here and now"—is a form of meditation. Living with Parkinson's, I'm forced to be more mindful of the present moment. Things that were once automatic are not automatic anymore. I can't just hop out of my car and run up a flight of stairs without hesitation. I need to see the stairs, focus my concentration on the task at hand, and then climb them with purpose. That's mindfulness. I have put my attention in the moment to accomplish the task.

My dedicated practice is like a form of training for my mind that helps make these moments of practical mindfulness come more easily throughout the day and my various activities. Extending that basic concept of mindfulness into other areas of life is a form of meditation.

For me, mindfulness ebbs and flows throughout the day. While I do set aside time at the beginning and end of each day to practice intentional meditation, it's really throughout the day that I can see the benefits of those dedicated practices, not during the practice itself. Meditation can be spiritual, or it can be secular. How you approach it has much to do with your worldview and what you hope to get out of the experience.

Meditative practices and mindfulness, in general, help me specifically to calm my overloaded Parkinson's mind. Five years ago, if I had ten things to do during my day, I would have become overloaded with distractions and suffered brain freeze. Now, I find that it's become much easier. First, I appreciate how anxious Parkinson's can make me, so I know that I need to counteract that somehow. Second, by practicing mindfulness, I have learned how to quiet my mind and focus on accomplishing one thing at a time before I turn to something else. This might sound simplistic, but it works for me. I find that I can get through whatever tasks the day holds with less stress and more ease.

I don't know if people who don't have a Parkinson's-affected brain can fully understand the anxiety and feelings of overwhelm that rush in when, as a person with Parkinson's, you're faced with an extensive menu of choices. It's like your brain freezes, wondering what you're going to decide. In situations like this, mindfulness helps me sort out, prioritize, and complete tasks or make choices. The better I understand anxiety and how it takes root in my mind, the less I'm carried away by the anxious thought process. Going into a social situation if I'm tired after a long day of flexing my brain and my vocal cords, if my voice quality is poor and my thought process is muddy, is a sure recipe for anxiety. But if I've planned my day right and managed my schedule so that I show up to a dinner party rested and with a bit of reserve in the tank, I am much better equipped to handle a challenging social situation. When I put the components in place that help me be mindful, organize my thoughts, and manage my energy, I have a great foundation to handle and enjoy that dinner party or any other social situation.

Meditation and mindfulness take practice, intention, and work. Sometimes people tell me, "I don't have time," or, "I can't quiet my brain." Just start where you are today, and begin training every day. Pretty soon, you'll start seeing the fruits of your labor, and it will get easier. When mindfulness begins to come more naturally, you'll appreciate how many times throughout the day you rely on this simple technique to clear your mind and live well.

About Davis Phinney

As an Olympic Bronze medalist and Tour de France stage winner, Davis Phinney has celebrated the most victories of any cyclist in American history. After nearly 20 years in professional cycling, he launched a successful second career as a television network sportscaster. In 2000, after years of feeling not quite right and a seemingly endless battery of tests, he was diagnosed with young onset Parkinson's at age 40.

Today, as the founder of the Davis Phinney Foundation, he is a passionate and outspoken role model for living well with Parkinson's. He speaks to thousands of people with Parkinson's every year through his work with the Foundation.

»

Davis' journey, learning to redefine victory post-Parkinson's, serves as a powerful example for others living with the disease. Though the day-to-day challenges of Parkinson's are always present, he practices what he preaches and encourages others to join him in getting up, getting out, and being active each day, savoring the Moments of Victory® as they come. Davis lives in Colorado with his wife, Connie Carpenter Phinney, and is the proud father of two grown children, Taylor and Kelsey.

"How Can I Manage my Emotional Health?"

By Joanne Hamilton, PhD, ABPP-CN

Living well with Parkinson's starts with addressing the health of the body and the mind. In the past ten years, there has been heightened focus by researchers and healthcare providers on the non-motor symptoms of Parkinson's. We now realize that depression, anxiety, suspicion, hallucinations, and aggression affect a large percentage of the people we serve. Moreover, we now recognize that these symptoms, not tremor, not rigidity, and not motor slowness, cause the most significant distress among people living with Parkinson's. They are also a common reason for a move out of the home and into a care community.

Too often, healthcare professionals fail to assess for emotional symptoms of Parkinson's. There are many reasons for this. Some providers do not realize that serious psychological issues—including depression, anxiety, and hallucinations—affect millions of individuals living with Parkinson's. Some providers may not feel comfortable asking questions about intimidating topics like suicide or irrational thoughts. Some providers mistakenly believe that you will spontaneously bring these issues up. Our failure as providers to ask challenging questions perpetuates the stigma that these symptoms of Parkinson's are unusual, or worse, unimportant.

Neither is true.

WHEN TO SPEAK UP

We are slowly getting this word out to providers and people living with Parkinson's. But like with most aspects of healthcare, being your own advocate is critical. It is essential to recognize when emotional symptoms need to be addressed. First, it is natural to feel some sadness, worry, and grief related to the challenges of Parkinson's. However, when sadness and loss of pleasure start to interfere with your day, your desire to get out of bed, or your relationships with your family, it is time to speak up. If feelings of worry, fear, and dread are continuously rolling in your head, making it hard to sleep or eat and keeping you from relaxing, it is time to speak up. If you are bothered by visions that others cannot see or thoughts that others do not share, it is time to speak up. If you are spending more time thinking about death and suicide, if you plan to end your life or start to settle your affairs, it is time to speak up.

How? You may be embarrassed to tell someone about your experiences. That is understandable because these are tough topics. Making an appointment with your healthcare provider is an excellent place to start. Telling your provider that you have been bothered by difficult thoughts can start the conversation.

Describe in your own words what you are experiencing. Do not be concerned if you do not know the "lingo." Be open about the frequency and severity of the problems. You are not being judged, you are not "crazy," and you are not alone. Remember, 30% or more of the Parkinson's community experience these same problems. A comprehensive evaluation can significantly improve your quality of life.

MANAGING YOUR EMOTIONAL HEALTH

Medication

There are many ways to manage these symptoms and promote good emotional health and wellness. Your healthcare provider may suggest medication, especially if the problems are becoming dangerous. Many people have misconceptions about how these drugs work, so it is important to have a collaborative relationship with your physician. Tell your physician what concerns you about these medications. Are you worried that they are addictive, that they will affect your motor symptoms, or that they will change your personality? Ask your physician what you should expect from the medications. Remember, antidepressants can take four to six weeks, on average, to reach their full effectiveness. Discuss the benefits and potential risks of the medications. Realize that there are many classes of medications, each with its pros and cons. There is even a new type of medication to treat hallucinations and unusual thoughts that may not affect your motor symptoms. In some cases, your healthcare provider might not feel that they have enough expertise in these emotional matters to develop an optimal treatment plan; so, they might ask you to visit a mental health specialist. I encourage you to request this consultation if you have questions about your treatment plan. This is how you start to develop a solid wellness team.

Talk Therapy

Medication is not the only treatment path for serious emotional issues. There are well-validated methods of talk therapy that can treat depression and anxiety as effectively as medication. Cognitive behavioral therapy, Acceptance and Commitment Therapy, and Interpersonal Therapy are each proven to improve emotional functioning.

> *Once you tell others about your diagnosis, you are free to heal. Until then, it's like a big secret—although most people probably already know something is wrong—and you spend your energy holding that secret. Once you open up about your Parkinson's diagnosis, you can fight it with the support of others in your life."*
>
> — JILL ATER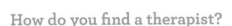

How do you find a therapist?

Ask your physicians, ask your spiritual leader, or ask your friends. ⬈ WebMD.com has an excellent article entitled "How to Find a Therapist" that explains the difference between all the different mental health providers and offers strategies to find one in your area and for your needs. Do not be afraid to "interview" your therapist because you must find one whom you feel understands you and with whom you can have a meaningful, collaborative relationship.

Physical Activity

As we've explained throughout this manual, exercise is essential for promoting emotional (and physical and cognitive) health and wellness. The Physical Activity Guidelines Advisory Committee from the Department of Health and Human Services (2008) concluded that exercise can protect against the harmful effects of stress, minimize the risk of developing anxiety and depression, and enhance emotional well-being. Since then, numerous studies have shown that exercise is as effective as antidepressants for some people who experience depression. As we've stated before (and will state again and again, because it's so important!), find exercises you love and do them regularly.

Social Activity

Social involvement can enhance mood, reduce stress, and prevent boredom. As isolation increases, so does the risk of major depressive disorders and anxiety. People may become more isolated because they have stopped driving, feel embarrassed about their motor symptoms, have trouble with speech, or have moved to a new community. COVID-19 dramatically worsened social isolation for everyone, including people managing Parkinson's, and movement disorder specialists found that in people with Parkinson's, motor symptoms, cognitive symptoms, and behavioral challenges worsened during the pandemic. Our experiences during this exceptional period highlight the fact that humans are social animals and that lack of interaction impacts our entire system.

> *There is nothing quite like living with COVID to reinforce the value of community. While Zoom has made a dent in my desire for connection, there is nothing quite like in-person meetings and classes. Most of us have experienced the bonds that are formed by seeing people regularly. It is often said that every*

213

Parkinson's-related class becomes a mini support group and that the enduring connections may be more important than the content delivered. Being with people with Parkinson's motivates me to keep going, even when my energy level may be lagging."

— RICH WILDAU

Stress Management

We all need to think about our emotional well-being and the harmful effects of stress on our bodies and minds. Not all of us manage stress exceptionally well. Fortunately, there are stress management techniques you can learn. Many larger healthcare organizations now include Integrative Medicine departments that can help you get started. There are opportunities to practice mindfulness, prayer, meditation, tai chi, yoga, and belly breathing in the community. And never underestimate the power of laughter, especially when you share your laughter with someone who may need a good laugh, too.

Parkinson's is a challenging condition that affects the whole self. Taking a proactive and positive approach to all the symptoms of Parkinson's will improve your quality of life and emotional well-being. In the same way you would address your tremor if it started to interfere with your eating, why not address your emotional symptoms when they start interfering with your sleep, appetite, relationships, activities, and general quality of life?

214

About Joanne Hamilton

Joanne Hamilton is the director of adult neuropsychology at Advanced Neurobehavioral Health of Southern California and resident neuropsychologist at the Parkinson's Disease and Movement Disorders Center at Scripps Clinic. Dr. Hamilton received her bachelor's degree from Stanford University and her doctorate in clinical psychology with a specialization in neuropsychology from the San Diego State University/University of California, San Diego joint doctoral program in clinical psychology.

She completed her postdoctoral fellowship at the University of California, Shiley-Marcos Alzheimer's Disease Research Center and was licensed to practice neuropsychology in 2003.

»

Dr. Hamilton became a diplomat in clinical neuropsychology from the American Board of Professional Psychology in 2010. She was a research neuroscientist at the Shiley-Marcos Alzheimer's Disease Research Center, studying cognitive changes associated with Lewy body spectrum disorders, including Parkinson's and Dementia with Lewy bodies, until 2012.

"How Can I Manage the Shame I Feel about What Parkinson's Is Doing to Me?"

By Steve Emerson, MA

It is indeed a rare and unusual human being who has not experienced shame at some point in their life. More often than not, shame manifests itself as feeling "less than" or embarrassment due to an event or action, usually in a social or interpersonal context. For example, one might legitimately feel shame in their community if they were caught shoplifting, and it is made public. Other forms of shame are not necessarily illegitimate but result from the fear of being perceived as unable to meet certain expectations. This is precisely the type of shame people living with Parkinson's are likely to experience.

CAUSES OF SHAME

As someone living with Parkinson's, feelings of shame can be common. You may fumble for your wallet in a busy checkout line or have difficulty handling utensils in an upscale restaurant. You may be unable to enunciate your words with friends in a conversation. Maybe you used to excel on the golf course and can no longer achieve the balance necessary to even stand over the golf ball. You may have been the primary breadwinner for your family and are now unable to work in your chosen profession due to debilitating fatigue or other Parkinson's symptoms. Your difficulty with physical movement may force you to change how you engage in intimacy with your spouse or partner.

I've experienced shame in every single one of these situations after being diagnosed with Parkinson's. Even after spending years as a professional counselor with deep working knowledge about shame, I wasn't prepared for how once shame sets in, my stress level skyrockets, and the very Parkinson's symptoms causing me shame in the first place go from bad to worse.

The good news is that shame can be made fleeting and insignificant. And this isn't only for those of us living with Parkinson's, but for anyone experiencing embarrassment or other stress-producing emotions simply because of how we believe we are being perceived. You see, the common thread that is always present when shame rears its ugly head is fear. And fear can only survive in an environment of silence. Fear-based shame is rarely discussed in an open, candid, and authentic setting. But when it is, something magical happens. The monster under the bed gets exposed, and we experience freedom. This is the primary reason I rarely miss an opportunity to let people know I am living with Parkinson's and offer to answer any questions they may have. Almost immediately, I feel something that is quite the opposite of shame, and that feeling is a sense of empowerment.

MOVING FROM SHAME TO EMPOWERMENT

There are many tools available to change shame to empowerment. These include support groups, self-education, open conversations with loved ones, and volunteering for an organization devoted to helping folks with Parkinson's live great lives like the Davis Phinney Foundation. Look, I get it; for many of us, these require action and aren't necessarily easy to do. But if the goal is to end the silence, then noise needs to be made! For some of us, it may be speaking in front of a large group at a conference. For others, it may be a quiet conversation with your spouse. Even your choice to read this *Every Victory Counts* manual is a start; this book is crammed with tools to convert shame to empowerment. If a 1,000-mile journey starts with a single step, then it is an excellent step to take. Take yours now.

216

About Steve Emerson

Steve Emerson was diagnosed with Parkinson's in 2007 at the age of 49. A former mental health therapist and current professional Christian life coach, Steve routinely meets with individuals and families living with Parkinson's and serves as a guest speaker for various organizations and events on the topic of living well with Parkinson's. For Steve, living well begins with attitude, and the building blocks of maintaining a strong, positive attitude include "exercise, good nutrition, prayer, and getting into the stream of life, even when I don't feel like doing so."

"I have come to learn that the more I give, the more I get," Steve says. "I hope to become increasingly able to educate and support those living with Parkinson's, their care partners, and the community at large that it is entirely possible to live a full, enriching, and wonderful life not only with Parkinson's, but with any of life's obstacles that may arise."

"What Role Can Spiritual Practice Play in Living Well with Parkinson's?"

By Rabbi Rena Arshinoff, PhD, BCC

Body, mind, and spirit are human components that are intertwined. The concept of spirituality is complex and sometimes used interchangeably with religion, yet religion refers to an institutionalized set of dogma, practices, and rituals of a particular faith. Spirituality does not; instead, it is about well-being, one's sense of wholeness, connection to others, and the search for one's place in the universe. For some people, spirituality includes religion, but not for all. Everyone has a personal spirituality, but people living with a chronic illness can, understandably, overlook their sense of wholeness and connection and focus on physical symptoms and medications. Spiritual care, therefore, must be given special attention.

The Hebrew word "shalom" means peace. Another word from the same root is "shalem," which means wholeness. Wholeness is experienced by the many gifts life offers, such as love, friendship, morality, contributions, and shared ideas. Together, shalom (peace) and shalem (wholeness) bring contentment to our lives. Easier said than done with Parkinson's.

The Webster-Merriam dictionary defines "body image" as "a subjective picture of one's own physical appearance established both by self-observation and by noting the reactions of others." How we look affects our sense of self; how we feel about ourselves influences our identity and quality of life. Body image in Parkinson's has a powerful influence on one's sense of dignity and wholeness. People may struggle with their identity wondering, "Who am I now?" and questioning their value as physical symptoms change or appear. In his book *Facing Illness, Finding God*, Joseph Meszler wrote: "Even this new person in the mirror we do not want to accept has meaning and value to God." People living with Parkinson's may wonder if they are being "punished" by God or may express anger at God and sometimes feel guilty about having such thoughts. It is acceptable to be angry at God.

Spirituality for some people does not include God. For some, spirituality may come from the outdoors or a world cause. Whatever it means for you, spirituality is important in living with Parkinson's, a condition that entails losses on many levels that need to be grieved. Loss is accompanied by suffering, and suffering can be accepted through spirituality if not completely explained. In his book about his time spent in concentration camps during World War II, *Man's Search for Meaning*, Viktor Frankl wrote about the meaning of suffering:

> *We must never forget that we may also find meaning in life even when confronted with a hopeless situation when facing a fate that cannot be changed. For what then matters is to bear witness to*

the uniquely human potential at its best, which is to transform a personal tragedy into a triumph, to turn one's predicament into a human achievement."

Can one turn the predicament of living with Parkinson's into a human achievement? Without a known cure for Parkinson's, you may feel disconnected and lost at times. Talk and think often about important roles you have had and still have. Grieve your losses, and feel your sadness, anger, worry, or jealousy. A Jewish concept teaches, "Do not separate yourself from the community," — remain involved with your community and in your world. Go to day programs, exercise programs, and activities that involve being with others. Isolation is the first step to social withdrawal, so it is important not to let it happen. Friendship is an essential spiritual experience that brings wholeness to all parties involved; maintain friendships because they are so very fulfilling. For some, attending religious services brings joy and contact with others. It may be challenging to get to a service or, once there, hard to stay for an entire service. If so, have members of the religious community visit you at home. Asking for a session with clergy or a counselor can bring profound insight as you speak about topics challenging to share with family.

Some people with Parkinson's worry about being a burden to their family; this can cause great spiritual angst. Meszler asks this question: would we consider God to be a burden? As you are an image of God, you are not a burden. He writes, "You are a creation of God, capable of inspiring others. You have a unique perspective on life that is worth sharing." Others living with Parkinson's benefit from sharing with you, just as you benefit from them.

Remember that spirituality is an important element of living well with Parkinson's. Your sense of spirituality can be expressed and honored in many ways, but it almost certainly involves love and gratitude for the people in your life. Express to loved ones your appreciation for their help and love, and express your frustrations. Martin Buber spoke of the space in relationships where trust and sharing occur: this space is where we find the Divine. Sharing both your love and your sorrow, your joys, and your concerns with those important to you will help bring them and you shalem (wholeness) at the same time.

About Rena Arshinoff

Rena Arshinoff obtained her nursing training in Montreal. She completed a Master of Health Science degree in epidemiology at the University of Toronto and worked for 20 years in clinical research before entering rabbinical school in 2003. She earned a PhD in palliative care from Lancaster University in England focusing on Parkinson's.

»

Following rabbinic ordination in 2008, she trained in hospital chaplaincy. She currently works with the Krembil neuroscience program as the spiritual care provider with that program at Toronto Western Hospital of the University Health Network, and at Baycrest as rabbi and chaplain with the palliative care and rehabilitation programs. Her main areas of interest are spiritual needs in Parkinson's and movement disorders, professional grief and bereavement, and healing in children and adults. She volunteers with Bereaved Families of Ontario with the children's program and the infant loss program as a group facilitator and professional advisor. She does rabbinic work in the community with Jewish Family and Child Services and Darchei Noam Congregation and lifecycle events and teaching in the area of bereavement.

"How Can I Find My Happy Again?"

By Edie Anderson

When I was diagnosed with Parkinson's, I was anything but happy. Like so many others following diagnosis, I allowed depression and despair to fill my heart. In the world of chronic illness, we call this a "pity party" — an odd term because it's not a party at all as there's only one guest, no games, and no cake! Almost everyone I've met on my Parkinson's journey has been to one of these parties. While some stopped in briefly, I was trapped for a year before I found the "exit," and once I was out, I was happy again.

How?

I found happiness in applying the Bible principles of love, compassion, and generosity. This not only brightens my day but helps balance my physical, mental and spiritual health to live well. I eat healthy food for physical strength, I dine on creativity to ensure emotional stability, and I feed on God's word and pray for peace of heart—this is the combination that works for me!

How exactly do I take in spiritual nourishment?

I make it a daily routine. As a morning person, I am at my best early in the day, and two things energize me: a prayer and a good strong cup of coffee. I also read and meditate on a few chapters of the Bible every morning—this keeps me focused on the important things in my life.

I express my thanks and my needs. When I'm sick, lonely, or depressed, I pray for comfort and guidance to cope with my situation. That is what I should do; however, I don't just pray when things are bad. That's like never saying anything nice to a friend, and who wants to be friends with a grump? So, I take the time to express my appreciation for the blessings I enjoy every day. When a butterfly flits into my garden, or I find a treasure at the beach, I view them as gifts from God, and I offer a few words of thanks right away. Expressions of gratitude make me smile, and that feels good.

I share my appreciation for the good things I enjoy with others. While we each have to establish our own relationship with God, it is also healthy to share our faith and hope with others; being part of a spiritual family promotes love, joy, and peace. We are all on a journey in this life, and when the road gets bumpy, it's not only good to have others to lean on for help; it's a provision that was intended for our benefit.

For me, spirituality isn't just a formality that demonstrates what I believe, but it defines who I am and is woven into every aspect of my life. As a woman of faith, I look forward to the fulfillment of God's promises of making my life better—that's called HOPE, and it's the best medicine for living well with Parkinson's. Living with Parkinson's is scary, but HOPE is more powerful than fear and helps me face the future with optimism. To push back against the progression of Parkinson's takes a great deal of energy, and if I were to rely on my own strength, I would quickly tire out. I rely on a higher source for the energy to thrive, as stated in my favorite scripture: "He gives strength to the faint one and plentiful vigor to the powerless. And young men will faint and tire and men in their youthful prime will stumble down, but those who hope in Jehovah will have freshening strength, take wing like eagles run without tiring, walk without fainting." (Isaiah 40:29-31 Byington version)

As a person with Parkinson's, the idea of walking without falling down is a positive message from God, and my relationship with Him is what keeps me strong and resilient in the face of struggle, uncertainly, and pain. It's what keeps me connected to the people I love and allows me to laugh in the face of Parkinson's. My spiritual routine allows me to address my physical and mental needs in a balanced way. I have good days and bad days, but I don't have dark days because I found my Happy and made it Happen!

About Edie Anderson

Edie Anderson was diagnosed with Parkinson's in 2013 at the age of 60. She developed Parkinson's symptoms after undergoing several surgeries and chemotherapy in her earlier battle with breast cancer. After a year-long "pity party," Edie found the help she needed through a local support group where she met another person living with Parkinson's who shared his passion for exercising. "I became a workout junkie," she says. "I have benefited physically, mentally, and emotionally from my active lifestyle."

»

Now retired, Edie is passionate about helping others with Parkinson's discover the benefits of exercise to live well. She teaches at a variety of support groups and other Parkinson's educational events about developing a proactive approach to wellness. Edie and her husband, Scott, split their time between the Blue Ridge Mountains of Virginia and the sunny southern coast of Florida. Snowbirding is an integral part of Edie's wellness program because the Florida sunshine warms her heart, body, and mind, helping her stay active year-round.

CHAPTER 13 – SOCIAL CONNECTIONS, RELATIONSHIPS, AND COMMUNITY

OVERVIEW – RELATIONSHIPS

Positive relationships and supportive environments play a significant role when it comes to facing adversity. The better our relationships, the better our health, outlook on life, and belief in our own self-efficacy and resilience. When we have solid relationships, we feel less stress and are more capable of overcoming challenges.

This doesn't change with a Parkinson's diagnosis.

Although Parkinson's can affect relationships over time, for many people, these impacts are often positive. Couples and families who cope most successfully tend to understand and prepare together for the challenges of Parkinson's.

In this chapter, we'll discuss how your relationships might change with people close to you and offer advice for navigating relationship highs and lows. Then we'll take a close look at how your relationships and connections correspond with social capital and why staying connected to your friends, family, and community is so important when you're living with Parkinson's.

> *I have six brothers, so there are a lot of assumptions, but also a lot of support in the family. I try to keep them informed but wonder how much information is too much. I've learned to address the big things, not the little things. I tend not to talk about the daily challenges or depression because we are so far apart geographically."*

— BRIAN

COMMUNICATING ABOUT PARKINSON'S

Keep in mind as you explore this chapter that one of the most critical components of any strong relationship is ongoing, open dialogue. Whether it's with your spouse or partner, your children, your friends, your medical providers, or others with whom you are close, communication is essential to living well with Parkinson's.

With whom and when you should share your diagnosis is a very personal decision, and it depends on many different factors. Before talking openly about their diagnosis, many people worry about:

- The added stress on their children
- Not being able to explain the many unknowns about Parkinson's
- Being treated differently by family, friends, and peers
- Receiving too much attention due to the Parkinson's
- Losing a job or friendships
- Being misunderstood or left out
- Feeling vulnerable
- How talking about the diagnosis makes it seem more real
- How it will impact career, benefits, etc.

If you feel these concerns, ask your physician to refer you to a social worker or another professional with whom you can discuss your fears or worries. You may feel less anxiety if you learn how to begin talking about Parkinson's with your family and friends without fully revealing your diagnosis. Understanding more about the early stages of Parkinson's can also ease the process of telling others about your diagnosis. The more you know, the easier it will be to talk with others and alleviate their fears on your behalf.

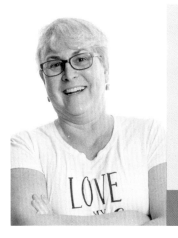

> **My kids are so aware of other people's needs because of my Parkinson's. They are both very empathetic and socially conscious – they'll automatically help older people with groceries, doors, etc. Part of it is that they're boys with good manners, but a larger part of it is that they grew up having to help their own mom with those things."**
>
> **— JILL ATER**

Plan what you want to share and what you wish to keep private. Going into these conversations with a clear intention will give you agency and control, which can help put you and the person you're talking to at ease. Plan, too, whether this communication will be in person, by phone, or via writing.

You can also prepare by thinking beforehand about people's questions and the answers you'll give. For example, people may have misconceptions about Parkinson's. They may think it's fatal, that it just causes people to shake, or that it's only an "older person's disease." So, you might want to prepare to respond to those myths with facts to avoid an overly emotional discussion that leaves you exhausted.

The people who care about you will want to know how they can help, and as a result, they may ask a long list of questions to show their concern for you. Again, you might think in advance about the answers you want to give to questions such as, "How can I help?" or "What will this mean for you in the long run?" Stay calm, be honest and forthright, but if the conversation grows overwhelming, gently tell them so and suggest you talk about it more at another time.

Finally, give yourself and others time to process. Although people may have noticed differences in you and reached their conclusions, your diagnosis may still be a shock to them. Make sure to allocate enough time for them to digest what is happening.

PARKINSON'S AND CARE PARTNER RELATIONSHIPS

Whether your care partner is your spouse or partner, child, parent, or friend, your relationship with this person will transform throughout your Parkinson's journey.

Soon after your diagnosis, your care partner may quickly embrace the role and seek to do as much as possible. They may deal with the uncertainty of diagnosis by controlling of medical appointments, treatment decisions, and lifestyle changes. They may be vigilant about monitoring your movements, carefully noting any changes from day to day. Conversely, some partners choose to deal with the uncertainty and fear accompanying diagnosis by distancing themselves and avoid getting involved with medical appointments or treatment decisions. Others take a middle-of-the-road approach, balancing their involvement in a way that allows you to remain in primary control.

> " *Even though I am very active in my local Parkinson's community, I've made it a priority to keep up with my groups and friends who are outside of Parkinson's.*"
>
> — BRENDA

There is no right or wrong approach. Talk with your care partner about your own concerns and how you would like to handle Parkinson's together. Decide the extent to which you want your care partner involved in your treatment, and remember that your care partner can be a powerful advocate for you in many circumstances, from medical appointments to get-togethers with friends.

For more about Parkinson's care partners, be sure to check out the 📖 *Every Victory Counts Manual for Care Partners*.

COMMUNICATE, COMMUNICATE, COMMUNICATE

We cannot say it enough: Communication is the cornerstone of every healthy relationship. This is especially true when someone in the relationship is living with a chronic condition like Parkinson's.

As you read earlier in this manual, Parkinson's can impact your voice, facial expressions, and mood. All of these can affect how your care partner may "see" you as you communicate with them. If you're suffering from depression or apathy, it may appear to them that you just don't care. Parkinson's can also blunt your facial expressions, a condition referred to as facial masking. As a result, your partner may not be able to tell what you're feeling based on outward cues. You may also experience softer, more monotone speech, which can sometimes cause care partners and friends and family to assume you're uninterested or uninvested in what's going on around you.

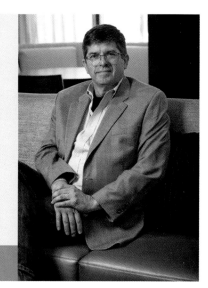

> " *I was head-down focused on my job all the time, and the energy I had left, I spent at home rather than volunteering. It took Parkinson's to shake me out of my complacency. The things I think are important and the way I choose to spend my time have changed. I don't think Parkinson's is a gift, but it's made me focus more on things that are important as opposed to things that are urgent and demanding my attention.*"

— COREY KING

Many members of your integrated care team can be instrumental in helping with these communication concerns. A speech-language pathologist can help you manage voice, facial masking, and other communication symptoms. (Remember, one of the main goals of speech therapy includes improving a person's ability to communicate effectively and to improve communication in social interactions.) If you experience depression, anxiety, and/or apathy, a mental health specialist can advise on therapies and medications that can help.

And, of course, advocating for yourself and letting people know that some of what they're seeing is symptomatic of Parkinson's will foster greater understanding and stronger relationships.

> *The friends I've made in the Parkinson's community are very aware of what I deal with every day. It's nice to have people understand that in a social setting."*
>
> — BRENDA

YOUR RELATIONSHIP WITH YOUR SPOUSE OR PARTNER

Many people receive their Parkinson's diagnosis with their partner sitting next to them; however, for those whose partner isn't there, it's important to tell them in a timely manner so that you can plan to move forward together. Even if you want to protect them from the truth or you're worried about how things might change, being open with them is critical. You and your partner can grow to understand Parkinson's by asking questions and seeking information together. Your partner or significant other may also have pertinent questions that you haven't thought of or offer a different perspective that can help you see your diagnosis in a new way.

Your partner can also become a resource and an advocate for you. Once you have told them, they can help facilitate further disclosures of your diagnosis. For example, it may be particularly challenging to tell your children, but telling them together can make it easier. They may also help you practice for future conversations and determine what you do and don't want to share with specific people.

INTIMACY AND PARKINSON'S

The emotional impact of a Parkinson's diagnosis can interfere with the desire for sexual intimacy, both for the person with Parkinson's and their partner. You both may be too distracted to initiate sex or participate with any interest. Discussing emotions isn't always easy, and it may take time to adjust and adapt to the idea of living with Parkinson's.

On the other hand, some people experience an enhanced sex drive after being diagnosed. This may be a reaction to the unknown future, or it may also be a side effect of certain medications, especially dopamine agonists. As you may remember from Chapter 6, sexual dysfunction is a pervasive problem in Parkinson's, and it may take a multidisciplinary approach to achieve the best outcome for you and your partner. Specialists who can help include gynecologists, urologists, sex therapists, counselors, and primary care physicians.

If you're concerned about sexual intimacy, talk about it with your partner. Look at it as an opportunity for you to connect on an emotional level. Make time for this discussion and remember that intimacy is an important part of your relationship. A counselor can help you and your partner navigate these changes.

DESIGNATE PARKINSON'S-FREE ZONES

Although Parkinson's is part of your life, it's important to spend time together and with friends when Parkinson's isn't the most important person in the room. Take time to connect with your partner in ways you did pre-Parkinson's. Did you spend Friday evenings at dinner parties with friends? Were Wednesday mornings set aside for your shared runs or yoga practice? Did you have daily routines like watching a game show together, taking a walk after dinner, enjoying coffee together first thing in the morning? Think about the everyday activities that brought you joy before your Parkinson's diagnosis, and make sure you're still taking time to do them together while talking about something other than Parkinson's.

Of course, some of these activities will change. Not everything will continue the way it did before Parkinson's was a part of your lives. Adapt, stay flexible, make new traditions, accept limitations, but remember that Parkinson's is a *part* of your life, but it's not your whole life. Focusing on the big picture will help you take care of yourself, your partner, and your relationship together.

> *There is no doubt in my mind that connecting with others is essential to living well with Parkinson's. I find great benefit in a small bi-weekly lunch group that offers lively conversation with no questions barred. I also attend a local support group and connect with one or more online groups. The bottom line is this: connecting to others helps me thrive, not just survive, with Parkinson's."*
>
> — LORRAINE WILSON

It is often easier to designate a "Parkinson's-free zone" in your home than in social settings or large gatherings. With the best of intentions, many friends and acquaintances may spend quite a bit of time asking how you're feeling and encouraging you to talk about your life with Parkinson's. Although these questions show that they care, you or your partner can step in and turn the conversation away from Parkinson's by asking friends about their own lives, their families, current events, and community news. By shifting the topic to something other than Parkinson's, you can keep it from being the center of attention.

TALKING TO CHILDREN ABOUT PARKINSON'S

YOUR RELATIONSHIPS WITH YOUR CHILDREN

One common Parkinson's challenge for people with children is deciding when and how to share the news of your diagnosis. The way you share your diagnosis with your children will vary based on their age and maturity level. No one knows your children better than you do; so, you probably know what they can and can't handle. With children of all ages, take time to check in with them about what they're thinking and feeling. Giving them opportunities to put their concerns into words can help them make sense of their feelings and allow for a more open and honest dialogue.

Children Seven and Younger

Begin by mentioning symptoms they may have already noticed. You might ask, "Have you noticed that my hand is sometimes shaky or that I've been walking slower? We talked to the physician, and it turns out that I have something called Parkinson's."

Give them the basic facts. Let them share what they have noticed, talk about things that might change, and stress that medication and other treatments will help you feel better. Be clear and consistent in what you say, and don't let the conversation go on too long. Remember, children pick up on a lot and will often mirror your demeanor. Maintain a positive attitude and make sure they know it's okay for them to go on as before.

> " *I remember my youngest son was in late elementary school when I came and did a presentation for his class. One of the kids in the class asked him why I was shaking so much, and my son became really upset and embarrassed. He'd grown up seeing me tremor, so for him it wasn't anything abnormal."*
>
> — JILL ATER

Children Ages Eight to Fourteen (Approximately)

Explain the diagnosis in a simple, factual way and don't overburden them with excessive scientific terms or non-motor symptoms like hallucinations that might seem scary. If you sense they are worried that they somehow contributed to your Parkinson's, reassure them that it is not their fault and that you're still the same person.

Be prepared for questions but try to keep the conversation brief and positive overall. Retaining as much normalcy as possible and giving them a sense of control will help them process your diagnosis. Be ready for them to ask questions, either in the moment or later, especially if they decide to research Parkinson's on their own. If they do that, be sure to stress the importance of seeking out reliable sources and how to do that. (We'll talk more about this in our final chapter.)

> " *Our girls are really supportive and interested, and I know they're going to be there for us in the future. It's mostly emotional support, caring, and love."*
>
> — NANCY HOVEY

Teenagers and Adult Children

After learning about your diagnosis, older children will often focus on what they can do. Depending on where you are in the process, you can either assure them that nothing much is changing or suggest some specific actions they can take to help. For example, you may suggest they can help by cooking dinner once a week or by holding you accountable for completing an exercise goal every day. Leave the dialogue open and communicate with them as your health changes or you experience new symptoms, so they know you want them to be in the loop.

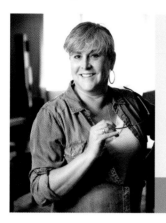

" *As the kids got older, we basically just answered any questions they had. If they asked, we answered. Otherwise, we tried not to make Parkinson's a central focus of their lives. They were regular kids growing up and we wanted to protect that for them."*

— JILL

With Grandkids

If you have grandchildren, you can follow the guidelines we shared above to tell them about your diagnosis, or you might choose to rely on your children to help guide the conversation. Either way, it's important to have a clear understanding with your own children as to how much your grandchildren can and should be told about Parkinson's. They will know better than you do how much their children can process and understand, so be sure to communicate with them before sharing the diagnosis with your grandchildren.

" *I see Parkinson's as both a blessing and a calling. I found it to be a blessing mainly because of the incredible people I've met through it. The people in the 'Parkiesphere' I've met are literally worldwide friends I can call on and get encouragement from daily. As far as a calling, I've found that one of the things I'm good at is gathering information and sharing it with people. It's something I enjoy, and it's an opportunity to share information that's accurate and timely to help people have a better quality of life."*

— JOHN ALEXANDER

PARENTS, FRIENDSHIPS, AND PARKINSON'S

RELATIONSHIPS WITH PARENTS

Telling your parents about your diagnosis may be difficult, especially if you're caring for them in some way and don't want to burden them. Some parents have reactions of guilt at not having protected their children from something like Parkinson's. Encourage them to focus on what you need now. Try to keep your routines consistent and be honest about where

228

you are on your journey with Parkinson's. Even if you're helping them, you can still be open and honest about your own experience.

RELATIONSHIPS WITH FRIENDS

After a Parkinson's diagnosis, many people wonder when to tell their friends and how it might change those relationships. While some people may feel tempted to retreat and keep to themselves rather than confiding in friends, social isolation is not the answer. While it's important to give yourself time before telling your friends that Parkinson's is now one part of your life, remember and remind them that it is just one part. Keep taking part in the activities and get-togethers you enjoyed before diagnosis. Be patient when friends ask questions and designate "Parkinson's-free zones" if doing so helps you feel more comfortable when with friends.

> " *Some people said all the wrong things. In the end, we made many new friends who did not know Davis before Parkinson's. That has helped us tremendously."*
>
> — CONNIE CARPENTER PHINNEY

Remember, too, that you are now part of a community of other people who truly get you. Many people in our community say that the new friendships they've made with others living with Parkinson's are the silver lining of their diagnosis. In Parkinson's support groups, exercise classes, conferences, and other social gatherings, you can find a group of people who understand what you're experiencing and who will be there to support you every step of the way.

As they learn more about Parkinson's, children and friends of all ages often feel inspired to get involved with advocacy, fundraising, and events. Numerous people in our community have told us that their family members love to hold bake sales for Parkinson's, fundraise through cycling events or other activities, and connect with other care partners and people living with Parkinson's in person and through online events. Invite your family and friends to participate in whatever activities call to them.

> " *I don't wish Parkinson's on anyone, but I wish everyone could have the opportunity to experience the things that I have experienced with Parkinson's, and more importantly, experience the love, compassion, and generosity coming from wonderful family, friends, and strangers that I am able to experience these things with!"*
>
> — CARL AMES

"How Can I Help my Kids Understand Parkinson's?"

By Michelle Lane

When I was diagnosed with Parkinson's in 2000, I first thought of my three children and of how my diagnosis would impact them. How would I tell them? Would I be able to help my daughter fix her hair and make-up? Would I be able to walk at their graduations and weddings?

At first, I chose not to share my diagnosis with my children, but I soon realized that I had to tell the older two who were nine and six at the time. Their first question was, "Are you going to die?" I reassured them that Parkinson's was not fatal but that sometimes I might need help with small tasks. At the time, neither child asked many questions, and both seemed relieved to know that I was "okay."

As time went on, I could see small but distinct ways that my announcement changed their behavior. When my son Kyle and I would go shopping, he would hold only my left hand. When I asked him about it, he said he was trying to stop the shaking. Erik decided that he would become a scientist and create a bracelet and anklet that would prevent people with Parkinson's from shaking.

As I considered how to help my boys understand Parkinson's, I received some excellent suggestions from my movement disorder specialist. Upon his request, my husband and I brought the boys on a "special" physician's appointment. The physician showed us pictures of the brain, explained the disease in simple terms, and told all of us what it is like to live with Parkinson's.

While this visit was invaluable to my children and me, I continued to see signs of their struggle with my diagnosis. They were unsure how to answer children at school when they asked them why their mom shakes so much, and I continually had to reassure them that I was not going to die. At one point, we decided to seek outside counseling from a psychologist for one of the boys who was having a particularly difficult time adjusting. He taught us tools for coping with this change we found helpful.

For my daughter, Rachel, who was only two years old when I was diagnosed, Parkinson's raised different issues. Rachel and I both had a difficult time dealing with my inability to pull up her long, thick brown hair in a ponytail and have her look like the other girls her age. At first, I asked the stylist to cut her hair short, but now, with adjustments and help from other family members, Rachel is learning to do ponytails on her own. It's just one of the many examples of simple things that Parkinson's can take away from you but that you can take back with a little teamwork.

This ponytail problem, however, turned out to be minor compared to what was to come. Just this year, at age seven, Rachel hit me with a bombshell that I will never forget. I was sitting on my porch enjoying a cool day when she sat on my lap, placed her arms around my neck, and asked, "Why do you have to have Parkinson's?" I tried to explain, but she kept saying, "I want you to be like you were before. It just isn't fair because Kyle and Erik got to see you like you were before, and I never have."

It made me realize that my daughter had many questions that she was trying to understand. We held each other, and she asked what the word "cure" meant. We talked about this, and then she asked the inevitable question: "Is Parkinson's contagious?" I told her that it was not and that I would be around for a long time to answer any other questions she had. I also set up a phone call with my physician so he could have the same conversation with Rachel that he had with my boys.

Of course, my children continue to have questions. When Rachel was seven, she asked me how old I was when I started shaking. I replied that I was 30, at which point she asked if she too would start shaking when she turns 30. As I assured her that she would not, it reminded me that the questions about my Parkinson's probably wouldn't end. But at least I know I am here for my children and plan to be for a long time.

My advice for dealing with Parkinson's is to keep the faith and recognize the strength of your family. Expect that they will have questions and be open to suggestions on how to deal with them. Remember that we are all in this together, and only together will we win this war on Parkinson's.

2021 Update: My children are now in their twenties. My grandson Chandler is three, and he asks, "MiMi, are you stuck? I will help you and tell others to step back. I have this!"

About Michelle Lane

Michelle Lane was diagnosed with Parkinson's in June of 2000 at the age of 32. Since then, Michelle has become one of the foremost advocates in her home state of Louisiana by starting the first young onset Parkinson's support group in New Orleans, beginning The Parkinson's Association of Louisiana (PAL), and championing numerous fundraising efforts, including Louisiana Walks for Parkinson's. Michelle, a Davis Phinney Foundation Ambassador, wants to live well with Parkinson's by showing and explaining to those diagnosed that you can still lead a productive and active life. She wants people to take "can't" out of their vocabulary and replace it with "yes, I can."

"How Does Parkinson's Impact Friendships"?

By Cidney Donahoo, MEd

Recently, during my Parkinson's Voice Project speech training, I was asked to read (with INTENT, of course) the song/poem with the well-known line of "make new friends but keep the old, one is silver and the other gold." I remember this song well from my childhood; we even had it written on a plaque in our house while I was growing up. When I was young, I didn't quite understand if the new friends or the old friends were silver or gold. I guess I just knew that friends were important.

There are various obstacles that a person with Parkinson's can face when it comes to friendships, both with making new friends and keeping "the old." Friends from before diagnosis may not understand Parkinson's (and a newly diagnosed person with Parkinson's also may not understand these complexities). Apathy, fatigue, cognitive changes, and other symptoms may be difficult for both the person living with Parkinson's and their friends to understand. This can be a challenge when you have difficulty just trying to figure out what it is and what to do about it. What do you share with friends, and what do you keep to yourself?

Some friends may find a Parkinson's diagnosis too much to process. That's okay. Just be where you can with them. Others may not completely understand but will be by your side, nonetheless. Treasure the friendships wherever they are. Some will fade, and again, that's okay. Give grace to those friendships and let them go where they naturally will. The others, the ones who stick around even though they don't understand, are "gold."

Doom and gloom do not need to follow a Parkinson's diagnosis. Everyone reacts differently, but in getting to know hundreds of people with Parkinson's, I have noticed that there's usually a period where denial or shock or disbelief sets in. Most people will keep the diagnosis to themselves and possibly a few close family or friends. This is normal. Don't get stuck there, though. Making new friends who understand what you're experiencing can be the balm that nourishes your soul.

Where do you find these new friends who, like you, are living with Parkinson's? How can they help? Look to your local resources to find a Parkinson's group nearby where you can meet people on a similar path. Many local Parkinson's organizations will have support groups; try to find one that reflects who you are. Exercise groups can also become a great source of community and friendship. Fellow members of Rock Steady Boxing, Pedaling For Parkinson's, Dance for PD, and other groups may become your new friend group.

The value of having friends with Parkinson's is that they "get it." They offer a safe place for you to be yourself. You will laugh, cry, and have solemn moments with these new friends. You may come from vastly different backgrounds, and yet one thing, Parkinson's, will bind you.

These new friendships very likely will become the silver lining in your Parkinson's diagnosis.

I don't know what I would do without my Parkinson's friends. They have become some of my closest friends, even though many of them live many thousands of miles away. It's like that old friend you haven't spoken to in a very long time, but when you get together, it's like no time has passed; you're laughing and joking as though you've never been apart.

So, as the song says, make new friends and keep the old. You will find a lovely journey through life as you embrace new friends who can help support you, and you will be a support to them in return. That sounds like a "gold" medal to me.

About Cidney Donahoo

Cidney Donahoo was diagnosed with Parkinson's in 2010 at the age of 47. She became involved in the Parkinson's community through cycling after participating in a tandem bike exercise study with Dr. Jay Alberts. She went on to ride RAGBRAI in Iowa with the Pedaling for Parkinson's team and Ride the Rockies in Colorado with the Davis Phinney Foundation team. Cidney continues to cycle, often riding tandem with her husband Pat, and has since added yoga, strength training, and boxing to her exercise regimen. Exercise helps her stay healthy and manage her Parkinson's symptoms. A Davis Phinney Foundation Ambassador, Cidney's mission is to "leave no Parkinson's person behind" by increasing the information and peer-to-peer support in her community. Cidney is a retired educator and co-founded a local support group for people with young onset Parkinson's in the Las Vegas area.

OVERVIEW - COMMUNITY

Many people living with Parkinson's, especially in the early days of their diagnosis when so much is new and unknown, being trying on a brand-new identity while also doing their best to keep their old one intact.

Maybe you can relate.

I am a big believer in the value of getting involved with your local Parkinson's community. Let's face it, we all share a common challenge, and there are going to be times in this journey when you'll need support in one way or another, or you can be that person for someone else."

— STEVE HOVEY

You read all the great things people are doing while living with Parkinson's, but you wonder and often doubt if that can be your reality too. As a person with Parkinson's, you may want to share your diagnosis because it's such a relief to finally have a name for what you've been feeling and experiencing, yet you fear how others will view you once they know. You know you may need some help now or someday soon, but the idea of being a burden is enough to keep quiet and vow to do it all on your own.

Also, certain Parkinson's symptoms that are especially visible such as tremor, shuffling, facial masking, and more lead some people with Parkinson's to isolate themselves. By limiting your contact with the outside world, you have less explaining to do, and you can avoid situations that make you feel like you aren't part of the "healthy club" anymore.

The problem with disconnecting is that social isolation can exacerbate your symptoms, put you at risk for developing other health problems, increase your chances of experiencing depression, accelerate cognitive decline, and decrease your quality of life. Taking control of what you can control can make a significant difference in how well you live with it.

> *It gives me a lot of emotional strength to be in a group of people with Parkinson's. It's nice to hear others talk about their experiences with Parkinson's because I don't feel so alone."*
>
> — BRENDA

THE POWER OF CONNECTION AND COMMUNITY

So, what can you do to avoid the temptation to isolate and get reconnected to the world around you?

Before we offer suggestions, let's first define social isolation and its relationship to loneliness. Many people have used these terms interchangeably, but research indicates that decoupling them may allow for greater insight, even if they are ideally researched simultaneously.

> *Being of service has allowed me to transition into a second career after being diagnosed with Parkinson's at 48. In Act 1, I was a midwife honored to help bring new life into the world. In Act 2, I write, speak, and podcast about wellness, hoping to inspire others to consider a mindset of ability with mindfulness, joy, and wellness."*
>
> — KAT HILL

Social isolation is characterized by having a small social network and infrequent participation in social activities. Loneliness, on the other hand, is a personal interpretation of a psychological state. It's about perceiving that you have a lack of social support. So, someone who is socially connected could still feel very lonely. And someone who does not have any social connections may not feel lonely at all.

Now that we know what it is, here's what being socially connected can do for you.

Benefits of Social Connectedness

People who are more socially connected...

- Have more access to information
- Have more access to transportation options
- Receive more emotional support
- Are more influenced by and likely to pursue healthy behaviors
- Have more financial resources
- Take advantage of community programs
- Experience better physical and mental health
- Manage stress, change, and loss in more productive ways
- Bounce back from physical setbacks more quickly
- Are less likely to engage in risky behaviors
- Seek out opportunities to help others in ways that give them physical and mental health benefits as well

So, why is it that with all of the evidence pointing to the benefits of social connectedness, is it so hard for some people to come out of hiding?

Because putting yourself out in the world as someone with Parkinson's isn't easy.

If you are using isolation as a way of coping with a diagnosis of Parkinson's, here are a few actions you can take to become more connected and live well today.

> " *I was not open to the idea of sharing my Parkinson's diagnosis at first. It did not take long for me to realize that I had nothing to be ashamed of, and the more people I told, the more support I received."*
>
> — LORRAINE WILSON

How to Build (or Rebuild) Social Connections

If being more socially active makes you feel anxious, start small. (If it makes you so anxious you can't move forward, please consider reaching out to a therapist who can help you through it.)

One way to start small is by making a deal with yourself to take one action a week or to do one new activity each month. There's no value in putting pressure on yourself. Choose an activity that challenges you to stretch but doesn't put so much stress on you that you can't reap the rewards of doing it.

The good news is, if you're like many of the people we've worked with who have moved from being socially isolated to feeling like engaged members of their community, once you get a taste of what it feels like to make more connections, you'll feel noticeably better and more eager to keep doing it.

" *Being a Davis Phinney Foundation Ambassador has been the best example of the reciprocity between giving and receiving. Each person or organization I have contact with gives me a chance to give back while helping deepen my interpersonal and community relationships. Definitely a two-way street!"*

— WENDY ANN MILLER

Ways to Connect

- Ask a friend or neighbor to join you for coffee or tea
- Attend a Parkinson's support group meeting (or start your own)
- Attend a church or spiritual service
- Adopt and train a pet
- Offer to teach people or share your skills and expertise with others
- Seek a teacher for a new skill or craft you'd like to learn
- Volunteer (maybe even become a Davis Phinney Foundation Ambassador)
- Take a class at your local community center, YMCA, or library
- Take up a physical activity you've always wanted to try or used to do and then invite someone to do it with you
- Join Team DPF to connect with others and participate in a fundraiser to raise money for Parkinson's
- Set a goal related to exercise or nutrition and connect with others who have similar goals at your local gym or through active online communities
- Take a vacation
- Try a Parkinson's-specific exercise class in your area
- Join the Tremble Clefs or another singing group
- Ask someone to help you learn a new technology

- Research or ask someone in your area to help you find all of the various paid and free transportation options in your community
- Move into a community with people in similar life stages (over 55, senior living, active, etc.)
- Ask for help
- Reconnect with your purpose or find a new one for this new stage in your life
- Eat a meal with someone
- Join a book/cooking/supper/chess/coloring club
- Take a museum tour

The important thing to remember is that you are not alone. Throughout the world, millions of other people living with Parkinson's experience many of the same worries, thoughts, and symptoms as you do. Find your community. Lean on them. Lift them up. Allow them to lift you up. Celebrate their victories and celebrate yours.

> " It can be hard to do, but you have to find friends or get a hobby or take a painting class – do something outside of everything that places demands on you."
>
> — SHERYL

"How Important Is Community to Living Well with Parkinson's?"

By Al Condeluci, PhD

Any of us who have experienced or have supported someone who has Parkinson's know that one of the biggest risks, along with the daily challenges, is that the condition will lead to social disconnection from friends and families. If this begins to happen, further compromise to health, safety, and overall well-being are accelerated. Today, we know that social isolation can be as lethal to a person's health and well-being as smoking two packs of cigarettes each day!

People living with Parkinson's and their families can maintain, and even add, social connections in their lives, regardless of the condition or other compromises they might experience. My first strong recommendation for social well-being is that folks stay as active as possible in their communities, despite their possible hesitations. Although this can be challenging, as Parkinson's has physical and/or cognitive ramifications that can get in the way of community engagement, one of the most important facets of community engagement is that it promotes an opportunity to maintain and grow social connections for the members who belong. These connections and friendships are often referred to by sociologists as "social capital." These connections provide an amazing amount of positive residue for people.

WHAT IS SOCIAL CAPITAL?

Social capital refers to the connections and relationships that develop around a community and the value these relationships hold. Like physical capital (the tools used by communities) or human capital (the people power brought to a situation), "social capital" is the value brought on by our relationships.

> " *Social capital is those tangible substances that count for most in the daily lives of people: namely goodwill, fellowship, sympathy, and social intercourse among the individuals and families who make up a social unit...The individual is helpless socially, if left to himself...If he comes into contact with his neighbor, and they with other neighbors, there will be an accumulation of social capital, which may immediately satisfy his social needs and which may bear a social potentiality sufficient to the substantial improvement of living conditions in the whole community. The community as a whole will benefit by the cooperation of all its parts, while the individual will find in his associations the advantages of the help, the sympathy, and the fellowship of his neighbors."*
>
> — L.J. HANIFAN (1916)

Renowned Harvard sociologist Robert Putnam defined the concept of social capital as: "referring to connections among individuals-social networks and the norms of reciprocity and trustworthiness that arise from them...[It] is closely related to...civic...virtue...A society of many virtuous but isolated individuals is not necessarily rich in social capital."

Other sociologists suggest that social capital is enhanced by social currency. This idea is how social fodder links people together. For example, a popular person who is the life of the party might be regularly included in activities. To this extent, he is strong in social capital. His jokes and storytelling, the items that make him popular in the gathering, are the social currency he exchanges. All of us, regardless of the situation, bring social currency to our relationships.

Think about the many communities with which you are involved. People who might be different from you in many ways surround you—your family, your work team, your church, your clubs, your associations—but the commonality of the community tends to override the differences you have and create a strong norm for connections. The exchange is based on social currency. Further, these relationships become helpful to you in a variety of ways. Sociologists call this helpfulness "social reciprocity," which is the core of the value we reap from our relationships. You scratch my back, and I will do the same for you.

The fact that social capital keeps us safe, sane, and secure cannot be understated. Most of us tend to think that institutions or organizations are key factors to safety. Places like hospitals or systems like law enforcement are thought to keep us safe, but the bold truth is that these systems have never really succeeded in keeping people safe or healthy. Rather, it is the opportunity for relationships that community offers us and the building of social capital that is at the core of safety or health. Simply stated, your circles of friends and the reciprocity they create are the most important element to your safety. As stated earlier, it has been suggested that social isolation, or the opposite of social capital, is a key determinant of our health. So, what are the things you should consider to maintain or build new friendships?

REGULARITY OF EXCHANGE

Cultures and communities have many features, but one key ingredient that is critical to friendship is regularity. For a community to be viable and to build trust in relationships, it must have some regular points of contact and connection. For a family community, this might be annual reunions or the celebration of holidays together. For a religious community, regularity may be found in weekly services and holy days for celebration. For organizations, the frequency could be found in regular staff meetings or stakeholder gatherings. For clubs, groups, or associations, regular meetings or gatherings can formalize the group as a community.

The more people come together, the more they find other ways that they are linked. That is, when a person first joins a community, they are drawn by the common interest of the group; as they stay regular in attendance, they will find other similarities with people in the community and create a deeper sense of bonding.

SIMILARITIES/COMMONALITIES

Other features of a community include the notions of consent, creativity, and cooperation. Years ago, sociologist Robert Nisbit suggested that a community thrives on self-help and equal consent. He felt that people do not come together merely to be together but to do something together that cannot be done in isolation. Others identified community for its sense of interdependence. John McKnight from Northwestern University described community as a cooperative association driven toward a common goal.

Indeed, if we think about communities that we know, they all work toward some identified goal that the members agree upon. From teaching people new skills to saving souls, addressing a common problem, and launching a government—all these ventures capture the power of community and then, through their behavior, create a culture. The most vibrant and successful of these communities are the ones that have built more social capital between and among members.

THE GATEKEEPER

The final key variable to building relationships in community is that of the gatekeeper. These are people who either open or close the gates of the community. They can advocate for or shun a new member, leading to an endorsement or an indictment for the newcomer. The key is to find or identify a gatekeeper to help guide your entry into the new group. When this happens, the gatekeeper, who the group already accepts, sanctions the newcomer in the eyes of the other members of the community. This type of valorization creates a social influence with the group that makes it easier to make new friends.

WHAT CAN YOU DO?

Here are four actions you can take to stay connected in your community:

1. **Think about things you like to do or are interested in.** For my family, when supporting my dad in his Parkinson's experience, we identified his interest in jazz music.

2. **Explore your community to see if there are any clubs, groups, or associations that correspond to your interest.** For my dad, he discovered a group in our town known as the "Pittsburgh Jazz Society."

3. **Once the group is found, explore the elements of the group around things like when and where they meet, what you need to do to become a member, and how they behave when they meet.** We learned these things when I did a reconnaissance of the group without my dad being present.

4. **Identify a gatekeeper who can help with introductions to other members.** For us, this happened when I did the reconnaissance and discovered that there were other members in the Jazz Society who were from our hometown.

Certainly, getting a diagnosis of Parkinson's is life changing. When my dad was diagnosed, we were all taken aback and wondered what the future would hold. Still, living with Parkinson's (or any other type of chronic disease) does not mean that you must now drop out of community, or that you can only be friends with other people with Parkinson's.

We know that community engagement nurtures social capital. The value reaped by these relationships provides amazing opportunities for us to be healthier, happier, and have a stronger sense of self. So, get out there in the community. Relationships are waiting for you—all you must do is seize them!

"Why Should I Get Involved in My Community?"

By Karen Jaffe, MD

You would think that being a physician would have given me a leg up in knowing what to do after I was diagnosed with Parkinson's. The truth is... it didn't.

I was 48 years old and knew no one else with this diagnosis. In fact, it was a full year before I met anyone else walking in these Parkinson's shoes.

I now know that I was not the only one being told early on to think twice about attending a support group. The notion that seeing people more symptomatic than me could be unsettling was a warning I took seriously. In hindsight, this was a missed opportunity for connection.

Going at it alone only added to the stigma attached to Parkinson's that keeps many of us silent. With the constant worry about getting worse and thus, being found out, it wasn't long before I had, in my head, become the person with Parkinson's who happened to be a physician, instead of the physician who happened to be a person with Parkinson's.

With the support of my family, in time, I let go of my Parkinson's secret and began to engage with others in the Parkinson's community. One of my greatest strengths as a physician was my ability to listen and offer guidance. As I began to do this for other newly diagnosed people with Parkinson's, I discovered my inbox was suddenly full of people whose stories were identical to mine: scared and alone, often keeping their diagnosis secret and knowing no one else with Parkinson's. Many were not sure what to ask their physician. Almost everyone wanted to know what I was doing to stay well. Looking back, I see now that these conversations were the spark for my dream of opening a center to help people to live well with Parkinson's.

Propelled by the easing of symptoms that exercise gave me, my recommendation for others was robust activity whenever possible. But for most people, especially those who were not avid exercisers, the lack of organized exercise programs specifically designed for people with Parkinson's proved to be a barrier. I had a hunch that what people were looking for did not exist: a place where there was no stigma, a place that defined community.

In 2013, I joined forces with four other like-minded people in my hometown of Cleveland: my founding partners, Allan Goldberg, Lee Handel, Dr. David Riley, and Ben Rossi, to begin the design and implementation of InMotion, a wellness center for people with Parkinson's (⊙ beinmotion.org).

InMotion provides our local community of people with Parkinson's and other movement disorders a place to turn for physical, emotional, and spiritual support where the stigma of Parkinson's is left at the door, and everyone is encouraged to take charge of their well-being. The center offers various exercise classes such as dance, cycling, and boxing, to name just a few of the activities that help clients strengthen their bodies. InMotion also has art and music therapy and a drumming circle to soothe the mind and spirit. A peer program and separate support groups for people living with Parkinson's and their care partners complement the classes. InMotion also hosts expert presentations to help bring the latest movement disorder research and news to light.

The wellness center provides a common ground along with fresh energy and hope, which reinvigorates entire families. Every day, many newly diagnosed people that have not even thought about exercising in years enter our circle of support, creating new friendships and building community.

We face Parkinson's together with grit and determination. We sweat, sing, laugh, and occasionally, we even help each other up off the floor. What makes this group so special is that we know that it is working. The impact is evident in our improved outlooks, better health, and more knowledgeable and invigorated Parkinson's community.

Perhaps hearing my story has you thinking how you, too, might become a Parkinson's advocate. Fortunately, the Parkinson's community knows how to roll up its sleeves and get things done. There are many things within your reach if you feel inspired to try. I have friends who started support groups where none previously existed. Groups bring many voices to the table, and from there, ideas become reality. There are a growing number of specialized Parkinson's exercise programs to choose from, some of the more widely known including PWR4Life®, Dance for PD®, Rock Steady Boxing, Pedaling For Parkinson's, and Delay the Disease™. Consider bringing an existing program into your area and expand offerings as interest grows. I know many people who have been given space for their Parkinson's classes at their local YMCA, in boxing gyms, and in community centers simply because they asked. It turns out that folks can be quite generous.

My best advice for how to begin making a difference in your community is this: share your story. Almost everyone knows someone who is living with Parkinson's, many of whom are looking for someone to talk to. Be the one who starts the dialogue in your community, and that might lead to something bigger than yourself.

About Karen Jaffe

Karen Jaffe is a retired OB/GYN and Parkinson's advocate. She was diagnosed with Parkinson's at the age of 48. She is a member of the Michael J. Fox Foundation's Patient Advisory Council and the Brain Health Initiative at the CWRU-SOM in Cleveland, Ohio. She and her husband, Marc, founded Shaking With Laughter, a nonprofit foundation that has raised one million dollars for Parkinson's research.

Today she spends much of her time at InMotion. InMotion is a center for Parkinson's and other movement disorders that strengthens lives through a holistic approach of education, exercise, and healing arts. She was the recipient of the Red Cross Heroes award, the Irene Zehman award for Volunteerism, the World Parkinson's Program International Parkinson's Community Service award, and the University Hospital Neurological Institute Champions for Parkinson's award.

MEET OUR AMBASSADORS

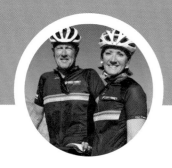 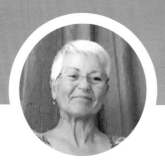 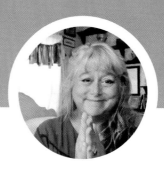 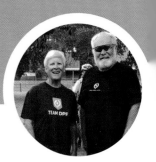

When we created our Ambassador Leadership Program in 2015, we did so because we recognized that, more than anything, our community members want more connection to people who truly understand what it means to live with Parkinson's. We hear so often that the support of our Ambassadors goes far beyond resources and advice. Our Ambassadors offer people a safe place that allows for real processing and change to happen.

The experience and wisdom our Ambassadors bring to the Parkinson's community is transformative, and we hope you will **reach out to them throughout your journey with Parkinson's**. Connect with an Ambassador in your area or reach out to anyone you think you would connect well with, regardless of location.

  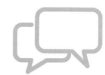

Ask questions   **Discover new resources**   **Get advice on how to live well with Parkinson's**

 Learn more and reach out to one of our Ambassadors at dpf.org/ambassadors.

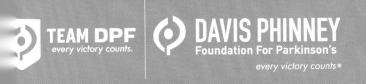

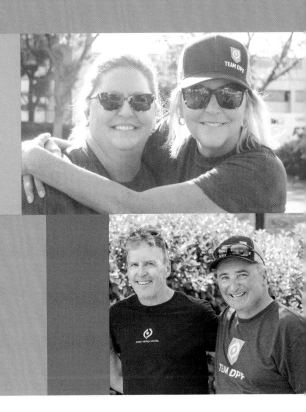

MAKE EVERY VICTORY COUNT

Team DPF, our fundraising community, provides opportunities for people with Parkinson's, care partners, friends, and family to walk, run, bike, and raise funds in a number of ways to support the mission of the Davis Phinney Foundation and make it possible for us to offer resources like the *Every Victory Counts*® manual for free to our community.

The possibilities are endless. Learn more about how you can join the Team!

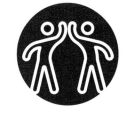

Connect with your community

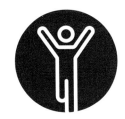

Set (and achieve) meaningful goals

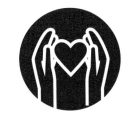

Make a real difference for people living with Parkinson's

Learn more about how you can get involved at **TeamDPF.org.**

CHAPTER 14 – GENERAL HEALTH AND WELLNESS

OVERVIEW

An essential aspect of living well is to separate your Parkinson's symptoms from other health-related issues. Many aspects of health unrelated to Parkinson's will impact you throughout your life. It's important to maintain a close relationship with your primary care physician and stay up to date on preventative screenings to sustain your overall health.

PRIMARY CARE PHYSICIAN (PCP)

As we highlighted at the beginning of this manual, your PCP will play an important role in problems unrelated to Parkinson's, monitor your general health, and make sure you stay up to date on preventive medical screening tests. A PCP also provides general health education and will work with you to diagnose and treat your general medical problems and ensure that you receive routine dental and vision care. Managing your healthcare without a PCP is like an orchestra playing without a conductor. Your PCP may help identify potential medication interactions and assist you in finding additional specialists if needed.

If you do not have a PCP, now is the time to get one. Ask friends, family, or other people with Parkinson's for recommendations. A physician assistant (PA) or nurse practitioner (NP) can serve as your general healthcare provider as well. Choose one who listens, respects your input, and with whom you feel comfortable. If you're starting from scratch, it's a good idea to schedule an interview or "get to know you" visit with a few different providers to find the best fit for you.

> **" My primary care doctor is the heart of my wellness team. He has cared for my health the longest, referred me to a local neurologist and a regional movement disorder specialist, and stays informed about my disease progression."**
>
> — LORRAINE WILSON

Questions you might want to cover during this "get to know you" visit include:

- Do you currently have any other patients who have Parkinson's? How many?

- What is your experience in treating people with Parkinson's, and for how many years have you been doing it?

- Do you work with movement disorder specialists? Do you have a recommendation for one?

- What is the role of rehabilitation for people with Parkinson's?

- Where do your patients with Parkinson's receive their rehabilitation therapy?

- Since Parkinson's research is rapidly progressing, can I share new information, research, or updates about my Parkinson's or treatment with you?

- What is your philosophy regarding prescribing various treatments, including medication, occupational or physical therapy, counseling, diet, and exercise for Parkinson's symptoms?

Avoid waiting until you have a problem or are sick before you see your PCP. Schedule a yearly examination to focus on your current medical problems, detect new problems, and/ or prevent future problems. Keep your PCP updated on any changes in your Parkinson's symptoms and treatment, as this may influence how other problems are treated and help avoid medication interactions. Many of the tools on the ⮕ *Every Victory Counts* website will help you do this.

Listed below are just a few of the medical concerns or preventative measures important to people with Parkinson's. (This is not a complete list but serves to reinforce the critical role your PCP has in your general health.)

PREVENTION

Preventative care, which includes regular health tests and screenings, is important for everyone, and some screenings are especially crucial for people living with Parkinson's. This kind of care includes everything from immunization vaccines to cancer screenings, blood pressure checks, cholesterol tests, and regular vision checks. Here, we'll look at some of the preventative care services you should discuss with your care team.

BONE HEALTH

Bone health becomes increasingly important as we age and become less physically active. Bones can become thinner and weaker as we grow older, increasing the risk of fractures from falls. Other changes associated with aging and Parkinson's are flexed posture, spine and joint arthritis, and pain. Osteoporosis (bone loss) and osteopenia (bone thinning) are treatable bone conditions that can harm bone health, especially the spine. Ask your physician about a bone density scan for early detection of osteoporosis or decreased bone density. This is important for both men and women.

Vitamin D is needed to help your body absorb calcium for strong bones. If you don't spend much time outdoors or always use sunscreen while you're outside, your vitamin D levels may be low due to minimal sun exposure. (The paradox here, of course, is that sunscreen is highly recommended for people with Parkinson's because of increased risks for skin cancer, but wearing it blocks your body from absorbing vitamin D from the sun. Talk to your physician for personalized recommendations about appropriate sun exposure for your needs.)

Parkinson's itself can also be associated with lower vitamin D levels, and because vitamin D helps your body absorb the calcium needed for strong bones, it is important to monitor your vitamin D levels. A blood test can determine your vitamin D level and whether supplementation would be appropriate.

DENTAL HEALTH

Regular dental exams and cleanings are important to ensure you have healthy teeth and gums. At these appointments, often scheduled every six months, your dentist can check for cavities, plaque, tartar, and gum disease and ensure that you are properly caring for your oral health. See the article at the end of this chapter for more information about dental health.

VISION HEALTH

Even people with perfect eyesight should schedule regular eye exams as part of their preventative care routine. These exams are essential for screening for eye diseases and preserving your vision. Typically, an eye exam includes visual acuity tests (sharpness), depth perception tests, eye alignment, and eye movement. Your eye physician may also use eye drops to dilate your pupils, allowing them to check for common eye problems such as diabetic retinopathy, glaucoma, and age-related macular degeneration.

Ali Hamedani, MD, MHS, instructor in neurology in the Division of Neuro-Ophthalmology at the University of Pennsylvania, says these are important for people with Parkinson's to keep in mind for two reasons: first, up to half of all vision loss in the US is preventable or treatable with early detection through annual eye exams, and second, vision loss has a disproportionate impact on people with Parkinson's: it increases the risk of falls, hip fractures, depression, anxiety, hallucinations, and dementia.

The American Academy of Ophthalmology recommends that all adults over 65 receive a comprehensive eye exam every one to two years. The recommended frequency of eye exams is every two to four years for age 40-54 and every one to three years for age 55-64. If you have a history of diabetes or are at an increased risk of glaucoma (for example, if you have a family history of glaucoma), you should have an eye exam every year regardless of age.

There are several different types of eye physicians. Ophthalmologists are physicians who have completed four years of medical school followed by four years of residency training in ophthalmology. They are experts in all aspects of eye disease, and most of them also perform surgery to treat eye conditions (cataracts, for example). Optometrists are healthcare providers who complete physician training in optometry but who have not attended medical school. They perform routine eye exams and prescribe glasses or contact lenses. If they detect a problem (such as glaucoma), they often refer to an ophthalmologist for further management, and they do not perform surgery. As Dr. Hamedani discusses later in this chapter, neuro-ophthalmologists are either neurologists or ophthalmologists with expertise in visual symptoms from neurologic disease. They provide guidance on specific visual symptoms related to Parkinson's (for example, double vision) but generally do not provide other routine eye care.

SKIN HEALTH

Skin cancer is the most common cancer in the US, and melanoma, one type of skin cancer, has been consistently linked to Parkinson's. Melanoma, which is treatable if caught early, can be dangerous if not detected until the later stages, so it's crucial that people with Parkinson's focus on skin protection and regular skin cancer screenings. During these screenings, a dermatologist will check your skin for moles, birthmarks, or other marks that are unusual in color, size, shape, or texture. If skin cancer is suspected after a screening, your physician will perform a biopsy to remove cells from the suspicious mark on your skin. A pathologist will then study the cells or tissue under a microscope to check for damage or disease.

LUNG HEALTH - SMOKING

Smoking is directly associated with heart disease, lung problems, and cancer. It also can reduce your stamina, making exercise and your everyday movements more difficult. Smoking harms your brain and bone health. If you need to kick the habit, there are various medications, nicotine supplements, and behavioral therapies available to help.

HEART HEALTH

Your heart supplies blood to vital organs, including your brain. Blood pressure control, diabetes care, screening for control of high cholesterol, dietary changes, weight management, and regular aerobic exercise are all important tasks that you and your PCP may work on together so you can maintain a healthy heart and brain. In general, what is good for your heart is also good for your brain.

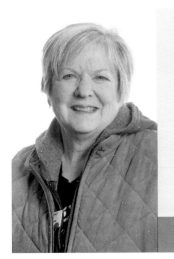

" *I tell each and every person I come in contact with that I have Parkinson's. From the receptionist who checks me in, to the maintenance staff who spread the de-icer on the sidewalk to the nurses who need to provide my medications on time, everyone knows. I have done my job when I hear from out in the hallway, 'Here's the ice cream for the lady with Parkinson's in room nine!'"*

— CAROL CLUPNY

HOSPITAL STAYS AND PARKINSON'S

In Chapter 7, we discussed important medication information to keep in mind during hospital stays. Here, we'll tell you where you can find helpful worksheets and checklists you can take with you to the hospital, as well as other information that can keep you feeling your best during and after your stay.

PREPARE YOURSELF FOR CHANGING SYMPTOMS

Your motor symptoms can worsen when you are coping with a medical illness in addition to your Parkinson's; so, during a hospital stay, you might not be able to move as well as you usually can, and you might find that some symptoms, such as tremor, dyskinesia, and freezing, worsen. Similarly, confusion and hallucinations can occur or worsen in the setting of medical stress or as a result of new medications, such as narcotics for pain or sedatives for sleep, anxiety, or agitation. Being aware that these symptoms might appear or worsen can help you feel more prepared and, just as importantly, inform others about what might occur and how to treat your symptoms.

WORKSHEETS AND HOSPITAL PREP

On our ⮕ *Every Victory Counts* website, you'll find several documents to help you capture and share medical information. A few to complete and take with you during your hospital stay include 📄Prepare for Your Hospital Stay, 📄Medical Summary for Your Physician's Appointment, and 📄Daily Medication Log.

Make sure you arrive at the hospital with a complete and updated list of your medications, dosages, and the times of day you take them. Be sure your hospital care team understands how important it is that you take your Parkinson's medications on time.

Also, take the 📄Current Symptoms Summary with you, which will help your hospital care team understand and recognize your symptoms. This will also explain why it is so vital for you to get your medications on time. Remember, you or your care partner should strongly voice your need to receive your medications on schedule.

Wear a medical alert bracelet if you have serious medication, latex, or tape allergies or if you have a surgical implant. If you have a stoma for enteral suspension or have had deep brain stimulation surgery, include the manufacturer's phone number on the medical alert bracelet in case of emergency.

BE YOUR OWN ADVOCATE

Sometimes, treatments in the hospital cause difficulty swallowing or eating. If this is the case, ask your providers about taking dissolvable carbidopa/levodopa instead of regular pills.

During your stay, ask for a physical therapy, occupational therapy, or speech therapy consult as illness and prolonged bed rest can weaken your body and affect daily activities. Also, consider asking to see a social worker, especially if you have questions about community resources, special needs after discharge, or changes in living arrangements. Chaplain services are available in most hospitals and are there to support you, no matter what your spiritual needs or beliefs. If you have had a severe illness or surgery, ask your neurologist and physician about inpatient (hospital-based) rehabilitation or home health services that may include social work, nursing, or dietary and rehabilitation services.

> *My healthcare career spanned 35 years. One of my physician friends once said, 'You're much more knowledgeable about your Parkinson's than I am. I can take care of heart attacks, trauma, sepsis, respiratory failure with no issue. But I might see one Parkinson's patient in my ER in a year, and I don't readily recall what limited knowledge I have about Parkinson's.' One of my roles was as the dietitian who oversaw the nutritional care for patients in critical care. One of my patients, admitted over the weekend for sepsis, had recovered but remained unresponsive, was unable to eat, and was immobile. His family stated that he had been interactive with family, ate normally, and moved about readily prior to admission. He was scheduled for a brain MRI the next morning to determine the reasons for his change in status. I reviewed his medical record and spoke with his nurse (the best RN in the ICU) and asked him to contact the hospitalist for an order to restart one of his home Parkinson's meds. The nurse replied, 'He's NPO (no food by mouth) and unresponsive.' I insisted and an order was obtained and the medication was given. The next morning, I found the patient up in a chair at his bedside, eating breakfast, conversing with his family. His MRI was canceled, he transferred out of Critical Care, and was discharged home the following day. This example is why each of us needs to be our own advocate so that we receive our medications on time (our schedule), with the correct dose, every time. Hospitalists, intensivists, ER docs, nurses, and pharmacists may not have a good knowledge of Parkinson's; they do not mean to cause us harm, but the necessary rules in hospitals don't always work for people with Parkinson's. While work is ongoing to better meet our needs while hospitalized through changes to our electronic medical records, we must remain diligent to ensure we are not given medications that can harm us and that our personal medication schedule is followed on time, every time.*"

— MARTY ACEVEDO

QUESTIONS TO ASK BEFORE DISCHARGE

- Have my neurologist and primary care physician been notified of my condition while I've been in the hospital?

- When should I next visit my primary care physician?

- Should I receive additional rehabilitation, such as physical therapy?

- What tests, procedures, or new diagnoses have I received?

- What medications have been changed (if any) and why?

- How do I get a copy of the hospital records sent to my physician?

HOSPITAL TIPS FOR PEOPLE WITH ENTERAL SUSPENSION CARBIDOPA/LEVODOPA OR DEEP BRAIN STIMULATION (DBS)

Be sure your physicians and nurses are informed about your enteral suspension or DBS. In some cases of DBS, MRI and diathermy cannot be performed without risk of serious injury to you. Use the 📄DBS Medical History form in the Worksheets and Resources section of our ⤢ *Every Victory Counts* website to provide your hospital care team with the appropriate information about your DBS if a surgery or procedure must be performed.

PARKINSON'S AND ANESTHESIA

Because anesthetic medications can interact with Parkinson's medications, and because Parkinson's puts people at a higher risk of experiencing side effects from anesthesia, your care team must understand these risks. Most people with Parkinson's tolerate anesthesia well. Still, special considerations are required, especially related to the timing of medications before and after surgery and the potential for neuropsychiatric problems, such as psychosis and confusion, following anesthesia.

Typically, it is not recommended to stop taking your Parkinson's medications before receiving anesthesia. To ensure you continue to receive your medications on time during procedures requiring extended anesthesia, your hospital care team may be able to administer carbidopa/levodopa through a nasogastric tube. As we have stressed, you or your care partner must stress to your hospital team how crucial it is to receive your medications on schedule.

Talk to your care team to see if you can avoid general anesthesia, which puts you completely to sleep. Instead, you could consider receiving local anesthesia, which numbs only one or a few body parts and tends to cause fewer side effects. Know, too, that if you experience worsening or new symptoms, such as psychosis, following anesthesia, this is typically short-lived. For questions about side effects and other risks, be sure to communicate with your physician, anesthesiologist, and other care team members.

"How Can my Dental Health Impact my Parkinson's?"

By Jane Busch, DDS

Regular visits to the dentist are, of course, important for all of us. As a dentist, I encouraged my patients to brush, floss, and see me regularly. For a person who has Parkinson's, good dental care is even more critical. That's because Parkinson's can impact the mouth and jaw and make dental care more challenging. I know this well, being both a retired dentist and a person living with Parkinson's.

HOW DOES PARKINSON'S AFFECT DENTAL HEALTH?

Research is currently exploring whether Parkinson's can directly increase the risk of periodontal disease (tooth or gum decay). What we do know is that decay can be caused by poor oral hygiene, either due to inadequate oral hygiene related to loss of dexterity or from conditions like dry mouth.

Then, there are the general effects of Parkinson's. Fatigue, apathy, and depression may make it difficult to even make or keep a dental appointment.

Rigidity, tremor, and dyskinesia can occur not only generally but orally and facially. This can lead to jaw discomfort, cracked teeth, tooth wear, and denture instability. In addition, rigidity and tremor of the hands causes a loss of dexterity, leading to oral hygiene issues. Dyskinesia may cause tooth grinding.

AT YOUR DENTAL APPOINTMENT

Your dentist specializes in treating your mouth, but it is tied in with the rest of your body's systems. Thus, the dentist must have a complete picture of your medical status. The information you provide in the medical history form is important. The more your dentist knows about you, the better care they can provide. Tell your dentist about your overall health, the degree to which Parkinson's affects you, and all the medications you take (both prescription and non-prescription). Your dentist might consider consulting your neurologist to inquire about disease stage, cognitive impairment, drug interactions, and treatment modifications. For example, people with Parkinson's who take MAO-B inhibitors need to limit the amount of epinephrine received via local anesthetics because it can raise blood pressure. A consult with your neurologist is most likely warranted, especially for elective general surgery, as it may be recommended to stop this medication prior to surgery. Your dentist will also evaluate the potential for drug interactions and avoid prescribing pain medications that are contraindicated.

Some Parkinson's symptoms can make dental check-ups more involved. For example, difficulty in swallowing, or dysphagia, is a big concern. This problem often causes decreased cough reflux, which increases the risk of aspiration. Discuss swallowing challenges with your dentist, as there are precautions they can take, such as using barrier protection or more diligent suctioning, to keep water and debris from reaching the back of your throat.

In addition, some motor symptoms present challenges at the dentist's office. It is more challenging for a dentist to work on a patient whose jaw is constantly moving or is so rigid that they can't open their mouth wide enough. Something as simple as the timing of medications can make your dentist's job easier and make you more comfortable.

Ask your dentist to keep the dental chair more upright to assist in swallowing. Plan shorter, morning appointments that are about 45 minutes in length. Schedule the start of the appointment about 60-90 minutes after taking your Parkinson's medication (or the amount of time it typically takes for your medication to begin optimally managing your symptoms). After dental treatment, rise from the chair gradually to prevent dizziness caused by orthostatic hypotension (OH). Ask your dental team to provide all instructions verbally and in writing.

Consider using our 📄Dental Worksheet as you prepare for your appointment and bring the 📄Medical Summary for Dentists to help educate your dentist about Parkinson's, both of which can be found on the ↗*Every Victory Counts* website.

HOW OFTEN SHOULD YOU SEE YOUR DENTIST?

I recommend more frequent check-ups for people with Parkinson's and a tooth cleaning at least every six months (every three months, if there is gum disease). Even if you wear dentures, routine visits are necessary to screen for oral cancer and evaluate the fit of your dentures. Restoration of oral health is best completed in the early stages of Parkinson's. If possible, replace old fillings, crowns, bridges, and ill-fitting dentures before your symptoms progress. Consider dental implants, especially for overdentures. Dental implants are metal substructures embedded in the upper or lower jawbone to which an overdenture can be attached. These stabilize the denture from the dislodging forces caused by chewing and swallowing, which helps the denture last longer.

DENTAL HOME CARE

Oral hygiene at home starts with your toothbrush. Your toothbrush should have a large handle to grip and soft bristles. A small brush head reaches the corners better. Electric toothbrushes work well, and some even have timers to remind you how long to brush. Ideally, brush after every meal for two minutes, and be sure to brush your tongue. Try a "one-handed" strategy, using the stronger side of your body. If you can't brush after a meal, rinse your mouth with water. Replace your brush every three months or when the bristles show wear. Floss once daily, preferably at bedtime. Floss aids ("floss swords") can be helpful, though you might need help from a care partner.

An over-the-counter fluoride rinse helps prevent decay, but you must be able to swish and spit. Your dentist may prescribe fluoride gels applied with a toothbrush or sponge applicator for serious decay issues. Periodontal disease may be treated with a prescription anti-microbial rinse containing chlorhexidine.

If you wear dentures, clean them daily. You may brush them or use a soaking cleanser. You should leave your dentures out at night.

As a dentist, I treated patients with Parkinson's. Now I, too, am living with Parkinson's. My teeth are important to me, as is my overall health. I encourage you to be committed to your dental health and consider it an essential part of your overall wellness.

About Jane Busch

Jane Busch is a former practicing dentist in Cross Plains, WI, and a current fitness instructor, focusing on Parkinson's. She completed her undergraduate degree at the University of Wisconsin-Madison and earned a bachelor's degree in dentistry and a Doctor of Dental Surgery at the University of Minnesota School of Dentistry-Minneapolis. After completing her education, Dr. Busch worked in a private dental practice for nearly 17 years, leaving in 1999 to become director of education for the Academy for Excellence in Dental Technology, an academic training program for dental technicians through D&S Dental Laboratory, Inc. For several years, she also was a post-graduate dental instructor at Madison Area Technical College.

Dr. Busch is a member of several professional societies, including Omicron Kappa Upsilon National Dental Society, the American Dental Association, the Wisconsin Dental Association, and the Dane County Dental Society. She is the founder, CEO, and chair of the LIFE Foundation (Lifestyles Initiative for Fitness Empowerment), a community-based health initiative fostering healthy lifestyles with evidence-based strategies.

"How Can Parkinson's Impact my Vision?"

By Daniel Gold, DO and Ali G. Hamedani, MD MHS

Research has shown that visual symptoms are extraordinarily common in people living with Parkinson's. Visual symptoms may occur due to changes in the front of the eye due to dry eye, changes in the retina (the part of our eyes that senses light), or changes in how our eyes move together. At the same time, many other things can affect vision, including diseases such as age-related macular degeneration, glaucoma, and cataracts, which increase with age. Distinguishing between visual symptoms caused directly by Parkinson's versus one of these other conditions can be difficult.

HOW VISION WORKS

Vision plays such a critical function that a substantial portion of our brain is made up of pathways that connect our eyes to the visual areas of our brain and the areas that help process this visual information (e.g., color, shape, size, motion). The primary purpose of the front part of our eyes (the cornea, lens, etc.) is to produce the clearest possible image, which is then transmitted to the back part of the eye, called the retina. The retina is made up of nerve cells that communicate via visual pathways using the neurotransmitter dopamine. In addition, we have two eyes with overlapping visual fields, which enables our brain to see the world in three dimensions and process complex visual information.

HOW PARKINSON'S IMPACTS VISION

Symptoms related to Parkinson's can be specific: eyes can feel dry, gritty/sandy, and may burn or have redness. You may experience crusting on the lashes, lids that stick together in the morning, sensitivity to light, or dry eye. On the other hand, symptoms can be non-specific: you may notice your vision just isn't what it used to be, and you have difficulty seeing on a rainy night, in dim lighting, or while reading, etc.

Vision problems can bring many practical challenges. For example, difficulty with color vision and loss of contrast sensitivity (the ability to differentiate an object from its background) can make reading signs or walking down patterned stairs difficult. Problems with motion perception and clarity of vision can affect driving.

Many of the visual symptoms experienced by people living with Parkinson's are mild, and overall visual function can remain quite good with routine examinations by an eye care professional. However, multiple, small abnormalities in combination may become problematic and cause more significant symptoms.

COMMON VISION PROBLEMS

Blurry vision and difficulty with color vision. Blurry vision may be related to dopamine depletion in the back of the eye and within the visual connections through the brain. This may be partially corrected with dopaminergic medications, though medication effects are usually subtle regarding vision, so you may not notice them.

Visual processing difficulty. This refers to the orientation of lines and edges, as well as depth perception. This can take different forms, including:

- Troubles with peripheral vision: distracted by objects and targets in your peripheral vision

- Difficulties perceiving overlapping objects

- Difficulty copying and recalling figures (e.g., intersecting pentagons)

- Difficulties detecting whether motion is occurring and in which direction

- Difficulties recognizing faces, facial expressions, and emotions

Dry Eye. Dry eyes are a consequence of decreased blinking and poor production of tears. Dry eye can be worsened by certain medications prescribed for Parkinson's, such as trihexyphenidyl or Artane. Dry eye improves with liberal use of artificial tears and good eye/eyelid hygiene. Of note, dry eye doesn't always feel dry! Sometimes it feels like watering, and other times it just feels like blurring or being out of focus.

Double vision due to convergence insufficiency. Convergence insufficiency is a common problem that can interfere significantly with a person's ability to focus on an object as it moves closer to them. This can be diagnosed during a routine examination by your eye care professional and often presents as seeing side-by-side or "double" images when reading. Other symptoms often emerge while reading or doing close work and include headaches, eye strain, blurry vision, short attention span, constant adjusting of the distance of a book, and loss of place on the page.

When double vision is experienced, the person living with Parkinson's should cover each eye individually. If double vision resolves when covering *either* eye, this is probably a convergence problem. If there is still double vision in one eye when the other is covered, this is often due to dry eye or an optical/refractive disturbance.

To help with convergence problems, consider:

- Occasionally, eye exercises like "pencil push-ups" can help with convergence problems. Pencil push-ups involve slowly moving a small object, like the tip of a pencil, from arm's length towards the nose, repeating 20 or so times a few times a day for a few weeks. There's no clear protocol or prescription for this, and it is usually much more effective in younger people recovering from head trauma, such as concussions.

- You could try an old trick of covering one eye or putting Scotch tape over one lens of your reading glasses to ensure only one eye is being used at a time.

- Regarding glasses, reading glasses are preferable to bifocals or progressives since they provide a greater area of visibility for reading. Your eye physician can also fit reading glasses with prisms to help with double vision due to convergence insufficiency.

257

Hallucinations. Hallucinations can result from Parkinson's itself or be exacerbated by medications used to treat Parkinson's. While it never hurts to inform your eye care professional about hallucinations you are experiencing, you should discuss these in detail with your neurologist. For an in-depth look at hallucinations and Parkinson's, see Chapter 5.

UNCOMMON VISION PROBLEMS

- **Blepharospasm.** Involuntary, forceful eyelid closure. May sometimes respond to carbidopa/levodopa dose adjustment or be treated with botulinum toxin injections around the eyes.

- **Apraxia of eyelid opening.** Difficulty voluntarily opening the eyes in the absence of spasms that force the eyes closed.

- **Vertical eye movement limitations.** Most common with progressive supranuclear palsy. People living with this disorder may be messy eaters or have significant difficulty walking downstairs due to eye limitations in looking down.

TAKE ACTION TO LIVE WELL

While there are no proven ways to prevent most ocular conditions from developing, routine visits with an eye care professional can lead to early recognition and treatment of eye issues before they harm your quality of life. Between you, your neurologist, and an ophthalmologist, most visual complaints can be handled. However, when symptoms remain unchanged and unexplained, consultation with a *neuro-ophthalmologist* is probably warranted.

A neuro-ophthalmologist is either a neurologist or an ophthalmologist with fellowship training in neuro-ophthalmology. Neuro-ophthalmologists have a unique appreciation for the intersection of the eyes and the brain and perform comprehensive testing in the office to determine where a visual or eye movement problem could originate. Once the location of the disturbance is identified, diagnostic testing (when appropriate), treatments, and therapies can be customized depending on the individual and their concerns(s).

While your eye care professional may not be aware of common ocular symptoms that people living with Parkinson's experience, explaining the kinds of situations and triggers that bring on eye symptoms is usually enough for your physician to know where to look during the examination (e.g., front part of the eye, back part of the eye, movements of the eyes). Keeping a journal or diary of symptoms can also be helpful for both you and your physician.

As we have stressed throughout this manual, you are more than your Parkinson's. Just as you make time for the activities that help you live well with Parkinson's, prioritize your general health to maintain or even improve your quality of life throughout your life.

About Daniel Gold

Daniel Gold, DO, is an assistant professor of neurology, ophthalmology, otolaryngology – head & neck surgery and neurosurgery at The Johns Hopkins School of Medicine in Baltimore, Maryland. He is a neurologist with fellowship training in neuro-ophthalmology. Dr. Gold has additional training in vestibular neurology and also sees patients with dizziness and imbalance. He is the director of Urgent Neurology, and has a particular interest in the rapid diagnosis and treatment of acute neuro-ophthalmologic and vestibular disorders.

Dr. Gold completed his DO at the University of Medicine and Dentistry of New Jersey – School of Osteopathic Medicine. He completed his residency in neurology at the University of Maryland and his fellowship in neuro-ophthalmology at the Hospital of the University of Pennsylvania.

About Ali Hamedani

Ali Hamedani is a neuro-ophthalmologist and movement disorder specialist at the University of Pennsylvania. He earned his Bachelor of Science in Biology at Yale University and his MD at the University of Maryland School of Medicine. He also holds a master's degree in epidemiology from the Johns Hopkins Bloomberg School of Public Health. Dr. Hamedani joined the faculty after completing his neurology residency and fellowship training at the University of Pennsylvania. Dr. Hamedani's primary clinical focus is neuro-ophthalmology, which is the study of visual symptoms from neurologic disease, and he has a particular interest in visual dysfunction in Parkinson's and other movement disorders. His research uses national health surveys and administrative claims data to understand how vision affects outcomes and quality of life in Parkinson's and other patient populations.

CHAPTER 15 – LONG-TERM CARE AND FINANCIAL PLANNING

OVERVIEW

Long-term care planning is a task that resembles many other proactive strategies discussed in this manual. Being proactive and discussing the situations you may face in the future is a positive endeavor and paves the way to your best future. Ask members of your wellness team about their experience with people with Parkinson's who find they need long-term care. Their insights can help as you think about future needs and how to plan ahead.

For instance, if falling becomes one of your mobility challenges, living in a multi-story home adds to the risk. For this reason, many people with Parkinson's transition to a one-story home before it becomes necessary. This way, making a move can be about simplifying life and the positive experience of creating a new home, rather than a negative reaction to a crisis or to a forced move due to safety concerns. Some people prefer to live closer to metropolitan areas to reduce drive time and for easier access to medical services, municipal services, and activities. While moving may not be the right solution for you, talking through the issues related to Parkinson's before problems occur gives you and your family time to think without the added stress of urgency.

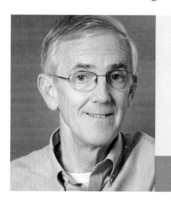

> " *It's the instability of what the future may bring, but we've still got to learn and keep digging for answers. We can't let uncertainty frighten us. We've got to be serious about it, but we've also got to keep our sense of humor.*"
>
> — MIKE

HEALTH-RELATED LEGAL PREPARATIONS

An important aspect of long-term care planning is getting your health-related documents in order. Once the documents are completed, they will be there when you need them.

The following are typically included in long-term healthcare planning:

- **Durable Power of Attorney.** A legal document allowing you to give someone else the authority to make financial and legal decisions for you if you are incapacitated

- **Medical Power of Attorney.** A legal document designating a person who will have the right to make healthcare decisions for you if you are incapacitated by illness or accident and unable to do so for yourself

- **Advance Care Directive.** A document prepared in advance, giving specific instructions about your healthcare wishes if you are unable to give those instructions yourself

Having both a medical and financial power of attorney will make it much easier for your loved ones to work with hospitals, physicians, banks, or anyone else who will potentially be involved in your care. You should also talk with your partner or family member about your end-of-life wishes. The Family Caregiver Alliance offers additional information and guidance on these topics at caregiver.org.

> *Planning is very, very important. Anybody with Parkinson's thinking about retiring should sit down with a financial advisor and look at how to scale things so you're living at a level within your means. Social security is a lot further off for someone with young onset Parkinson's."*
>
> — STEVE HOVEY

UNDERSTANDING YOUR PARKINSON'S PROGRESSION

The discussion about needing help at home or about assisted living should occur well before an event leaves you in crisis mode and compromises your ability to process options calmly. Have a thoughtful discussion with your physician and care partner about your prognosis so you'll have a good understanding of when your Parkinson's reaches a point where you require increased supervision. Your providers can let you know when a higher level of medical help at home or when a move to a care facility would be advisable. For instance, the onset of hallucinations and paranoia that cannot be addressed by medication may signal the need for constant supervision. If blood pressure becomes erratic and treatment options do not address the issues, a home nurse or nursing home placement may be advised. Cognitive and mood-related symptoms typically require more hands-on care than some of the mobility challenges of Parkinson's. It's crucial for you and your family to anticipate and recognize worsening symptoms that are unlikely to improve with medication therapy. This knowledge will prepare you to take appropriate steps when care needs to increase.

Many of the advanced symptoms of Parkinson's can be managed at home with the appropriate assistance; however, be aware that your care partner may take the brunt of increasing demands. Plan together for the onset of some of the more demanding symptoms and encourage your care partner to investigate respite care services so they can get the break they need to recharge. These actions will reduce some of the strain of the difficult decision-making associated with advanced Parkinson's.

> *"You could live for many years and not need this, and yet you don't know – you could have cognitive factors or depression that prevent you from making the decisions you would have when you were at your best. Getting this information early on is very important."*

— JOHN ALEXANDER

"How Can I Plan for the Financial Impact of Parkinson's?"

By Donald L. Haisman, CFP, MBA

At first, the day seemed like a routine visit to a physician's office. Then, after a sunny, two-and-a-half-hour drive to the Cleveland Clinic Florida, a neurologist said to my wife, "You have Parkinson's."

I hardly remember the drive back. Between the discussions the two of us were having, my inner voice kept asking, "What now?"

I was supposed to be an expert planner. For three decades, I was a Certified Financial Planner. I flashed back to the many meetings with families over the years, where I had provided my list of "to-dos" for them to accomplish so they would be prepared for various unforeseen events. Now, on that drive back, I was mentally checking off that "to-do" list while looking not into the eyes of a client but into a mirror in my mind. Was I a cobbler with no shoes, or had I followed my own financial planning advice in my own life? One of those unforeseen life events had just happened to me, to my wife... to us.

> *My Parkinson's encouraged my husband to retire earlier to spend time with and take care of me. He was working all day and then coming home to take care of both me and the kids, which was a lot. He does the laundry, the housework, the finances. Like many husbands, he's always done some of those, but now it's on a totally different level. When I do help, it's not with the same energy at the same level I used to."*

— JILL ATER

Once you receive a diagnosis of Parkinson's, you need to prepare your to-do list. Since I am a US citizen, I am familiar with US legal protections and procedures. If you reside elsewhere, the basic planning concepts still apply, although you might need to investigate the specifics in your country. Here are the items that I recommend you consider:

262

1. Complete Advance Directives and Other Legal Preparation

This should be quite high on your list, probably even number one. Your legal preparation should consist of various documents that will lay out your plans now that Parkinson's is in your family picture. A friend of mine who is an estate planning attorney reminded me that in addition to a will and maybe a trust, it is very important to have a Durable Power of Attorney and a Designation of Healthcare Surrogate in place to avoid guardianship. If you live in the US or Canada, this collective group of legal documents is frequently called advance directives. If you live elsewhere, familiarize yourself with the legal documents that allow you to designate a loved one to make healthcare decisions on your behalf, should you become unable to do so yourself. US residents might also want to review Medicaid benefits and determine how those fit into the plan.

> *Witnessing a relative go through a major health scare without having legal paperwork describing his wishes caused his wife and family turmoil. It made me very glad my husband and I have planned, so our choices in difficult times are known."*
>
> — CAROL CLUPNY

Your advance directives will lay out the foundation of your estate plan, which is an orderly plan for your family for the future. Do not rely on legal documents that you created years ago since changes to the laws and statutes where you live are common. Your legal documents need to be updated to comply with those changes and the new reality of your life. If you are considering relocating due to Parkinson's, consider having your legal documents drawn in your intended eventual place of residence because much of your planning will be specific to that area, especially legal documents.

I have often run across the situation that the person living with Parkinson's was previously named to be a legally responsible party, like a trustee or maybe custodian of a child's education fund. With the new diagnosis, this responsibility may better be transferred to another person.

2. Appraise Your Financial Situation

This can be done by listing all the items of value that you and your family own or in which you have any financial or legal interest. This might be all investments, real estate, retirement accounts, business interests, hobbies of value, or automobiles. Make a note of the legal owner of each item or collection. Locate the deeds.

Locate all insurance policies. This includes life, disability, long-term care, homeowners, and auto (also known as property and casualty). Do not forget that general liability or "umbrella" liability policy, if you have one.

Now here is a difficult question: who or what OWNS the policies? Yes, most insurance policies have owners, and this is critical to know. The owner has control of the policy. In that same vein, who or what is the beneficiary of those policies? This is probably one of the most overlooked financial planning issues. Are the beneficiaries (and the owners) appropriate now? Also, know that most insurance policies have a person you can designate to be notified if premiums are not being paid. It is probably a good idea to implement this service.

Your retirement plans require special attention because they have distinct and unique rules and tax ramifications. Beneficiary designations are of particular importance here, and also remember to name secondary beneficiaries.

> " *Anyone with Parkinson's has to face the reality that life could change – maybe not for a long time, but financial planning becomes much more important than before. The clock moves faster than you'd anticipated. I recently left my job of 15 years, though I didn't anticipate fully retiring quite yet, so I've had to look at other options.*"
>
> — JOHN ALEXANDER

3. Organize

Gather all your original legal documents. Include a detailed list of all your valuable assets, along with the ownership information. If you and your wellness team have prepared a healthcare plan, include a copy of that as well. Collect and store your insurance policies in one place, along with your list of current beneficiaries for all retirement plans and insurance policies.

Finally, tell your executor or a trusted friend or family member how and where to access all this information. If your files are stored electronically, be sure to provide them with all passwords.

> " *I was invited to speak to a cohort of physical therapy students about medications. We spoke of this drug and that, possible side effects, and changes in effectiveness over time. It was all quite clinical until I revealed that I had Parkinson's and explained about my drugs, the number of pills I took daily and at what intervals, the timing of carbidopa/levodopa with regard to meals (protein), and the out-of-pocket expense. They were dumbstruck at the cost of my Medicare and supplemental insurance coverage ('Isn't Medicare free?') versus the cost of medications. I let them know that my social security is currently less than one-third of my pre-retirement income. I added that my*

annual social security 'raise' was not keeping up with the rising costs of my supplemental insurance plans, let alone any new wonder drugs coming down the pike that would have potential to make my life better if I could afford the drug. I wanted to leave them with a positive thought, so I reminded them that as future professionals, they were looking at a reasonably good income and needed to make financial wellness a goal from day one."

— LORRAINE WILSON

4. Ask for Help

I know that all this seems like a monumental task to organize, coordinate, and administer. Remember how important it is that people living with Parkinson's have a devoted care partner or group of care partners and a team of medical professionals so they can have the best outcome? This same concept applies to your financial planning. You should consider a team of "financial" care partners to assist you.

Who should you consider to be on your financial team? Your financial team should be made up of the following functions (Specific US-based designations in parentheses):

- Accountant (ideally a Certified Public Accountant, CPA)
- Attorney who specializes in estate planning
- Financial planner (ideally a Certified Financial Planner-Professional, CFP)
- Investment advisor (many times this is also the CFP)
- Insurance agent (ideally a Certified Life Underwriter, CLU)

Share your honest concerns with those professionals on your team; they likely have years of experience assisting families in your situation.

Someone on your team needs to be the coordinator of all these professionals. This is very important because these disciplines overlap and contribute to your estate plan. Of the professionals I have suggested, the CFP is most likely to have the overall training, experience, and background to be your coordinator. Often, if you start with a CFP, they can refer you to others, if necessary.

5. Take It One Step at a Time

This sounds like a lot of work, and it is. However, once you get organized and develop a plan with your financial care partners, you will feel peace of mind, and it is well worth the effort. The goal is to get your entire financial house in order, simplify your financial life, and make smart money decisions so you can focus more on things you enjoy doing to live well today.

About Donald Haisman

Donald Haisman is the managing director of Carnegie Investment Counsel in Fort Myers, FL, and is the president of Haisman Wealth Management, Inc. He shows successful families and organizations, many with charitable intent, how to simplify their financial lives and make smart money decisions, so they can achieve their goals and fulfill their values. He does this by helping them get their financial house in order and keeping it that way forever.

Mr. Haisman has previously served as the president of multiple organizations, including the Financial Planning Association, the Institute of Certified Financial Planners, the International Association for Financial Planning, and the Estate Planning Council of Lee County. He has also served on the Planned Giving Board of the Lee County American Cancer Society and the National Committee on Planned Giving.

Donald Haisman holds an MBA in finance, an undergraduate degree in mechanical engineering, and is a CFP. He has produced and hosted hundreds of radio shows on various financial and investment topics, been a guest lecturer on cruise ships, and is an occasional "on-air" guest at Waterman Broadcasting local NBC-V2 discussing current financial matters. Mr. Haisman has also authored multiple articles and presented on money management, investing, and charitable giving.

266

"How Can Home Caregivers Improve Health and Quality of Life for People with Parkinson's and Their Families?"

By Bud Rockhill, MBA

At some point, your Parkinson's may progress to the point that you need additional help at home. The timing and type of help depend on your medical condition, family situation, and financial resources. Still, it's worth understanding the types of assistance that are available in advance, especially since the need for outside support can arise with little notice.

There are two basic categories of home assistance, and the process of finding help and the availability of financial support for each are very different. The two types are:

1. Home Healthcare – Medical care provided at home

2. Homecare – Assistance with non-medical Activities for Daily Living (ADL), such as bathing or meal preparation

HOME HEALTHCARE

As the term indicates, home healthcare is the provision of medical care by a medical practitioner at home.

Some of the different types of home healthcare services include:

- Physician care
- Short-term nursing services
- Lab tests
- Medication/pharmacy services
- Physical therapy services
- Occupational therapy services
- Speech-language pathology services
- Medical social work
- Home health aide services
- Companionship
- Nutritional support and meal delivery

In many cases in the US, home healthcare services are covered by Medicare or Medicaid with a physician's prescription. Medicare has an excellent website that provides information you can use to learn about home healthcare and find and evaluate potential providers. You can find the most current information available by visiting ☐ medicare.gov.

To get the most value from the information on the site:

- If you have a Medicare health plan, check it for information on home healthcare benefits
- If you have Medical Supplement insurance, make sure to talk with your physician in advance so that your bills are paid correctly

If your physician or referring healthcare provider decides you need home healthcare, they should give you a list of agencies that serve your area. If they suggest an agency or give you a list, they must tell you whether their organization has a financial interest in that agency.

As with many things in our lives, a recommendation from a trusted source can often be the most efficient way to start the process. Then you can use the information provided on the Medicare website to do a more detailed evaluation.

267

Your physician or medical group may also provide recommendations. It is legal and appropriate for you to ask if the recommended agency is the owner or is affiliated with your physician's group or hospital, and they are obligated to tell you.

The agencies available to you will depend on your insurance plan; so, please make sure to check whether your insurance covers the agency you're interested in. This information should be on the website, but you will want to call your insurance plan to be sure.

Home healthcare is typically provided for 30, 60, or 90 days; based on your physician's orders and insurance plan, the number of visits per week and the length of each visit will vary—such as three times per week for two hours per visit. In most cases, home healthcare does not include full bathing or household activities like laundry.

HOMECARE

A second type of assistance you can receive in your home is homecare, which provides in-home assistance for activities of daily living (ADLs) that are not medical in nature. ADLs are the necessary daily activities people must be able to do to continue to live independently.

There are several variations on the list, but there are five basic categories that are often referenced as ADLs:

1. Personal hygiene, including bathing/showering, grooming, nail care, and oral care
2. Dressing and undressing
3. Eating
4. Maintaining continence, with both the physical and mental capacity to use a restroom, including getting on and off the toilet
5. Transferring – the ability to stand up from a seated position, get in and out of bed, and walk independently (including with a walker or cane)

Medicare and Medicare Supplement plans usually will NOT cover homecare. However, a long-term care policy often does include it. (Note that long-term care is not the same as long-term disability). Also, some Medicare Advantage programs may include homecare coverage.

While long-term care policies were more popular 10 or 20 years ago, people who have this type of policy should review the terms to see what is covered and if homecare is included. The specific coverage will vary by policy, with some having a daily dollar limit and some having a total limit. For example, a policy might limit the daily reimbursement to $100 per day and the total reimbursement over the period for which homecare is provided to $5,000.

Many of these policies require the individual to pay the homecare expenses out of pocket before the reimbursement from the long-term care policy begins. This period is called the "elimination period," which is basically the deductible the policy owner is responsible for paying before any insurance reimbursement will kick in. Please make sure that whoever is managing your care decisions and finances researches your options thoroughly and understands the policies and expenses before hiring a homecare agency.

SELECTING A HOMECARE AGENCY

Finding a homecare agency is an important and personal decision. It's estimated that more than half of all caregiving is provided by a family member. Of the other half, care or help is often provided by a neighbor or friend.

Therefore, deciding to hire a homecare agency rather than relying on a family member, friend, or neighbor is difficult. It can be hard to admit that you need help and hard to allow strangers to have such personal interaction with a family member. Also, it results in additional expenses that can be difficult to come by.

However, it does not need to be an "all or nothing" decision. Sometimes, having a homecare agency is a great way to provide a short break, both mentally and physically, to the family member or friend who is the primary care partner.

There are several places to look for a homecare agency:

- As with home healthcare, your physician or medical group may also provide recommendations
- Many county websites have a department of health and human services or a department of aging that lists providers
- Religious organizations may have affiliated or referred agencies
- You may be able to find an "Aging Lifecare Specialist" whose job is to act as a "concierge" or resource manager to help you save time and provide referrals to trusted providers

Other considerations in evaluating and selecting a homecare agency:

- A reputable agency will have insurance, train their staff, and conduct background checks before hiring caregivers, whereas most care partners who are friends and neighbors will not have insurance or formal training.
- The most important considerations for most people in selecting an agency are the safety of the care recipient and the quality of care. Therefore, it may be prudent to choose an agency whose caregivers are employees rather than independent contractors. This employer-employee relationship provides you with additional protection because it ensures that the agency has worker's compensation and is responsible for paying its employees' payroll taxes.
- The federal government's classification of a caregiver includes employee status. Some people try to operate independently to avoid paying taxes, which could jeopardize the quality of care and create liability issues.

269

- In most cases, be aware that there will be more than one caregiver who serves you or your person with Parkinson's. Rarely will you have one dedicated person providing care. This provides some variety in personalities and can add to the social interaction. On the other hand, you or your care recipient may not get along with every caregiver; so, be sure to exercise your right to request a change if desired.

- In terms of reliability, an agency will be responsible for finding a replacement caregiver if the person scheduled cannot show up for an appointment. Friends and neighbors, on the other hand, have their own lives to manage and sometimes cannot prevent a last-minute schedule change. This can create unnecessary chaos in your home if it happens too often.

INTERVIEWING WITH THE HOMECARE AGENCY

It's essential to interview each homecare agency you consider. Here are a few things to consider:

- Before an in-person interview, conduct a phone conversation to learn the basics. This will also help you assess responsiveness, courtesy, clarity, and the ability to build a rapport over the phone.

- The first interview can be conducted at the agency office or the home (or both).
  - Some adult children will prefer to conduct the first visit at the agency so that they "pre-screen" the agency before introducing anyone to their parent.
  - A home visit allows the agency representative to assess the physical surroundings and understand the environment in which care will be provided.
  - The family should be ready to explain the medical status and physical capabilities or limitations of the person who will receive the care and have an initial list of services they need provided.
  - The family should also explain the daily routine of the person receiving the care— the goal should be to minimize any disruptions that could cause anxiety.
  - The agency may then be able to suggest other services that the family has not considered.

In evaluating and selecting a homecare agency, questions you may want to ask include:

1. What are the minimum number of hours per week required for a person to be employed as a caregiver?
2. What specific training is provided to caregivers about Parkinson's (or other neurological disorders)?
3. What types of checklists or standard procedures are provided and used by caregivers?
4. What type of feedback or reports will the family receive?

a. Is there a standard reporting procedure?

b. Families and caregivers can also benefit from having a care log—a notebook used by the caregivers to note things about the visit. For example, did the person with Parkinson's have trouble eating or refuse to eat? Did they take their medications?

c. Were there any physical/mental changes or general observations about temperament and interaction worth noting?

5. What are the basic rules of care and service?

a. Can a caregiver sleep if they are working overnight?

b. Can they eat?

c. How does the caregiver verify arrival and departure time? For example, some agencies use a call verification system, and the caregiver must call when they arrive and depart from the home.

d. Is the caregiver allowed to drive the person with Parkinson's to appointments or does the agency offer a separate service with a medical transport vehicle?

The family should discuss the amount of care they expect is needed and ask about costs and billing timing/procedures:

1. In the case of a chronic condition or very limited mobility, is 24/7 care needed?

2. With limited mobility, is one caregiver sufficient or will two be needed?

3. Is there a minimum number of hours per shift? Depending on geography, many caregivers may either have a long commute or rely on public transportation and to make it worthwhile, the agency may require a four-hour minimum shift.

4. Is there a long-term care policy in place? If so, the family should explain that the agency should coordinate billing.

5. What type of insurance and bonding is provided if the caregiver has an accident or believes something was stolen?

While the process may seem daunting and the costs intimidating, the goal is to make sure your care is safe, you receive your medications on time, you practice good hygiene, and you stay as engaged and as mobile as possible.

271

"Will I Need Long-Term Care? How Can I Plan for It?"

By Jessica Shurer, LCSW, MSW

Contemplating and planning for the future can be a daunting task, especially when something like Parkinson's keeps you from knowing exactly what to anticipate. Because of this, many people avoid exploring or having preemptive conversations around long-term care needs and options. However, sometimes this can lead to emotionally charged situations where you are faced with important decisions that need to be made more quickly than expected. Whether you are exploring professional in-home care or considering moving to a long-term care community, understanding the options in advance can help give you peace of mind, knowing you are better prepared for the "what ifs."

Do All People with Parkinson's Wind Up in a Facility? Are There Alternatives?

Many people with Parkinson's can have their care needs met in their homes, but this varies greatly and depends on many factors. Take time to reflect on what "aging in place" would mean for you and your partner or family over time. Many people with Parkinson's have increased needs as their symptoms change and progress; so, even if you are opting not to move to a long-term care facility, you may need to tap into additional support systems and resources to stay at home safely.

A good starting point would be to have an occupational therapist perform an in-home evaluation to determine if home safety modifications, such as installing a ramp, widening doorways, and adding grab bars, should be made. Think about whether such modifications are feasible in your home space, what those costs could look like, and what other safety measures might enhance your ability to live safely and independently with Parkinson's.

Consider if you would be willing to bring outside care services into the house and understand what options are available. For in-depth details about this, see the article above.

Besides homecare and home healthcare, adult daycare is another alternative. Adult day centers can be a great addition or alternative to in-home care, as they offer socialization, activity engagement, and monitoring and provide some respite for family care partners.

> **❝** *When my husband semi-retired, we built a house with a lot of adjustments to help me down the road. I didn't need all of them at the time we moved in, but I wanted them there for when I need them in the future."*
>
> — LINDA

What Are the Options for Long-Term Care Communities?

While the definitions can vary, it can be helpful to know the general options for long-term care community-based living:

#1 - Continuing care retirement communities (CCRCs). CCRCs offer multiple levels of care, including independent living, assisted living, and skilled nursing, all within the same community. For many CCRCs, you begin residence in the independent living area and move to the higher care levels with greater assistance and supervision as your care needs change. The policies and requirements vary regarding eligibility; it is common for CCRCs to require up-front "buy-in" fees and a physician's report stating that you will most likely remain independent for a certain number of years.

#2 - Independent living communities. These are often planned communities geared for those over 55. There may be services and amenities offered, such as transportation, meal service, and exercise opportunities, and some will offer "à la carte" contracted in-home care. For the most part, however, you are typically expected to live independently and safely without extensive assistance.

#3 - Assisted living. This level of care is customarily for those who need some assistance with everyday tasks. Residents in assisted living frequently require help with bathing, medication management, household tasks like laundry and meal preparation, and overall safety monitoring, but they may not need much help with mobility or eating. Family care homes often offer an assisted-living level of care but in a more intimate setting, typically with fewer residents and in a house setting.

#4 - Memory care. These care units cater to people with more complex care needs specifically related to cognitive impairment or dementia. This can include delusions or paranoia, disorientation, wandering, agitation, and difficulty with task follow-through (for example, understanding how to get dressed).

#5 - Skilled nursing. This level of care is most appropriate for people who need help with three or more activities of daily living. Additionally, a person may benefit from a skilled nursing facility if they need to follow a more complex medication regimen, have multiple medical diagnoses, or have more involved care requirements, such as a feeding tube, tracheostomy, pressure wound, or catheter.

When It Comes to Finding the Right Long-Term Care Setting for Myself or my Loved One, Where Do I Start?

- **Think about what level of care might be appropriate.** Consider what types of assistance with daily tasks you need. Also, consider what may be needed down the road to avoid multiple residence moves.

- **Reflect on your priorities for a long-term care community.** Think through a few main aspects of a long-term care community that you would prefer and that will meet your needs, lifestyle, and comfort level. Factors to be taken into consideration might include location in relation to family members, cost, quality of food, activities offered, staff turnover, on-site allied health clinicians who have been specifically trained in Parkinson's, and if other people with Parkinson's reside there.

- **Consult your healthcare team.** Ask your physician for their professional input. This can be a neurologist, primary care physician, or whoever is the is most familiar with your symptoms, treatment plan, safety concerns, and care needs. Your allied health care team may contribute their valuable perspectives as well. If you are considering a move to long-term care, your primary Parkinson's physician will benefit from having seen you recently in the event the facility asks them to complete paperwork.

- **If possible, visit at least two communities.** It would be beneficial to schedule a tour when you can ask questions and observe the staff and residents in action and view the living quarters, common areas, outdoor spaces, and surrounding neighborhood. Ask yourself if the residents look clean, happy, and engaged. Inquire about the staff's experience with caring for people with Parkinson's. Getting a feel for the living environment and services offered will help you decide which place is the best fit for you.

- **Check out the reviews.** Because government entities regulate assisted living and skilled nursing, you can often find lists of facilities and ratings online. Medicare has a nursing home comparison tool that can be found online, and many state- or county-level agencies, such as the state Department of Health & Human Services or Area Agencies on Aging, will provide credible information about reported quality of care at assisted living facilities and family care homes. Be aware that privately-owned care finders, social media-style review sites, and sites that accept paid advertising might not always project accurate assessments. You can also ask your friends, community members, and/or those in your Parkinson's support groups if they would share their personal experiences with a long-term care community. Keep in mind that experiences and chemistry with facilities are subjective, and your perspective might be different from what you hear or read.

How Much Will It Cost My Family?

Depending on the level and amount of care needed and where you live, long-term care costs can vary greatly. It is surprising for many to learn that most health insurance, including Medicare, does not cover long-term care. However, it can be covered by Medicaid, long-term care insurance, or veterans' benefits.

Organizations and county and state agencies sometimes offer limited in-home aide or respite programs or vouchers. However, most long-term care services, including facility-based and in-home care, are paid for privately. It can be financially feasible for some and cost-prohibitive for others. Financial advisors and elder law attorneys can also help you better understand what you can afford and explore asset protection options.

This Can Feel a Little Overwhelming at Times. Do You Have Any Other Recommendations When Making These Decisions?

Remember that you do not have to make these decisions alone. There are people who can support and advise you through the process, including family members and your healthcare team. While acknowledging that it may not necessarily be fun, it is extremely helpful to have candid discussions about long-term care decisions.

Reflect together on your support system to address Parkinson's care needs over time, including your primary care partner's physical and mental health. The clinical social worker at your neurology clinic or local aging resources, such as a senior center, long-term care ombudsperson, or Department on Aging, can often share tips and resources. You can also consider hiring a professional geriatric care manager to help you navigate your options. As part of the planning process, it can also be extremely helpful to complete a Healthcare Power of Attorney and Living Will so that you can designate someone to make medical decisions on your behalf if needed and document personal wishes around medical interventions and care.

For many, there is ultimately peace of mind that comes from embracing long-term care, especially when it's planned openly and in advance. For example, it is common for families to share that the quality of their time together improves after a move to long-term care facility because now their shared time can be spent enjoying one another's company instead of being focused on providing care. Another common circumstance we see when a family hires professional in-home care is that people with Parkinson's are pleasantly surprised with the companionship they get from forming a relationship with the caregivers, while family care partners often report improved mental well-being from assistance with daily tasks and having time to recharge. You may be surprised at how much you thrive when you open yourself up to opportunities for *interdependence*.

We recognize that guilt and a sense of lost independence are associated with shifting to residence in a long-term care community or bringing in professional in-home care. This is often a transition for everyone involved, and it is normal and understandable to struggle with different emotions. When making these decisions, allow space to process your feelings while also being aware of your limitations and practical needs. The biggest factor in deciding what type of long-term care accommodation is right is determining what support is needed for your well-being and safety, and what is sustainable for you now and in the future. Overall, what is important is that you know the options available so you can make informed decisions beforehand that will support your best possible quality of life.

Long-term care planning is a difficult undertaking. After all, who is excited for the day when we can't make decisions or are facing the end of our lives? However, by planning ahead with intention, you and your loved ones can rest assured that your needs and wishes are continually met. Prepare for your future now, as you live life to its fullest, so you can continue doing so for many years ahead.

About Jessica Shurer

Jessica Shurer is the Director of Patient and Carepartner Advocacy of CurePSP, whose mission and services are dedicated to the awareness, education, care, and cure of atypical Parkinsonism diseases—progressive supranuclear palsy, corticobasal degeneration, and multiple system atrophy. Prior to joining the team at CurePSP in October 2021, she served as the Center Coordinator & Clinical Social Worker of the Movement Disorders Center at the University of North Carolina at Chapel Hill, a Parkinson's Foundation Center of Excellence and CurePSP Center of Care. She had been in this previous position since graduating from UNC Chapel Hill with her Master of Social Work in 2012. Her clinical and research interests include the psychosocial needs of navigating neurodegenerative disease, integrated healthcare models, and palliative and end-of-life care.

Parkinson's Today and Beyond

■ CHAPTER 16 – LIVING WELL WITH PARKINSON'S TODAY

As Professor Bas Bloem said in his foreword, now is a time for hope for people living with Parkinson's. From innovative new treatments to increasing awareness of exercise's neurological benefits to encouraging advocacy initiatives, the Parkinson's field is rapidly changing for the better. You don't have to wait for the future, though, to begin living well with Parkinson's. Begin today. Here's what you can do, starting right now, to live well with Parkinson's.

**   ** *Wellness is a choice. No one can make you better until you want to be better."*

— JILL ATER

Listen. Pay attention to your body and report changes to your healthcare team. Listen also to family and friends who may see changes in you that you don't notice.

277

Think holistically. Every part of you is connected to and influenced by the other parts of you; so, it is important to address Parkinson's through the whole picture of lifestyle, nutrition, exercise, stress management, relationships, and personal and spiritual care and growth.

Be informed. Learn how personal and lifestyle habits can impact your Parkinson's symptoms. The more you know, the more empowered you'll feel to form useful habits to minimize your symptoms.

Be prepared. Organize your healthcare documents and other information important to your medical team. Prepare for your medical appointments to get the best results from your time with your physicians.

Be your own best advocate. Ask for a referral to a rehabilitation therapist if you haven't received one. Talk with your healthcare team about your goals and concerns. Make them aware of areas you want to improve. If you seek treatment early and are specific about symptoms or problems that are frustrating, you'll help your physician develop the most effective treatment plan for you.

Prioritize the symptoms you can change. This may mean taking medicines on time to limit symptoms or beginning rehabilitative therapy to improve posture or the volume of your voice. It may mean starting or renewing your commitment to daily exercise and may also include changing your lifestyle to promote overall health. You can't change that you have Parkinson's, but you can absolutely change how you live with it.

Learn to live with the symptoms you can't change. Although a combination of medications, complementary therapies, and lifestyle changes will help you manage Parkinson's symptoms, symptoms will still show up in different ways in your life. Start to learn different ways to live with the reality of symptoms as you manage them or ways to manage those symptoms that may be less responsive to the various therapies we've mentioned. For instance, if a bothersome tremor doesn't always respond to medications, try reducing the anxiety that can make your tremor worse. Practice deep breathing relaxation techniques and reduce stress as other ways to help manage tremor and explore additional ways to minimize stressors that worsen other symptoms.

Be engaged. Seek out support from people with whom you feel comfortable sharing your thoughts and concerns, such as family members, friends, or individuals from church or work. Support groups can be helpful, as are group exercise classes and gatherings with other people living with Parkinson's who encourage and inspire you.

" *For decades I knew wellness was multifactorial and found that I was usually at my best when I regularly focused on the 'fab four:' physical, spiritual, social, and emotional wellness. I am now convinced that the 'fab five' makes life even better. Creative wellness includes making art and/or appreciating the art of others. It increases the value I place on myself and others as we interact in this thing called life. I may not value or appreciate Parkinson's, but opening myself up to creative endeavors with and by persons with Parkinson's reduces stress and increases joy. Win-win!"*

— LORRAINE WILSON

Learn about clinical research trials that may be available to people living with Parkinson's. Many researchers seek to understand the impact medicines have on people in the early stages of Parkinson's before any other medicine has been started, and they are always looking for participants. Another especially important area of research is the study of neuroprotective therapies that can slow or potentially even stop the progression of Parkinson's. While participating in a research trial is not for everyone, you may be empowered by participating in the latest research and by potentially advancing the science of Parkinson's for the greater community. Learn more about Parkinson's research in our ⤤ *Every Victory Counts* **website** or research trials online at ⤤ **ClinicalTrials.gov** and ⤤ **FoxTrialFinder.org**.

Stay positive. A positive attitude focuses on what you can do, not what you can't. It fosters hope. If you're having a bad day, recall at least one victory you've had that day and know that tomorrow will bring another opportunity to live well.

Keep learning. New information about Parkinson's research, treatments, and living well is being released all the time. Visit the ⟳ *Every Victory Counts* **website (dpf.org/evc-hub)** to stay up-to-date and learn even more about Parkinson's throughout your journey.

After almost two decades of working to help people live well with Parkinson's, we know those three life-changing words—"You have Parkinson's."—don't have to mean giving up on the kind of life you imagined for yourself. Remember: your life's design plan is yours to make. Design it to be the best it can be. Stay active. Stay engaged. Stay informed. Stay in control of your destiny. And remember that you hold the power you need to live well.

Appendix

When you journey mindfully through your experience with Parkinson's, you will discover the activities, exercises, connections, and other actions that help you feel your best. We encourage you to keep an open mind and seek out new adventures. As you do, however, remember that not all advice is sound, and not all "experts" are the best guides to living well. We reached out to a long-time friend of the Foundation and movement disorder specialist Benzi Kluger for this section. As a powerful advocate of people living with Parkinson's, he shares this content with the goal of helping you get the very best care possible. Part of that involves making sure your medical bullshit detector always has a full charge.

"The Medical Bullshit Detector"

By Benzi M. Kluger, MD, MS, FAAN

When you have a serious illness like Parkinson's, it seems that everyone has some advice to make your life better or some promise of a new cure. The amount of information and misinformation inundating us can feel overwhelming. How can you tell who to trust and what to believe?

For as long as physicians and scientists have discovered medicines and treatments to help their fellow citizens, there have been scrupulous individuals trying to make a buck on counterfeit cures and overblown hype. Medical bullshit is misinformation meant to get you to either buy a worthless product or to follow baseless and potentially harmful advice. Medical bullshit for Parkinson's comes in many forms, ranging from bestselling self-help books on the latest miracle diet to unregulated claims on the bottles of supplements to actual medical physicians offering untested stem cell treatments.

Medical bullshit is a serious business that rakes in billions of dollars for those who profit from it. Unfortunately, there are also thousands of victims, people who were hoping for a miracle and ended up losing thousands of dollars on a worthless scam or, not uncommonly, suffering serious ill-effects from ingesting untested and unsafe products.

To try to combat bullshit, several authors have developed bullshit detectors—quick and useful rules of thumb—to recognize and avoid bullshit. The most famous of these may be Carl Sagan's "Baloney Detection Kit," described in his 1995 book *The Demon-Haunted World*.[6] But this idea goes back hundreds and thousands of years, with several ancient Greek skeptics seeking to create laws that might help one recognize deception more easily.

Fortunately, sniffing out whether a medical product has a high chance of being bullshit is not rocket science or brain surgery. Some tell-tale signs will act as signals to you to put your skeptic hat on. Below, I enumerate some of the more reliable clues that the hype, expert, or product in front of you is more likely to be misleading than helpful.

SEEING THROUGH THE HYPE

The following tips deal with hype—exaggerated and often misleading claims meant to sell a product, or in the case of news media, to attract readers and advertisers.

#1 - The "information" provided is tied to selling a product.

Many websites, videos, and books appear to offer information about a disease or health topic important to you. However, once you get past the headline, you find yourself immersed in an infomercial for a particular product, diet, or expert. When evaluating healthcare products, you should always ask yourself: what does the person recommending it have to gain by me doing this therapy? A common goal of bullshit is not to cure your illness but to get your money. This may occur by selling you books, supplements, tests, procedures, medications, stem cells, news, or an expert who wants to launch their medical celebrity career.

#2 - The promotions use terms like "revolutionary," "unbelievable," or "miracle."

Certain words should always set off your bullshit detector. Unfortunately, these terms are used to sell products; the media also use them to make their news stories sound exciting. News stories on medical advances are often overblown hype—compare how often you have heard a story headline like "scientists at the University of Smartsville may have discovered a cure for cancer"? (hint—a lot) vs. how often has a cure for all cancer been discovered (hint—never). Granted, some therapies truly are revolutionary. Some examples include penicillin, anesthesia, and handwashing. But, as you might expect, truly revolutionary ideas do not come along every day.

#3 - Initial findings are sent directly to the press without attempts at validation.

If you look back at medicine's history, many of our most significant discoveries came from chance observation or accidents. However, a core principle of science is validation - one must replicate and test initial observations before we can trust them. For example, in the late 1700s, Edward Jenner noted that milkmaids appeared protected from smallpox. Rather than publish a book about the Dairy Lifestyle or selling udder balm, he did two important things. First, he continued his observations until he recognized that cowpox exposure might be the key to preventing smallpox. Second, he and others carefully tested this hypothesis.[7] In contrast, many would-be medical saviors today never test their initial observations, much less carefully validate them, before trying to take them to the press and market.

#4 - Promotions use more resources on marketing than on validating its safety or effectiveness.

When one sees a frantic amount of energy and resources being used to promote a product, it often indicates an underlying lack of confidence in that product to sell itself. Often this advertising focuses on what life will be like with this product (relaxing on a beach, going to a party with beautiful friends) and not on the product itself. This is true not just for alternative medicines and supplements but prescription medications. Pharmaceutical companies have huge advertising budgets that target both consumers and physicians. For products that serve a unique need and work, they may not need to spend much money. But for products with cheaper alternatives or a need to manufacture demand, there is a greater motivation to advertise.[8, 9] There have been tragic examples of heavily advertised products that later turned out to have serious safety issues, possibly known but suppressed by the company.[10, 11, 12, 13]

#5 - The claims are inconsistent with what you know from reputable sources.

If something seems too good to be true, it probably is. If you stop to think about it, curing Alzheimer's would be a significant medical advance that would land one or more people a Nobel Prize. To cure Alzheimer's, one would have to a) find a therapy that cures the disease and b) test it to make sure that it is safe and reliably works. It would also help to understand what causes Alzheimer's, although one might find a cure through sheer blind luck. Given the vast amounts of research done by teams worldwide to understand and cure Alzheimer's, it seems highly unlikely that a lone individual would stumble upon it by chance or genius.

#6 - The promotion relies heavily on celebrities and celebrity experts.

Here is a general rule of thumb that applies to medical bullshit: when you lack substance, it helps to dress fancy and surround yourself with famous people. When it comes to putting things in your body that are meant to improve your health but could harm you, it often comes down to who the discoverer knows or can get to endorse their product. When it comes to science, the value of a famous person's opinion is a piece of data just like any other piece of data from a single subject—nearly worthless. Even true medical experts' views are not valued as highly by scientists as a well-conducted experiment in hundreds of people. An excess of famous people should clue you in to see if there is a lack of data.

#7 - The amazing findings are not cited or found outside of the product or expert's website.

Another crucial question: are there any independent sources also promoting this product? If not, you should probably move on. One of the principles of science is that facts can and should be independently verified. People who care about the truth want to see verification. People who want to sell you bullshit or have something to hide don't want their claims tested.

#8 - The promotion reports research studies but neglects to share the details of that research.

This happens most often with news stories. The headline reads, "Researchers at the Genius College Discover Cure for Parkinson's." When you read the full story (or go beyond the story to find the source of the article), you are very likely to run into one of the following scenarios:

- The research was performed on animals,
- The research is based on an observational study that found a correlation, and
- The research is a preliminary and small trial with no control group.

The bottom line is that none of these pieces of evidence are enough by themselves to conclude that something is safe and effective in people. The history of science is filled with examples of:

- Animal studies that found a cure for Parkinson's that never made it to people,
- Correlational studies that found something in the diet associated with lower risks of Parkinson's that failed to show benefit in clinical trials, and
- Small clinical trials, sometimes of very fancy treatments like stem cells and gene therapy, that were proven to be placebo effects.

SPOTTING UNRELIABLE EXPERTS

While it's true that you can't judge a book by its cover, you can often learn a lot by looking at its author. In the case of medical bullshit—whether that be a best-selling book, a "miracle supplement," or a "revolutionary new theory on health"—a careful glance at the person's real accomplishments and actions behind the message should, in many cases, put you on your guard. You will be surprised to see how often self-proclaimed experts have no actual claim to expertise. As you develop a nose for bullshit, you will find that simply the name of certain self-proclaimed experts may be enough to turn you away.

#1 - The expert calls themselves "a leading medical expert" or is endorsed by other "medical opinion leaders."

I have seen some of the world's most outstanding researchers speak, including several Nobel Prize winners. Many of these individuals truly needed no introduction because their work was so well known. However, they still got introduced. And when they did, the introducer listed their *impressive accomplishments*, things like their significant discoveries, illnesses they cured, people they trained, critical new ideas. None of them were introduced as, or called themselves, a "health expert," nor did they list a bunch of bestselling diet books, Oprah appearances, or drop names of other medical (or nonmedical) celebrities who they are friends with to support their credentials. If you pay attention to how experts are selling themselves, ask yourself, "Does this really matter?" Does writing a best-selling book prove you know what you are talking about?

#2 - The expert does not have the correct credentials.

Medical bullshit experts flaunt any credentials they have—diplomas, certificates, awards, publications—prominently on their website, flyers, books, and office walls. Having too many credentials may even be a clue to something amiss. Often a careful look will reveal that the credentials on display are not the credentials needed to claim expertise in a field. Some common examples include:

- Having training in one field and claiming expertise in another (e.g., a surgeon who writes a book on nutrition)
- Doing research in one field and claiming expertise in another (e.g., a physicist promoting stem cells)
- Highlighting the fancy school one went to but not what was studied (e.g., a Lyme Disease author who highlights they are a Harvard graduate but neglects to mention that they majored in English)
- Having a degree in a field you've never heard of or from a school you've never heard of (this, of course, could be just your lack of familiarity with a legitimate field or school, but it would be worth looking up)
- Buying or simply fabricating a fake degree

#3 - The expert brags about being rejected by the mainstream medical establishment.

The idea that there is a monolithic entity, "the medical establishment," is appealing to some people, but what does this really mean? If one is talking about the culture of medicine, there may be some interesting things to say about how healthcare professionals act or what they believe in different contexts. However, suppose one is claiming that ALL physicians, researchers, hospitals, or insurance companies get together to make collective decisions, particularly against a specific individual. In that case, that is simply creating conspiracies as a branding strategy. Don't be fooled. It is next to impossible to get healthcare professionals to agree on almost anything.

#4 - The expert tells you that their ideas or your diagnosis are "too complicated" to understand.

If you can't convince them, confuse them. When a so-called expert doesn't have evidence to support their claims, they often present some vague and fancy-sounding ideas and then add that the details are too complicated for any but the most brilliant experts to understand. They hope that people will just take their word for it rather than press for details. This goes with the notion that experts know things not just that most people don't know but that most people can't know. Pretending that one holds ideas that can't be understood or shared with others is akin to modern-day witchcraft. Real experts do society a disservice by not treating the person in front of them with respect and explaining things so they can understand. Some experts have a difficult time writing or speaking clearly. Some are purposefully trying to hide weak points in their research. And some may enjoy the power of being an unchallenged expert. None of these are good reasons not to explain ideas clearly.

Regardless of the reasons for not being clear, the result is the same—a claim to unjustified power for those in the Expertocracy that reinforces a message of helplessness for everyone else. Granted, certain things do require specialized knowledge. I don't understand the complex biochemistry and pharmacodynamics of many of the medications I prescribe. But I understand other essential things about them—the symptoms they treat, what dose to use, and what side effects to watch out for. Similarly, my patients don't need to know all the medical science underlying their symptoms (although I would be happy to share what I know if they are interested), but they should understand what treatments are available to manage their symptoms, how those symptoms may affect their lives, and how to plan for the future. I feel the mark of a true expert is someone who can clearly explain what needs to be known. As Albert Einstein said: "If you can't explain it simply, you don't understand it well enough."

#5 - The expert actively encourages fear.

Fear sells. Richard Leask, a representative of the California Chamber of Commerce, said, "if you can't convince 'em, confuse 'em: if you can't confuse 'em, scare 'em." As a healthcare provider, I do my best to balance being realistic with compassion. If I have bad news for someone, for example, that their disease is progressing rapidly, I have a conversation with them about it. They tell me what they want to hear, and I do my best to provide them with the information they need to make the best decisions possible. I also check in with them about difficult emotions, like fear or grief, and explore whether there may still be opportunities for meaning, connection, or joy. In contrast, the bullshit artist will focus on the worst, will fan the flames of your fear (often while pretending to offer understanding), and will lead you towards the one best choice for someone in your situation, which, coincidentally, happens to be what they are selling.

#6 - The expert is not part of a regulated or established profession or clinic.

Like medicine, counseling, or acupuncture, many professions have state boards that regulate the profession and handle licensing and testing. It is never a good sign when an expert dismisses these regulations. Sometimes the person behind the product introduces himself as a physician, which in the setting of healthcare implies a medical physician, but they really hold a physicianate in another field, perhaps philosophy or business. A somewhat newer phenomenon is a medical physician embracing a new branch of medicine (e.g., Functional Medicine, Alternative Neurologist) that does not have established training requirements. As with most of these clues, this doesn't automatically mean this person is a quack— some have taken a thoughtful approach to integrate alternative treatments, exercise, and nutritional choices with traditional Western medicine. However, many times they cross the line from a balanced approach to feigning knowledge or expertise that does not exist and is a harmful deviation from standard practice.

#7 - The expert doesn't take time to listen to you or examine you fully.

This comes up in two contexts. First, someone with the goal of selling you a product lets you talk, but only up to the point where they feel they have the information they need to move forward with their sale. Sometimes this can be subtle. The expert pretends to listen to you, to "understand exactly what you are going through," and then, once they have your confidence, they begin to talk more than listen.

In the second, a practitioner, often a physician or nurse, hurriedly sees you. Perhaps they are busy. Maybe they have their own agenda. Perhaps, at some point in your story, they make up their mind about what's going on and are now simply seeking to confirm it. In any case, you get a distinct feeling that you're not being seen or heard. Listen to this feeling. Recommending prescriptions or therapies without knowing your values or hearing your entire story can lead to dangerous situations and regrets.

#8 - The expert discourages you from getting a second opinion.

Getting a second opinion is never a bad thing. If patients ask me about getting a second opinion, I encourage it. Maybe I'll be proven correct, perhaps I'll have the opportunity to learn something, but most importantly, the patient can move forward knowing they have the proper diagnosis and treatment. When someone warns you against getting a second opinion or dismisses second opinions without really listening, they do you and themselves a disservice. They are also providing a clue that what they are selling may be more about them than you. No matter how confident or influential the physician, treating their ego should never take precedence over your health.

#9 - The expert asks you to stop conventional treatments.

People who don't know you or your medical situation should not make recommendations about how you take care of yourself. They certainly should not ask you to stop medications other physicians have prescribed. I am not talking about situations where a medication may be causing side effects or contributing to symptoms where stopping it may be perfectly reasonable. Instead, I am referring to cases where treatments that are working are stopped. For example, I've known patients with Parkinson's who were told to stop taking carbidopa/ levodopa, the single most effective medication for this condition, in favor of acupuncture, herbal treatments, dietary changes, or cannabis. Abruptly stopping this medication will not only worsen the symptoms of stiffness and tremor it was treating, but it could have disastrous consequences ranging from falls to a life-threatening condition called parkinsonism hyperpyrexia characterized by intense muscle spasms, fever, unstable blood pressure, and sometimes death. People who don't know what they don't know and who believe they know what they don't know are dangerous when they start making recommendations about your health.

Medical bullshit is everyone's problem. Please be responsible for what information you share with your friends and family. If you see something, say something—you don't have to call someone a liar, but you can question their facts and information. If you want to learn more about how to assess untested but highly marketed products and "cures" read, How to Avoid Unproven Products on our 🔗 ***Every Victory Counts** website.*

About Benzi Kluger

Benzi Kluger is the Founding Director of the Palliative Care Research Center and Neuropalliative Care Division at the University of Rochester Medical Center, where he also serves as professor of neurology and medicine. He is a pioneer in neuropalliative care, a field dedicated to the radical idea that improving the lives of persons affected by neurological illness requires seeing and treating them as whole people. He is constantly looking for opportunities to undermine heartless systems through subversive kindness.

Dr. Kluger created one of the first team-based neuropalliative care clinics in the world at the University of Colorado. He has published numerous papers important to the growth of this field. His research focuses on neuropalliative care, fatigue, and neurodegenerative illness (Parkinson's and Alzheimer's) with some brief excursions into other areas, including nutrition, acupuncture, and cannabis. Dr. Kluger's research has been funded by the National Institutes of Health, the Patient Centered Outcomes Research Institute, the Department of Defense, the Parkinson Foundation, and the Michael J Fox Foundation.

As a writer, Dr. Kluger's goals are to empower patients and give them the tools they need to navigate the medical industry for themselves and their loved ones. He has published several essays related to humanism in medicine and is currently working on a book to empower patients to save money, avoid dangerous healthcare decisions and debunk medical bullshit. If you'd like to read more from Dr. Benzi Kluger, visit his website at BenziKluger.com and on Facebook (@BenziKluger), Twitter (@BenziKluger), and LinkedIn (@BenziKluger).

287

■ ENDNOTES

1   Hardy, John. Genetic analysis of pathways to PD. (2010, Oct 21). *Neuron*, 68(2): 201-206.

2   Bronstein, Jeff, Carvey, Paul, Chen, Honglei, Cory-Slecta, Deborah, Dimonte, Donato, et. al. Meeting Report: Consensus Statement–Parkinson's Disease and the Environment: Collaborative on Health and the Environment and the Parkinson's Action Network (CHE PAN) Conference 26 – 28 June 2007. (January 2009). *Environmental Health Perspectives*, 117(1): 117-121.

3   https://www.healthandenvironment.org/our-work/toxicant-and-disease-database/ ?showcategory=&showdisease=794&showcontaminant=&showcas=&showkeyword=

4   Zeynep, S. Agim and Cannon, Jason R. (2015). Dietary Factors in the Etiology of Parkinson's Disease. *Biomed Res Int*.

5   Crane, Paul K., Gibbons, Laura E., and Dams-O'Connor, Kristen. (2016). Association of Traumatic Brain Injury with Late-Life Neurodegenerative Conditions and Neuropathologic Findings. JAMA *Neurol*, 73(9): 1062-1069.

6   Sagan, C. *The Demon-Haunted World: Science as a Candle in the Dark*. New York, NY: Random House, Inc.; 1996.

7   Rusnock AA. Historical context and the roots of Jenner's discovery. *Hum Vaccin Immunother*. 2016;12(8):2025-2028.

8   Frosch DL, Krueger PM, Hornik RC, Cronholm PF, Barg FK. Creating demand for prescription drugs: a content analysis of television direct-to-consumer advertising. *Ann Fam Med*. 2007;5(1):6-13.

9   Podolsky SH, Herzberg D, Greene JA. Preying on Prescribers (and Their Patients) - Pharmaceutical Marketing, Iatrogenic Epidemics, and the Sackler Legacy. *N Engl J Med*. 2019;380(19):1785-1787.

10 Moynihan R. Court hears how drug giant Merck tried to "neutralise" and "discredit" physicians critical of Vioxx. *BMJ*. 2009;338:b1432.

11 Maron BJ, Hauser RG. Perspectives on the failure of pharmaceutical and medical device industries to fully protect public health interests. *Am J Cardiol*. 2007;100(1):147-151.

12 Van Zee A. The promotion and marketing of oxycontin: commercial triumph, public health tragedy. *Am J Public Health*. 2009;99(2):221-227.

13 Hadland SE, Rivera-Aguirre A, Marshall BDL, Cerda M. Association of Pharmaceutical Industry Marketing of Opioid Products With Mortality From Opioid-Related Overdoses. *JAMA Netw Open*. 2019;2(1):e186007.

■ GLOSSARY

Acetylcholine: A brain chemical that acts as both a neurotransmitter and a neuromodulator and plays a role in muscle function, attention, arousal, memory and motivation. Acetylcholine is reduced in Parkinson's-related dementia.

Acetylcholinesterase inhibitors: Medications that block the breakdown of the neurotransmitter acetylcholine to help treat Parkinson's-related dementia.

Action tremor: Type of tremor that gets worse when trying to perform an action, such as picking up a coffee cup or eating with a spoon.

Activities of daily living (ADLs): Basic self-care skills, including eating, dressing, grooming, bathing and using the toilet. Occupational therapists often focus on improving ADLs.

Adaptive equipment: Devices used to assist with activities of daily living, such as bathing, dressing and using the toilet. Examples include tremor-management eating utensils, non-skid mats, adaptive writing utensils, button hooks, etc.

Advance healthcare directive: A legal document in which someone explains the actions that should be taken for their health if they are no longer in a capacity to make their own decisions. In the US, an advance healthcare directive has its own legal status.

Akinesia: Lack of movement caused by Parkinson's, such as loss of arm swing, that primarily affects walking or the hands and trunk area. A hallmark motor symptom of Parkinson's.

Alpha-synuclein: A protein found in the brain. While the role of alpha-synuclein in a healthy brain is unknown, alpha-synuclein clumps together in the brains of people with Parkinson's to form Lewy bodies, one of the hallmark features of Parkinson's. This has led to ongoing investigation into the role this protein plays in the development of Parkinson's.

Alternative brain pathways: Recruiting stronger brain circuits to execute similar functions that enables people to perform and gain strength in a difficult task. For example, people with speech problems may be able to sing or someone who struggles walking may be able to ride a bicycle.

Amantadine: A medication originally used to treat the common flu and later found to improve the symptoms of Parkinson's. Amantadine can be used alone or in combination with other Parkinson's medications. It is sometimes added specifically for the treatment of dyskinesia and can also improve freezing of gait. Also has a stimulant effect, which can help with fatigue.

Amino acid: The building blocks of protein.

Anticholinergics: A type of medication that interferes with the action of the neurotransmitter acetylcholine to try and restore the balance between dopamine and acetylcholine.

Anxiety: Excessive feelings of worry, nervousness, apprehension and unease. Can be associated with compulsive behavior or panic attacks.

Apomorphine: A dopamine agonist that helps improve motor function by stimulating dopamine receptors. It is a Parkinson's medication used to help with "off" episodes and to treat muscle stiffness, slow movements or movement difficulties associated with Parkinson's.

Art therapist: A type of therapist who uses art and creative expression as a healing tool to convey the inner self and emotions, strengthen concentration and executive function and reinforce mind-body connections.

Aspiration: When food or fluid enters the lungs.

Ataxia: A loss of muscle control or the ability to coordinate one's voluntary movements, such as walking. Ataxia signals the presence of an underlying condition and can affect various movements, leading to challenges with swallowing, speech and eye movement.

At-risk: A person who is "at-risk" of developing Parkinson's has known risk factors, for example, lifestyle or environmental risk factors or a genetic variant, but no detectable underlying pathology.

Basal ganglia: Clusters of neurons located deep in the brain that play an important role in movement. The basal ganglia includes the substantia nigra, and cell death in the substantia nigra contributes to signs of Parkinson's.

Benzodiazepines: A category of psychoactive medications used to treat anxiety and insomnia by slowing the central nervous system.

Biomarker: An early indicator that a person may have a disease, such as Parkinson's, that can be recognized before symptoms appear. Identifying biomarkers may lead to earlier interventions and treatment. Biomarkers could be a chemical, clinical, or physiological change or found via imaging.

Blood brain barrier: The membrane separating the blood and the brain; a tight physical barrier that normally keeps immune cells, chemicals, and drugs out of the brain.

Botulinum toxin: A neurotoxic protein that prevents the release of acetylcholine. Injections may help with dystonia. Commonly referred to as Botox.

Bradykinesia: The slowness of movement that can be caused by Parkinson's. One of the hallmark motor symptoms of Parkinson's.

Bradyphrenia: Slowed thinking that can be caused by Parkinson's.

Carbidopa: A drug given with levodopa. Carbidopa blocks the enzyme dopa decarboxylase, thereby preventing levodopa from being metabolized to dopamine. Since carbidopa does not penetrate the blood brain barrier, it only blocks levodopa metabolism in the peripheral tissues and not in the brain, thereby reducing side effects such as nausea while increasing the effectiveness of levodopa.

Care partner: Anyone who provides help or support to a relative or friend living with Parkinson's.

Caregiver burnout: A medical syndrome resulting from untreated caregiver strain that includes feeling overwhelmed, angry, irritable, sleeping poorly, fatigue, worsening medical problems, and/or self-medicating.

Caregiver strain: A medical syndrome resulting from the burdens and demands of caregiving.

Chronic: A condition of long duration. Chronic diseases typically appear gradually and progress slowly over time. The term does not imply anything about the severity of a disease. The opposite of a chronic condition is an acute condition.

Clinical trials: Experiments or observations done in clinical research on human participants. Clinical trials are designed to test the safety and efficacy of biomedical or behavioral interventions, including new medications, medical devices, and supplements.

Cognition: Mental processes including attention, remembering, producing and understanding language, solving problems, and making decisions.

Cognitive behavioral therapy (CBT): A type of treatment for anxiety and depression addressing behaviors and thought patterns. CBT is time-limited and skills-based and may be used alone or in combination with medication.

Complementary therapies: Non-medical treatments used in addition to conventional medical and surgical treatments, such as physical therapy, occupational therapy, speech-language therapy, music and art therapies, etc.

Complex carbohydrates: Long chains of sugar molecules that require more complex digestion and are more slowly absorbed; includes starch and fiber.

COMT inhibitors: A type of medication that prevents the COMT enzyme from converting levodopa into a form unable to be used by the brain. When levodopa is taken, a portion of the COMT enzyme converts into a useless compound. COMT inhibitors prevent this, thus making more levodopa available for the brain to use to counteract symptoms of Parkinson's.

Compulsive behaviors: The overwhelming and often repetitive drive to act in a certain way to ease an urge or reduce worry or tension. Often, this behavior can be out of character for the person experiencing it and can be a side effect of certain Parkinson's medications.

Constipation: Infrequent or hard to pass bowel movements. A common problem for people living with Parkinson's that can be helped by increasing water intake and fiber in the diet.

Continuous subcutaneous infusion of apomorphine (CAI): An ongoing stream of apomorphine delivered into the bloodstream through a needle into the skin, similar to an insulin pump. This treatment is designed to limit the amount of OFF time experienced. It is currently not available in the US, but is in advanced clinical trials.

Controlled release drugs: Special preparations of drugs that release the drug into the body slowly and steadily, rather than all at once. This helps to keep the amount of the drug in the blood stream at a steadier level than the "ordinary" version of the same drug.

DaTSCAN: A nuclear medicine scan that measures levels of dopamine nerve cells in the basal ganglia. While this scan cannot determine if someone has Parkinson's or not, it was approved by the FDA in 2011 to help differentiate Parkinson's tremor from Familial or Essential Tremor (ET). It is also not able to distinguish Parkinson's from other forms of parkinsonism, nor is it used to track symptoms or progression.

Deep brain stimulation (DBS): A surgical procedure involving the implantation of electrodes in specific areas of the brain that produce electrical impulses to help regulate abnormal impulses or affect certain chemicals or cells in the brain. DBS is used to help a variety of neurological conditions, most commonly the motor symptoms of Parkinson's, including tremor, rigidity, stiffness, slowed movement, and walking problems.

Dementia: A decline in cognitive function due to damage or disease in the brain beyond what might be expected from normal aging. Areas particularly affected include memory, attention, judgment, language, planning, and problem solving.

Depression: A mood disorder that causes a persistent feeling of sadness and loss of interest. Depression can affect feelings, behavior, and thinking, leading to various physical and emotional problems.

Designation of healthcare surrogate: A document naming another person as a representative to make medical decisions on one's behalf should one be unable to make them oneself. As in a living will, people can include instructions about treatments they do and do not want.

Dopa decarboxylase inhibitors (DDI): Parkinson's medications that block the actions of the enzyme dopa decarboxylase (DDC) to inhibit the metabolism of levodopa to dopamine in the bloodstream, allowing more levodopa to reach the brain and be converted into dopamine there. Includes carbidopa and benserazide.

Dopamine: A small chemical molecule that is one of the brain's neurotransmitters. It is found especially in cells within the substantia nigra and conveys messages in the brain to coordinate muscle movements. The motor symptoms of Parkinson's appear when 60-80% of the dopamine-producing neurons in the brain are damaged and unable to produce sufficient dopamine.

Dopamine agonist: A type of medication that acts like dopamine but is not actually dopamine. These compounds activate dopamine receptors and can be used in both the early and later stages of Parkinson's. Dopamine agonists can cause side effects such as confusion, sleepiness, sleep attacks, ankle swelling, hallucinations, and impulse control problems, like uncontrollable gambling, eating, obsessive behaviors, and sexual urges.

Durable power of attorney: A document appointing an agent (usually a trusted relative or friend) to carry out specific health, legal and financial responsibilities on behalf of another. There are two types of power of attorney: POA for healthcare and POA for finances. The POA for healthcare gives the appointed agent authority to make healthcare decision on behalf of someone. The POA for finances gives the appointed agent authority to make legal/financial decisions on behalf of someone. At the time the documents for POA are signed, the person establishing a durable power of attorney must be physically and mentally capable of making the decision to seek assistance.

Dysarthria: A motor speech disorder characterized by slow or slurred speech. Dysarthria results from impaired movement of the muscles used for speech production, including the tongue, vocal folds, lips, and/or diaphragm. The type and severity of dysarthria depends on which area of the nervous system is affected.

293

Dyskinesia: Uncontrollable, jerky, irregular, and involuntary movements.

Dysphagia: Difficulty swallowing.

Dystonia: Involuntary tightening or spasms of the muscles, often in the feet or lower legs, caused by a lack of dopamine.

Electrocardiogram (ECG): A test that measures the electrical activity of the heartbeat.

Employee assistance program (EAP): A voluntary, confidential program that helps employees navigate various life challenges that may affect their health, job performance and personal well-being.

End-of-dose wearing off: The phenomenon of medicine's effectiveness wearing "off" before the next dose, causing Parkinson's symptoms to re-appear or get worse before it is time to take the next dose of carbidopa/levodopa.

Erectile dysfunction (ED): The inability to achieve a sustained erection throughout intercourse. Can be a symptom of Parkinson's.

Executive function: Cognitive processes that allow one to plan, focus attention, remember, and multitask.

Facial masking: A condition resulting in reduced facial expression that may additionally cause softer, more monotone speech. The technical term for this is "hypomimia" and often this is referred to as "mask-like" or "masked" face.

Family Medical Leave Act (FMLA): A federal act in the US entitling employees to an unpaid, extended leave of absence for specified family and medical reasons. It also ensures that employer-provided health insurance continues during leave. There are specific criteria that must be met to qualify for FMLA.

Festination: The tendency toward smaller, faster steps that pitch a person forward.

Freezing of gait: Problems with initiating movements that often result in feeling like one's feet are glued to the floor. A motor symptom that is more common in later stages of Parkinson's.

Functional mobility: Ability to move around one's home and environment to perform daily activities, such as getting in and out of bed, bathing, sitting on and getting up from the couch or table, etc. Occupational therapists often focus on improving functional mobility.

Glutamate: An amino acid and the main excitatory neurotransmitter in the human brain. Glutamate plays a critical role in the development of the brain and helps with learning and memory. Excess glutamate in the brain is associated with neurological diseases like Parkinson's, Alzheimer's, multiple sclerosis (MS) and amyotrophic lateral sclerosis (ALS).

Glycemic index: A number measuring a food's effect on blood glucose after consumption. The GI represents the rise in a blood sugar level two hours after consumption and depends on many factors. GI is useful for understanding how the body breaks down carbohydrates.

Glycemic load: A measure related to the glycemic index that multiplies the glycemic index of a food by the carbohydrate content in the actual serving to put the glycemic index into appropriate context. For instance, watermelon has a high glycemic index, but a low glycemic load per the typical quantity consumed.

Gut microbiome: The complex community of microorganisms that live in the digestive tracts of humans and other animals.

Growth factors: Naturally occurring substances (usually proteins) that help maintain the health of neurons and encourage cell growth, proliferation, and differentiation. Some growth factors are being looked at to try to promote the survival of the neural cells that are degenerating in Parkinson's.

Hallucinations: The experience of perceiving something that is not actually there. Hallucinations may be a symptom of Parkinson's or a side effect of certain Parkinson's medications.

Hypertension: Abnormally high blood pressure.

Hypersexuality: A clinical diagnosis describing extremely frequent or suddenly increased sexual urges or activity. Can be a side effect of certain Parkinson's medications.

Hypokinesia: Small movements that can come as a result of Parkinson's. One of the hallmark motor symptoms of Parkinson's.

Hypomimia: The decrease in facial expressions resulting in a masked-like face that can come as a result of Parkinson's.

Hypophonia: Soft speech caused by Parkinson's.

Idiopathic: A type of condition arising from an unknown cause. The majority of people living with Parkinson's are considered to have "idiopathic" Parkinson's, meaning there is no clear and definitive genetic or environmental cause for developing the disease.

Impulsive behaviors: The inability to resist the temptation to engage in a certain activity. Often, these activities give an immediate sense of pleasure, such as eating, gambling, increase in sexual thoughts or feelings, etc. Can be a side effect of certain Parkinson's medications.

Impulse control disorders (ICDs): A set of psychiatric disorders characterized by an inability to control one's actions, particularly activities that could bring harm to oneself or others. This can be a side effect of certain Parkinson's medications. People taking dopamine agonists may experience ICDs, including compulsive gambling, eating, shopping, and hypersexuality.

Instrumental activities of daily living (IDLs): Activities that include caring for others and pets, financial management, driving, one's ability to be active in the community, health and medication management, meal preparation, leisure activities, shopping, safety, etc. Occupational therapists often focus on improving IDLs.

Insoluble fiber: A type of fiber found in many plant foods that does not absorb water and passes through the gastrointestinal tract without being digested. Found in foods such as whole grain breads, bran, cauliflower, artichokes, and potatoes, insoluble fibers helps bulk up stool and therefore can help reduce constipation.

Interdisciplinary care: Multiple healthcare professionals collaborating to provide care with a common perspective, often involving joint consultations. Sometimes referred to as "integrative care."

Leucine rich repeat kinase 2 (LRRK2): A large and complex gene that influences the production of proteins. Mutations in this gene are the most common cause of Parkinson's in the small percentage (~10%) of people with Parkinson's whose disease is linked to a genetic component. Mutations in the LRRK2 gene that can increase one's risk of developing Parkinson's are much higher in certain ethnic groups, such as Ashkenazi Jews, Basque, and North African Berbers.

Levodopa (L-DOPA): A chemical that is the precursor to dopamine and one of the oldest and most effective medications for Parkinson's. It can pass through the blood brain barrier where it is absorbed by dopamine nerve cells and converted to dopamine to replace lost dopamine in the brain.

Levodopa sparing strategy: Limiting the use of levodopa in an attempt to minimize wearing OFF problems and dyskinesia as Parkinson's progresses.

Lewy bodies: A pathologic hallmark of Parkinson's and dementia with Lewy bodies. Named for Frederic Lewy who first described them, Lewy bodies are seen microscopically as inclusions in neurons in several brain regions, including the substantia nigra.

Macronutrients: The three major food categories: carbohydrates, fats, and proteins.

MAO (monoamine oxidase): A family of enzymes with two subtypes: MAO-A and MAO-B. These catalyze the oxidation of amine molecules, replacing the amine group with an oxygen molecule. MAO-B inhibitors are a type of drugs (such as selegiline, rasagiline) that inhibit the breakdown of dopamine via MAO-B enzyme and do not cause abnormally high blood pressure (hypertension).

Mediterranean diet: A type of eating plan consisting of traditional foods consumed in Mediterranean countries, emphasizing plant-based foods like fruits and vegetables, whole grains, legumes, and nuts, as well as moderate consumption of poultry and dairy. The diet replaces butter with fats such as olive oil and canola oil and uses herbs and spices instead of salt to flavor food.

Micrographia: Small, cramped handwriting that can be a symptom of Parkinson's.

Micronutrients: Vitamins and substances found in food that are needed in smaller amounts to promote cell health and catalyze biochemical reactions.

Mind-body medicine: An approach to medicine based on the belief that thoughts and emotions can influence physical healing and well-being.

Modified barium swallow (MBS): A radiology procedure that can show the passage of food or fluids from the mouth to the stomach.

Monounsaturated fats: Type of fat that is liquid at room temperature but gets cloudy when refrigerated. Examples include olives and olive oil, canola oil, nuts and nut oils, and avocado. These oils are a better substitute for saturated fats, and can reduce cholesterol levels and improve insulin activity.

Motor fluctuations: A complication of levodopa therapy characterized by periodic reemergence of Parkinson's symptoms that are normally controlled when the medication is working.

Motor skills: The degree of coordination provided by the brain's control of the skeletal muscles.

Motor symptoms: Symptoms that involve movement, coordination, physical tasks, or mobility. These include resting tremor, bradykinesia, rigidity, postural instability, freezing, micrographia, facial masking, unwanted accelerations, stooped posture, dystonia, impaired motor dexterity and coordination, speech problems, difficulty swallowing, muscle cramping, and drooling.

Movement disorder specialist (MDS): A neurologist with additional training in movement disorders like Parkinson's, essential tremor, and ataxia.

Multidisciplinary care: Care given by multiple healthcare professionals, each approaching the patient from their professional perspective. This often involves separate, individual consultations.

Music therapist: A specialist who uses music to achieve therapeutic goals, including movement.

Neurogenic bladder: Problems with nerve control of the bladder, including urinary frequency and sense of urgency.

Neurogenic orthostatic hypotension (nOH): A type of orthostatic hypotension caused by a neurological disorder like Parkinson's or multiple system atrophy that triggers a sustained drop in blood pressure upon standing. Common symptoms include dizziness, lightheadedness, blurry vision, and occasional fainting.

Neurological conditions: A collection of disorders caused by damage or malfunctioning of the brain or nervous system.

Neurologist: A physician who specializes in the diagnosis, care, and treatment of disorders of the brain or nervous system.

Neuromodulation: The act of altering nerve activity through delivering a targeted stimulus in the brain, such as electrical stimulation. Neuromodulation devices use electrical signals, pharmaceutical agents, or other avenues to stimulate nerves and modulate the abnormal neural pathway behavior caused by a neurological disease. Approaches to neuromodulation range from non-invasive techniques, such as transcranial magnetic stimulation, to implanted devices, such as a deep brain stimulation system for Parkinson's.

Neuro-ophthalmologist: A neurologist or ophthalmologist with fellowship training in the field of neuro-ophthalmology. These specialists have a particular appreciation for the intersection of the eyes and the brain and perform comprehensive testing to determine the cause of visual or eye movement problems.

Neuroplasticity: Activity and experiences that cause the development of new nerve connections or the strengthening of old connections, resulting in improved brain function.

Neuroprotection: Mechanisms within the nervous system that protect neurons from dying as a result of a degenerative disease like Parkinson's or from other types of injury.

Neuropsychologist: A psychologist specializing in understanding the relationship between the physical brain and behavior.

Neurostimulator: A device that delivers electrical impulses through tiny wires placed in regions of the brain affected by Parkinson's.

Neurotransmitter: A chemical messenger in the nervous system that facilitates communication between two neuronal cells, normally across a synapse. The neurotransmitter is released from the nerve terminals on the axons. Examples of neurotransmitters include dopamine, acetylcholine, adrenaline, noradrenaline, serotonin, glutamate, and GABA.

Non-motor symptoms: Symptoms of Parkinson's that do not involve movement, coordination, physical tasks, or mobility. Common non-motor symptoms include loss of sense of smell, constipation, sleep disorders or disturbances, mood disorders, orthostatic hypotension, bladder problems, sexual problems, excessive saliva, weight loss or gain, vision and dental problems, fatigue, depression, fear and anxiety, skin problems, and cognitive issues.

Occupational therapist: A specialist concerned with assessing a person's home or work situation to determine ways to make life more manageable. Occupational therapists can also advise on aids and adaptive equipment that may make everyday life easier.

Omega-3 fats: A type of fat necessary for brain cell function found in walnuts, flaxseeds, pumpkin seeds, purslane, and cold-water fish.

Omega-6 fats: A type of fat that includes sunflower oil, safflower oil, corn oil, most seeds, and oil from grains.

ON-OFF fluctuations: The clinical states of Parkinson's while being treated with carbidopa/levodopa, which can often fluctuate after a few years of treatment. The ON state is when carbidopa/levodopa reduces Parkinson's symptoms. The OFF state is when the benefit has been reduced or lost. The most common type of OFF is referred to as "wearing OFF," and happens because of carbidopa/levodopa not lasting more than four hours after a dose. Sudden and unpredictable OFF states can also occur but are less common. OFF states usually will respond to another dose of carbidopa/levodopa.

Orthostatic hypotension (OH): A sustained drop in blood pressure that occurs after standing. OH can happen for a variety of reasons. When OH is caused by a nervous system disorder, like Parkinson's or multiple system atrophy (MSA), it is called neurogenic orthostatic hypotension (nOH). Symptoms can include lightheadedness, dizziness, or feeling as though one is about to black out.

Overactive bladder (OAB): A sense of urgency and needing to urinate quickly and/or frequently, even if the bladder is not full.

Palliative care: An approach to care of chronic illness that is holistic and team-based, shifting the focus from an individual patient to the patient together with their family. Palliative care places a strong emphasis on enhancing quality of life and integrating psychological and spiritual aspects. Hospice is a subset of palliative care, administered in the US in the last six months of life.

Parkinsonism: A general term for group of neurological conditions displaying movement changes often seen in Parkinson's, such as slowness of movement, rest tremors, muscle stiffness, and impaired speech. Not everyone who has parkinsonism has Parkinson's.

Parkinsonian gait: A slow, short-paced way of walking common in people living with Parkinson's. Often there is a tendency to shuffle and a decreased arm swing.

Parkinson-plus syndromes: A group of neurodegenerative diseases displaying the classic motor symptoms of Parkinson's (such as slowness of movement, rest tremors, and muscle stiffness), but with additional features that distinguish them from typical Parkinson's. Parkinson-plus syndromes include multiple system atrophy (MSA), progressive supranuclear palsy (PSP), dementia with Lewy bodies (DLB), and corticobasal degeneration (CBD).

Partially hydrogenated oils: Primary source of artificial trans fat in processed foods. In 2013, the US Food and Drug Administration (FDA) made a preliminary determination that partially hydrogenated oils are no longer Generally Recognized as Safe (GRAS) in human food.

299

Periodic limb movement disorder (PLMD): A sleep disorder involving repetitive movements, typically in the legs and feet, that occur about every 20-40 seconds and cluster into episodes lasting anywhere from a few minutes to several hours. These movements can be brief muscle twitches, jerking movements, or an upward flexing of the feet. PLMD often occurs in tandem with restless legs syndrome, with nearly three-quarters of people with RLS also experiencing PLMD.

Peripheral neuropathy: A condition caused by damage to peripheral nerves. This often results in weakness, numbness, and pain, usually in the hands and feet, but can also affect other areas of the body.

Physical therapist: A specialists who use physical means such as exercise and manipulation to help prevent or reduce stiffness in joints and restore muscle strength. Physical therapists can also advise on aids and equipment to help with movement problems.

Placebo: A simulated or inert form of treatment without known proven benefit on a symptom or a disease. A pill serving as a placebo is often called a "sugar pill." When placebos provide benefit, this phenomenon is called a "placebo effect." Placebos are employed in controlled clinical trials along with the active drug being tested. The difference in responses between the two drugs is considered the true effect of the active drug.

Polyunsaturated fats: Type of fat that is liquid at both room temperature and when refrigerated. Can be divided into two types: omega-6 fats and omega-3 fats.

Postural instability: General balance issues that result from how Parkinson's delays reflexes related to posture. Although this typically shows up as problems with balance, there can be many different causes for balance challenges in Parkinson's.

Preclinical: The preclinical stage of Parkinson's is defined by biomarkers. Underlying pathological changes are present but remain clinically silent: the patient may be "without signs and symptoms."

Prodromal: Underlying pathology is present in the prodromal stage of Parkinson's. Signs and symptoms are present but do not rise to the level of clinical diagnosis.

Receptor: A protein structure typically embedded in the cell membrane with which neurotransmitters and drugs interact.

Recreational therapist: Specialists who help people stay active in hobbies and play.

Rapid eye movement sleep behavior disorder (RBD): A sleep disorder that involves movement and abnormal behavior during the sleep phase with rapid eye movements, the stage of sleep in which dreaming occurs. In normal sleep, muscles are paralyzed during dreaming, except for eye movements. In individuals with RBD, the muscles are not paralyzed, so the dreamer is free to physically act out his or her dreams. RBD is common in people with Parkinson's and may precede the onset of motor symptoms.

Restless legs syndrome (RLS): A neurological disorder characterized by unpleasant sensations in the legs, like the feeling of ants crawling underneath the skin. These sensations usually occur in the late evening and during sleep. Walking around relieves the sensation, hence the term "restless legs." RLS interferes with sleep and is common in people with Parkinson's.

Rest tremor: A type of tremor that worsens when relaxing or resting.

Retropulsion: The tendency to fall backward, caused by postural instability.

Rigidity: A special type of muscle stiffness, which is one of the hallmark motor symptoms of Parkinson's. The muscles tend to pull against each other instead of working smoothly together.

Saturated fats: Type of fat that is solid at room temperature and found primarily in red meat, tropical oils (like coconut) and dairy. A diet high in saturated fats can increase cholesterol levels, one's risk of accumulating plaque in the arteries (called "atherosclerosis"), stroke, and heart disease.

301

Seborrhea: Flaky, white or yellowish skin forming on oily areas of the scalp, forehead, or ear. Can be an early, non-motor symptom of Parkinson's.

Selective serotonin reuptake inhibitors (SSRIs): A class of antidepressant medications that increases serotonin levels in the brain and can be used to treat depression and anxiety.

Serotonin: A neurotransmitter that contributes to feelings of happiness and well-being.

Serotonin-norepinephrine reuptake inhibitors (SNRIs): A class of antidepressant medications that increase the neurotransmitters serotonin and norepinephrine and are used to treat depression and other mood disorders.

Shuffling gait: Short, slow steps, with feet close to the ground or dragging along the ground. Often seen in people with advanced Parkinson's.

Simple sugars: Sugars that are only made up of one or two sugar units and can be used to fuel cells and provide energy to the brain. Simple sugars are absorbed quickly as they require little to no digestion. For instance, table sugar is a simple sugar comprised of the sugar units glucose and fructose.

Skin biopsy: a procedure during which your clinician anesthetizes one or more sites to remove small pieces of skin. Analyzing the skin with immunofluorescent technology has been found to be a reliable way to locate the presence of misfolded alpha-synuclein protein in the peripheral nervous system and visualize the health of the central nervous system.

Sleep apnea: A sleep disorder in which one's breathing stops and starts during the night. While sleep apnea is not more prevalent in people living with Parkinson's, it does occur more frequently as adults age.

Soluble fiber: A type of dietary fiber that absorbs water as it passes through the digestive system. Water transforms the soluble fiber into a gel-like substance, which softens the stool and helps it move more smoothly through a person's bowels.

Speech-language pathologist: A specialists trained to treat problems associated with speech and swallowing. Speech-language pathologists can also advise on communication aids.

Starch: A long chain of carbohydrates that is digestible by the body and must be metabolized before absorbed. Starch does not cause glucose to rise as quickly as simple sugars do, resulting in steadier energy.

Stem cells: Special cells with the potential to develop into several different cell types in the body. When a stem cell divides, each new cell has the potential to remain either a stem cell or become another, more specialized type of cell, such as a brain cell or red blood cell. Stem cells are currently being researched as a potential disease-modifying treatment for Parkinson's.

Substantia nigra: An area located in the midbrain that looks like a dark streak in brain tissue, hence the Latin name meaning "black substance." The substantia nigra influences movement and coordination and is additionally thought to also play a role in other functions and behaviors, such as learning, drug addiction and emotions. A large amount of the dopamine cells that die in the brain because of Parkinson's are located in the substantia nigra.

Subthalamic nucleus (STN): A small lens-shaped area of the brain (specifically located in the basal ganglia) involved in movement control. The STN is "overactive" in people living with Parkinson's and is a common target in deep brain stimulation for Parkinson's.

Supine hypotension: Low blood pressure that occurs when lying down. Common in people with neurogenic orthostatic hypotension (nOH).

Syn-One Test®: a convenient diagnostic aid utilizing skin biopsy that can be performed in your doctor's office. The Syn-One Test highlights misfolded, pathological alpha-synuclein proteins associated with Parkinson's, dementia with Lewy bodies (DLB), multiple system atrophy (MSA), REM sleep behavior disorder, and pure autonomic failure. Healthcare providers can use this test in combination with clinical exams and patient health history to make a specific diagnosis.

Trans fats: Type of fat found in two forms: naturally occurring in animals (such as meat and milk products) or made artificially by adding hydrogen to liquid vegetable oils. The primary dietary source for trans fats in processed food is partially hydrogenated oils. Trans fats raise LDL cholesterol levels and lower HDL cholesterol levels, increasing one's risk of developing heart disease, stroke, and Type 2 diabetes.

T.R.A.P.: Acronym for four primary Parkinson's motor symptoms: tremor, rigidity, akinesia/bradykinesia, and postural instability.

Tremor: Involuntary shaking, trembling, or quivering movements of the muscles. In Parkinson's, tremor is usually a resting tremor, which lessens with movement and is aggravated by stress. It can occur in any part of the body, although it often begins in one hand or arm. Although tremor is one of the hallmark motor symptoms of Parkinson's, not everyone with Parkinson's will experience tremor.

Visuoperceptual: Understanding the location of objects around oneself.

Xerostomia: Lack of saliva or dry mouth.

Young onset Parkinson's disease (YOPD): A diagnosis of Parkinson's under the age of 50.

■ INDEX

305

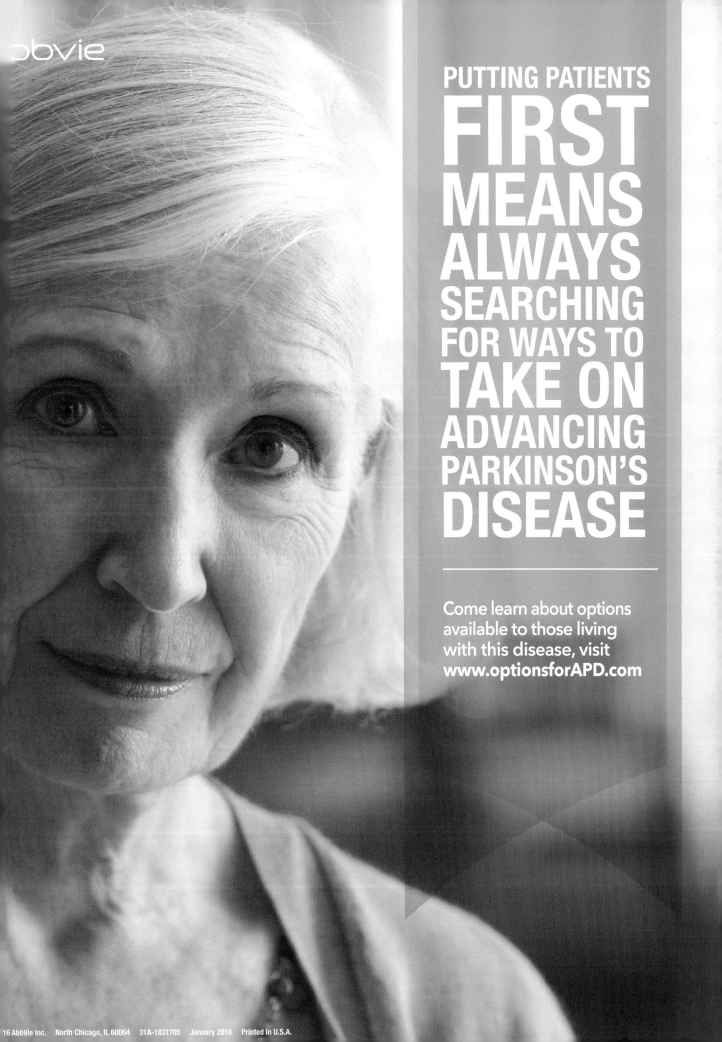

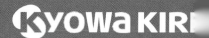

We work to help patient communities,
provide greater support to care partners, and
develop deep, strategic philanthropic partnerships
that improve the communities we operate in... that's

profound impact.

To learn more about us and our community commitment,
please visit **kkna.kyowakirin.com**

Scan to Read
"Burden and Benefit: Embracing the Du
of the Parkinson's Caregiving Experien

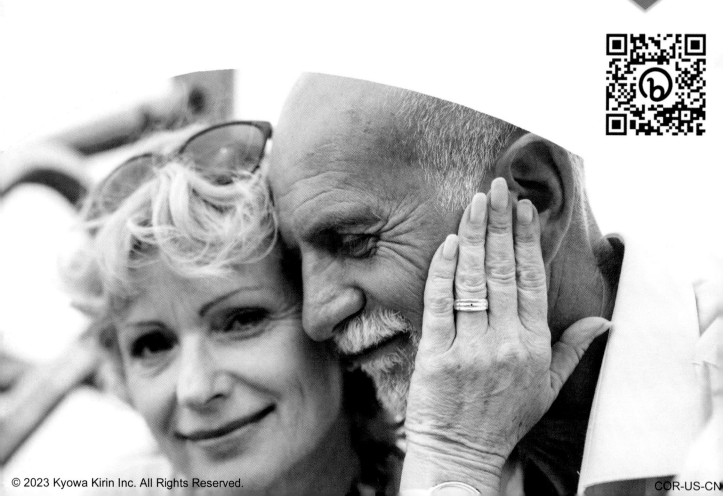

COR-US-CN

you getting enough out of Parkinson's medication?

serve more from your Parkinson's
ent. It might be time to speak with
octor about your Parkinson's treatment
-to better help you thrive.

**riving with Parkinson's starts with
"Good On" time.**

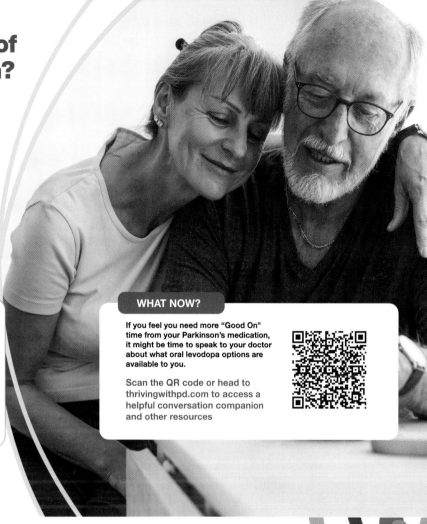

is "Good On" time important?

" time is when levodopa medication is working with
esia or with dyskinesia that does not interfere with
activities. Dyskinesia consists of those uncontrolled
ts, jerks, and twitches you may have experienced.
od On" time means doing more of what you love.

WHAT NOW?

If you feel you need more "Good On"
time from your Parkinson's medication,
it might be time to speak to your doctor
about what oral levodopa options are
available to you.

Scan the QR code or head to
thrivingwithpd.com to access a
helpful conversation companion
and other resources

Did you know the Davis Phinney Foundation now offers resources, programs, and community events in Spanish?

¡Página de recursos
educativos en español!

CONTACT US:
micomunidad@dpf.org

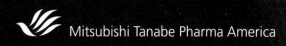

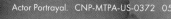
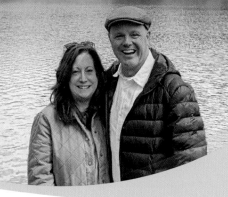

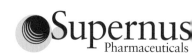

NOTES

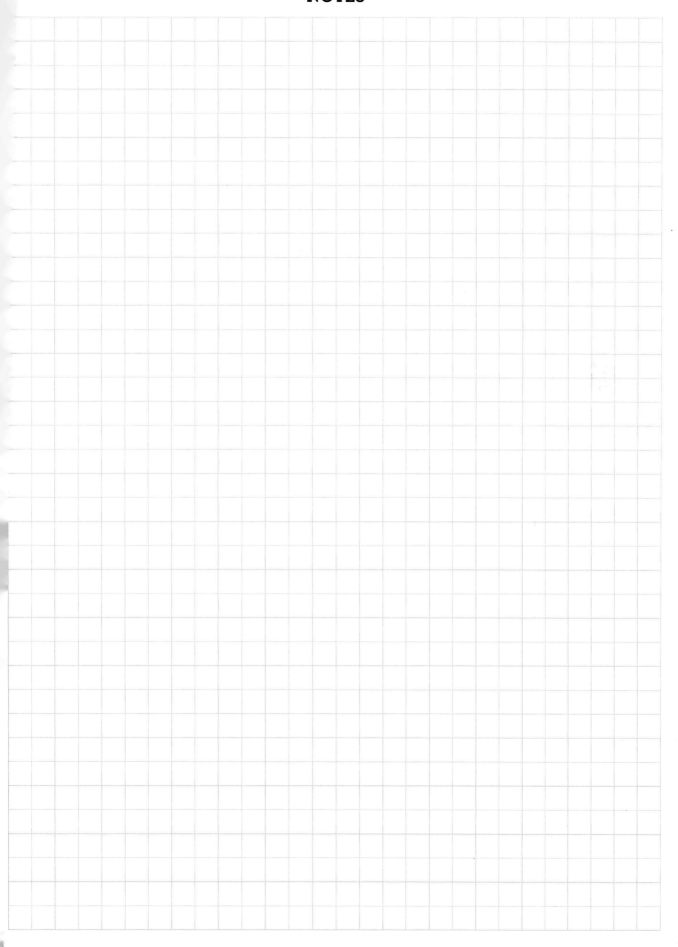